Recent Advances of Avian Viruses Research

Recent Advances of Avian Viruses Research

Guest Editor

Chi-Young Wang

MDPI Basel • Beijing • Wuhan • Barcelona • Belgrade • Novi Sad • Cluj • Manchester

Guest Editor
Chi-Young Wang
Department of Veterinary Medicine
National Chung Hsing University
Taichung
Taiwan

Editorial Office
MDPI AG
Grosspeteranlage 5
4052 Basel, Switzerland

This is a reprint of the Special Issue, published open access by the journal *Viruses* (ISSN 1999-4915), freely accessible at: www.mdpi.com/journal/viruses/special_issues/PH78913LM8.

For citation purposes, cite each article independently as indicated on the article page online and using the guide below:

Lastname, A.A.; Lastname, B.B. Article Title. *Journal Name* **Year**, *Volume Number*, Page Range.

ISBN 978-3-7258-3348-1 (Hbk)
ISBN 978-3-7258-3347-4 (PDF)
https://doi.org/10.3390/books978-3-7258-3347-4

Contents

About the Editor . . . . **vii**

Preface . . . . **ix**

Chi-Young Wang
Recent Advances of Avian Viruses Research
Reprinted from: *Viruses* **2025**, *17*, 99, https://doi.org/10.3390/v17010099 . . . . **1**

Maria Chaves, Amro Hashish, Onyekachukwu Osemeke, Yuko Sato, David L. Suarez and Mohamed El-Gazzar
Evaluation of Commercial RNA Extraction Protocols for Avian Influenza Virus Using Nanopore Metagenomic Sequencing
Reprinted from: *Viruses* **2024**, *16*, 1429, https://doi.org/10.3390/v16091429 . . . . **5**

Qingqing Xu, Yaoyao Zhang, Yashar Sadigh, Na Tang, Jiaqian Chai and Ziqiang Cheng et al.
Specific and Sensitive Visual Proviral DNA Detection of Major Pathogenic Avian Leukosis Virus Subgroups Using CRISPR-Associated Nuclease Cas13a
Reprinted from: *Viruses* **2024**, *16*, 1168, https://doi.org/10.3390/v16071168 . . . . **25**

Chao-Yu Hsu, Jyun-Yi Li, En-Ying Yang, Tsai-Ling Liao, Hsiao-Wei Wen and Pei-Chien Tsai et al.
The Oncolytic Avian Reovirus p17 Protein Inhibits Invadopodia Formation in Murine Melanoma Cancer Cells by Suppressing the FAK/Src Pathway and the Formation of theTKs5/NCK1 Complex
Reprinted from: *Viruses* **2024**, *16*, 1153, https://doi.org/10.3390/v16071153 . . . . **39**

Brian Harvey Avanceña Villanueva, Jin-Yang Chen, Pei-Ju Lin, Hoang Minh, Van Phan Le and Yu-Chang Tyan et al.
Surveillance of Parrot Bornavirus in Taiwan Captive *Psittaciformes*
Reprinted from: *Viruses* **2024**, *16*, 805, https://doi.org/10.3390/v16050805 . . . . **57**

Kelsey O'Dowd, Ishara M. Isham, Safieh Vatandour, Martine Boulianne, Charles M. Dozois and Carl A. Gagnon et al.
Host Immune Response Modulation in Avian Coronavirus Infection: Tracheal Transcriptome Profiling In Vitro and In Vivo
Reprinted from: *Viruses* **2024**, *16*, 605, https://doi.org/10.3390/v16040605 . . . . **78**

Ines Szotowska and Aleksandra Ledwoń
Antiviral Chemotherapy in Avian Medicine—A Review
Reprinted from: *Viruses* **2024**, *16*, 593, https://doi.org/10.3390/v16040593 . . . . **109**

Hoang Duc Le, Tuyet Ngan Thai, Jae-Kyeom Kim, Hye-Soon Song, Moon Her and Xuan Thach Tran et al.
An Amplicon-Based Application for the Whole-Genome Sequencing of GI-19 Lineage Infectious Bronchitis Virus Directly from Clinical Samples
Reprinted from: *Viruses* **2024**, *16*, 515, https://doi.org/10.3390/v16040515 . . . . **128**

Hongyu Ren, Sheng Wang, Zhixun Xie, Lijun Wan, Liji Xie and Sisi Luo et al.
Analysis of Chicken IFITM3 Gene Expression and Its Effect on Avian Reovirus Replication
Reprinted from: *Viruses* **2024**, *16*, 330, https://doi.org/10.3390/v16030330 . . . . **139**

Matteo Legnardi, Francesca Poletto, Shaimaa Talaat, Karim Selim, Mahmoud K. Moawad and Giovanni Franzo et al.
First Detection and Molecular Characterization of Novel Variant Infectious Bursal Disease Virus (Genotype A2dB1b) in Egypt
Reprinted from: *Viruses* **2023**, *15*, 2388, https://doi.org/10.3390/v15122388 . . . . **153**

Sheng Wang, Tengda Huang, Zhixun Xie, Lijun Wan, Hongyu Ren and Tian Wu et al.
Transcriptomic and Translatomic Analyses Reveal Insights into the Signaling Pathways of the Innate Immune Response in the Spleens of SPF Chickens Infected with Avian Reovirus
Reprinted from: *Viruses* **2023**, *15*, 2346, https://doi.org/10.3390/v15122346 . . . . **167**

Ishara M. Isham, Reham M. Abd-Elsalam, Motamed E. Mahmoud, Shahnas M. Najimudeen, Hiruni A. Ranaweera and Ahmed Ali et al.
Comparison of Infectious Bronchitis Virus (IBV) Pathogenesis and Host Responses in Young Male and Female Chickens
Reprinted from: *Viruses* **2023**, *15*, 2285, https://doi.org/10.3390/v15122285 . . . . **186**

About the Editor

Chi-Young Wang

Dr. Chi-Young Wang received his bachelor's degree in veterinary medicine from National Chung Hsing University, Taiwan. He earned his Ph.D. in animal virology and avian diseases at Auburn University, then spent a year doing postdoctoral research at the University of Alabama at Birmingham, where he studied genetics. He joined the faculty of National Chung Hsing University as an assistant professor of veterinary virology and avian diseases and was promoted to full professor in 2015. In 2023, he served as an editor for the Special Issue, titled "State-of-the-Art Avian Virus Research in Asia", in the journal *Viruses*.

Preface

Due to several epidemic outbreaks caused by numerous avian viruses, the threat of pathogenic avian diseases to human health and the food industry has become an emergent issue within the framework of One Health. Recently, experts around the world have developed various novel strategies, innovative approaches, and state-of-the-art techniques devoted to studying different aspects of these important avian viruses. The major mission for research teams is to maintain the health of humans and birds in order to ensure the safety of public health and a sufficient food supply for our community. Therefore, the accumulated knowledge regarding molecular virology, viral immunology, viral pathogenesis, epidemiology, antivirals, novel vaccines, and applications of avian viral vectors, established by various international expert research groups, has advanced the global understanding of these pathogens. This Special Issue includes all research aspects of avian virus research, which provides an exceptional example that will lead to more excellent studies in the future.

Chi-Young Wang
Guest Editor

viruses

Editorial

Recent Advances of Avian Viruses Research

Chi-Young Wang

Department of Veterinary Medicine, College of Veterinary Medicine, National Chung Hsing University, 250 Kuo Kuang Road, Taichung 40227, Taiwan; cyoungwang@dragon.nchu.edu.tw

The outbreaks of several epidemics caused by pathogenic avian viruses pose significant threats to the poultry industry. Nowadays, this problem also becomes an emergent issue to human health within the framework of One Health. Thus, more and more avian virologists have devoted themselves to exploring innovative approaches and strategies to study important pathogens, to gain the newest and valuable knowledge in order to assist in the control of those diseases. Therefore, several high-quality papers are assembled in this Special Issue.

The first paper in this Special Issue concerned avian influenza virus (AIV). The current AIV diagnostic process is to identify the virus via real-time reverse transcription–polymerase chain reaction (rRT-PCR). The virus is subsequently characterized by using whole-genome sequencing. This two-step diagnostic process takes days to weeks, but it can be expedited by using some novel sequencing technologies. The authors optimized a nucleic acid extraction setup from Oxford Nanopore Technologies for the rapid identification of AIV from clinical samples. The results showed that the magnetic-particle-based method was the most consistent regarding C_T value, purity, total yield, and AIV reads, and that it was less error-prone [1].

The second paper focused on the development of rapid, accurate, and cost-effective on-site diagnostic methods for the detection of avian leukosis virus (ALV) subgroups. The distinct trans-cleavage activity of Cas13, an RNA-guided RNA endonuclease, has been exploited in the molecular diagnosis of several viruses. The development and application of a Cas13a-based molecular test for the specific detection of the proviral DNA of ALV-A, B, and J subgroups were demonstrated. This novel system is based on the isothermal detection at 37 °C with a color-based lateral flow readout. The detection limit of the assay for ALV-A/B/J subgroups was 50 copies with no cross-reactivity with ALV-C/D/E subgroups and other avian oncogenic viruses, such as reticuloendotheliosis virus and Marek's disease virus. It will benefit ALV detection in eradication programs [2].

The third paper explored whether the p17 protein of oncolytic avian reovirus (ARV) mediates cell migration and invadopodia formation. ARV p17 activates the p53/phosphatase and tensin homolog (PTEN) pathway to suppress focal adhesion kinase (FAK)/Src signaling and downstream signal molecules, thus inhibiting cell migration and the formation of invadopodia in murine melanoma cancer cell lines (B16-F10). It also suppresses the formation of the TKs5/NCK1 complex. This work provided new information about the p17-modulated suppression of invadopodia formation by activating the p53/PTEN pathway, suppressing the FAK/Src pathway, and inhibiting the formation of the TKs5/NCK1 complex [3].

The fourth paper in the Special Issue explored the prevalence of parrot bornavirus (PaBV) in Taiwan. Among 124 psittacine birds tested, 57 were PaBV-positive, a prevalence rate of 45.97%. Most of the PaBV infections were adult psittacine birds with a low survival rate (8.77%). A year of parrot bornavirus surveillance presented a seasonal pattern, with a

check for updates

Received: 6 January 2025
Accepted: 10 January 2025
Published: 14 January 2025

Citation: Wang, C.-Y. Recent Advances of Avian Viruses Research. *Viruses* **2025**, *17*, 99. https://doi.org/10.3390/v17010099

peak infection rate in spring, indicating the occurrence of PaBV infections linked to seasonal factors. Severe meningoencephalitis and dilated cardiomyopathy in psittacine birds that suffered from proventricular dilatation disease were evident. PaBV-2 and PaBV-4 viral genotypes were found in the phylogenetic analyses [4].

The fifth paper in the Special Issue characterized the impact of infectious bronchitis virus (IBV) Delmarva/1639 and IBV Massachusetts 41 on chicken tracheal epithelial cells (cTECs) in vitro and the trachea in vivo. cTECs and young specific pathogen-free chickens were inoculated with IBV DMV/1639 or IBV Mass41, along with mock-inoculated controls, and the transcriptome was studied by using RNA-sequencing (RNA-seq) at 3 and 18 h post-infection for cTECs and at 4 and 11 days post-infection in the trachea. It was shown that IBV DMV/1639 and IBV Mass41 replicate in cTECs in vitro and in the trachea in vivo, inducing host mRNA expression profiles that are strain- and time-dependent. The different gene expression patterns between in vitro and in vivo tracheal IBV infection were demonstrated [5].

The sixth paper in the Special Issue characterized the impact of IBV Delmarva (DMV)/1639 and IBV Massachusetts (Mass) 41 on chicken tracheal epithelial cells (cTECs) and the trachea of chickens. cTECs and young specific pathogen-free chickens were inoculated with IBV DMV/1639 or IBV Mass41 and their transcriptomes were studied by using RNA-sequencing (RNA-seq) for cTECs and the trachea. It was shown that IBV DMV/1639 and IBV Mass41 replicate in cTECs and the trachea, inducing host mRNA expression profiles that were shown to be both strain- and time-dependent. The different gene expression patterns between in vitro and in vivo tracheal IBV infection were observed [6].

The seventh paper in the Special Issue studied interferon-inducible transmembrane protein 3 (IFITM3), which is an antiviral factor that plays an important role in the host innate immune response against viruses. In this study, the role of chicken IFITM3 in ARV infection was explored to show that this protein was localized in the cytoplasm. The homology analysis and phylogenetic tree analysis showed that the IFITM3 genes of different species exhibited great variation during genetic evolution, and chicken IFITM3 shared the highest homology with that of *Anas platyrhynchos* and displayed relatively low homology with those of birds such as *Anser cygnoides* and *Serinus canaria*. An analysis of the distribution of chicken IFITM3 in tissues and organs revealed that the IFITM3 gene was expressed at its highest level in the intestine and in large quantities in immune organs, such as the bursa of Fabricius, thymus, and spleen. Further studies showed that the overexpression of IFITM3 in chicken embryo fibroblasts (DF-1) could inhibit the replication of ARV, whereas the inhibition of IFITM3 expression in DF-1 cells promoted ARV replication. In addition, chicken IFITM3 exerted negative feedback regulatory effects on the expression of TBK1, IFN-γ, and IRF1 during ARV infection [7].

The eighth paper in the Special Issue examined how infectious bursal disease (IBD) is an immunosuppressive disease causing significant damage to the poultry industry worldwide. In Egypt, very virulent strains (such as genotype A3B2), responsible for typical IBD signs and lesions and high mortality, have historically prevailed. The present molecular survey, however, suggests that a major epidemiological shift might be occurring in the country. Out of twenty-four samples collected in twelve governorates in 2022–2023, seven tested positive for IBDV. Two of them were A3B2 strains related to other very virulent Egyptian isolates, whereas the remaining five were novel variant IBDVs (A2dB1b), reported for the first time outside of East and South Asia. This emerging genotype spawned a large-scale epidemic in China during the 2010s, characterized by subclinical IBD with severe bursal atrophy and immunosuppression. Its spread to Egypt is even more alarming considering that, contrary to circulating IBDVs, the protection conferred by available commercial vaccines appears suboptimal [8].

The ninth paper in the Special Issue combined transcriptome and translatome sequencing to investigate the mechanisms of transcriptional and translational regulation in the spleen after ARV infection. On a genome-wide scale, ARV infection can significantly reduce the translation efficiency (TE) of splenic genes. Differentially expressed translational efficiency genes (DTEGs) were identified, including 15 upregulated DTEGs and 396 downregulated DTEGs. These DTEGs were mainly enriched in immune regulation signaling pathways, which indicates that ARV infection reduces the innate immune response in the spleen. In addition, combined analyses revealed that the innate immune response involves the effects of transcriptional and translational regulation. Moreover, the key gene IL4I1 was discovered, which was the most significantly upregulated gene at both the transcriptional and translational levels. Further studies on DF1 cells showed that the overexpression of IL4I1 could inhibit the replication of ARV, while inhibiting the expression of endogenous IL4I1 with siRNA promoted the replication of ARV. The overexpression of IL4I1 significantly downregulated the mRNA expression of IFN-β, LGP2, TBK1, and NF-κB; however, the expression of these genes was significantly upregulated after the inhibition of IL4I1, suggesting that IL4I1 may be a negative feedback effect of innate immune signaling pathways. In addition, there may be an interaction between IL4I1 and ARV σA protein, and it was speculated that the IL4I1 protein plays a regulatory role by interacting with the σA protein. This study not only provided a new perspective on the regulatory mechanisms of the innate immune response after ARV infection but also enriched the knowledge of the host defense mechanisms against ARV invasion and outcomes of ARV evasion of a host's innate immune response [9].

The tenth paper in the Special Issue compared IBV pathogenesis and host immune responses in young male and female chickens. One-week-old specific pathogen-free (SPF) White Leghorn male and female chickens were infected with Canadian Delmarva (DMV)/1639 IBV variant via the oculo-nasal route while maintaining uninfected controls, and these chickens were sampled at 4 and 11 days post-infection (dpi). No significant differences were observed between the infected male and female chickens in regard to IBV shedding, the IBV genome loads in all organs, and lesions in all tissues. The percentages of B lymphocytes were not significantly different between infected male and female chickens in all of the examined tissues. The percentages of CD8+ T cells were not significantly different between infected male and female chickens in all of the examined tissues, except in the trachea at 11 dpi, where female chickens had higher recruitment when compared with male chickens. Overall, the sex of chickens did not play a significant role in the pathogenesis of IBV, and only marginal differences in viral replication and host responses were observed that suggested more severity in male chickens infected by IBV [10].

The final paper reviews the current understanding about the use of antiviral chemotherapeutics in both farm poultry and companion birds. Some antiviral drugs, repurposed drugs originally used as antiparasitic drugs, other substances exhibiting antiviral activity, and novel peptides were described. Despite some drugs without pharmacokinetic and safety data having already been widely used in daily practice, the possible direction of further research on these drugs remains to be highlighted [11].

In conclusion, this Special Issue offers appealing portraits of recent advances in avian virus research. Its contents, encompassing molecular virology, viral immunology, viral pathogenesis, epidemiology, and antivirals, indeed provide some state-of-the-art advances in this field that can contribute to sustaining the health of poultry and humans to ensure the safety of public health and a sufficient food supply for the community. It surely provides a stellar example that will result in more exciting studies on this area in the near future.

Conflicts of Interest: The author declare no conflicts of interest.

References

1. Isham, I.; Abd-Elsalam, R.; Mahmoud, M.; Najimudeen, S.; Ranaweera, H.; Ali, A.; Hassan, M.; Cork, S.; Gupta, A.; Abdul-Careem, M. Comparison of Infectious Bronchitis Virus (IBV) Pathogenesis and Host Responses in Young Male and Female Chickens. *Viruses* **2023**, *15*, 2285. [CrossRef] [PubMed]
2. Wang, S.; Huang, T.; Xie, Z.; Wan, L.; Ren, H.; Wu, T.; Xie, L.; Luo, S.; Li, M.; Xie, Z.; et al. Transcriptomic and Translatomic Analyses Reveal Insights into the Signaling Pathways of the Innate Immune Response in the Spleens of SPF Chickens Infected with Avian Reovirus. *Viruses* **2023**, *15*, 2346. [CrossRef]
3. Legnardi, M.; Poletto, F.; Talaat, S.; Selim, K.; Moawad, M.; Franzo, G.; Tucciarone, C.; Cecchinato, M.; Sultan, H. First Detection and Molecular Characterization of Novel Variant Infectious Bursal Disease Virus (Genotype A2dB1b) in Egypt. *Viruses* **2023**, *15*, 2388. [CrossRef] [PubMed]
4. Ren, H.; Wang, S.; Xie, Z.; Wan, L.; Xie, L.; Luo, S.; Li, M.; Xie, Z.; Fan, Q.; Zeng, T.; et al. Analysis of Chicken IFITM3 Gene Expression and Its Effect on Avian Reovirus Replication. *Viruses* **2024**, *16*, 330. [CrossRef]
5. Le, H.; Thai, T.; Kim, J.; Song, H.; Her, M.; Tran, X.; Kim, J.; Kim, H. An Amplicon-Based Application for the Whole-Genome Sequencing of GI-19 Lineage Infectious Bronchitis Virus Directly from Clinical Samples. *Viruses* **2024**, *16*, 515. [CrossRef] [PubMed]
6. Szotowska, I.; Ledwoń, A. Antiviral Chemotherapy in Avian Medicine—A Review. *Viruses* **2024**, *16*, 593. [CrossRef] [PubMed]
7. O'Dowd, K.; Isham, I.; Vatandour, S.; Boulianne, M.; Dozois, C.; Gagnon, C.; Barjesteh, N.; Abdul-Careem, M. Host Immune Response Modulation in Avian Coronavirus Infection: Tracheal Transcriptome Profiling In Vitro and In Vivo. *Viruses* **2024**, *16*, 605. [CrossRef]
8. Villanueva, B.; Chen, J.; Lin, P.; Minh, H.; Le, V.; Tyan, Y.; Chuang, J.; Chuang, K. Surveillance of Parrot Bornavirus in Taiwan Captive Psittaciformes. *Viruses* **2024**, *16*, 805. [CrossRef]
9. Hsu, C.; Li, J.; Yang, E.; Liao, T.; Wen, H.; Tsai, P.; Ju, T.; Lye, L.; Nielsen, B.; Liu, H. The Oncolytic Avian Reovirus p17 Protein Inhibits Invadopodia Formation in Murine Melanoma Cancer Cells by Suppressing the FAK/Src Pathway and the Formation of theTKs5/NCK1 Complex. *Viruses* **2024**, *16*, 1153. [CrossRef] [PubMed]
10. Xu, Q.; Zhang, Y.; Sadigh, Y.; Tang, N.; Chai, J.; Cheng, Z.; Gao, Y.; Qin, A.; Shen, Z.; Yao, Y.; et al. Specific and Sensitive Visual Proviral DNA Detection of Major Pathogenic Avian Leukosis Virus Subgroups Using CRISPR-Associated Nuclease Cas13a. *Viruses* **2024**, *16*, 1168. [CrossRef] [PubMed]
11. Chaves, M.; Hashish, A.; Osemeke, O.; Sato, Y.; Suarez, D.; El-Gazzar, M. Evaluation of Commercial RNA Extraction Protocols for Avian Influenza Virus Using Nanopore Metagenomic Sequencing. *Viruses* **2024**, *16*, 1429. [CrossRef] [PubMed]

viruses

MDPI

Article

Evaluation of Commercial RNA Extraction Protocols for Avian Influenza Virus Using Nanopore Metagenomic Sequencing

Maria Chaves [1], Amro Hashish [1,2], Onyekachukwu Osemeke [1], Yuko Sato [1], David L. Suarez [3] and Mohamed El-Gazzar [1,*]

1 Department of Veterinary Diagnostic and Production Animal Medicine, College of Veterinary Medicine, Iowa State University, Ames, IA 50011, USA; mpeixoto@iastate.edu (M.C.); hashish@iastate.edu (A.H.); oosemeke@iastate.edu (O.O.); ysato@iastate.edu (Y.S.)
2 National Laboratory for Veterinary Quality Control on Poultry Production, Giza 12618, Egypt
3 US National Poultry Research Center, Agricultural Research Service, US Department of Agriculture, Athens, GA 30605, USA; david.suarez@usda.gov
* Correspondence: elgazzar@iastate.edu

Abstract: Avian influenza virus (AIV) is a significant threat to the poultry industry, necessitating rapid and accurate diagnosis. The current AIV diagnostic process relies on virus identification via real-time reverse transcription–polymerase chain reaction (rRT-PCR). Subsequently, the virus is further characterized using genome sequencing. This two-step diagnostic process takes days to weeks, but it can be expedited by using novel sequencing technologies. We aim to optimize and validate nucleic acid extraction as the first step to establishing Oxford Nanopore Technologies (ONT) as a rapid diagnostic tool for identifying and characterizing AIV from clinical samples. This study compared four commercially available RNA extraction protocols using AIV-known-positive clinical samples. The extracted RNA was evaluated using total RNA concentration, viral copies as measured by rRT-PCR, and purity as measured by a 260/280 absorbance ratio. After NGS testing, the number of total and influenza-specific reads and quality scores of the generated sequences were assessed. The results showed that no protocol outperformed the others on all parameters measured; however, the magnetic particle-based method was the most consistent regarding C_T value, purity, total yield, and AIV reads, and it was less error-prone. This study highlights how different RNA extraction protocols influence ONT sequencing performance.

Keywords: avian influenza; metagenomic sequencing; nanopore sequencing; nucleic acid extraction

Citation: Chaves, M.; Hashish, A.; Osemeke, O.; Sato, Y.; Suarez, D.L.; El-Gazzar, M. Evaluation of Commercial RNA Extraction Protocols for Avian Influenza Virus Using Nanopore Metagenomic Sequencing. *Viruses* **2024**, *16*, 1429. https://doi.org/10.3390/v16091429

Academic Editor: Chi-Young Wang

Received: 24 July 2024
Revised: 21 August 2024
Accepted: 4 September 2024
Published: 7 September 2024

1. Introduction

Avian influenza is an infectious disease that significantly impacts human and animal health and the economy worldwide [1]. The disease is caused by a segmented negative-sense RNA virus, a member of the influenza A virus (IAV) genus (Orthomyxoviridae family), and it is classified into different subtypes based on its surface glycoproteins—hemagglutinin (HA) and neuraminidase (NA) [2]. Wild waterfowl are the main reservoir for viral strains and are a source of introduction of avian influenza virus (AIV) outbreaks to poultry. The 2015–2016 highly pathogenic avian influenza (HPAI) outbreak was considered the most impactful foreign animal disease in U.S. history at the time. However, the current 2022–2024 outbreak has already surpassed this outbreak in the number of affected animals, including dairy cattle [3,4].

The antigenic drift and shift of avian influenza viruses (AIVs) are a significant concern to both animal and human health, leading to constant viral monitoring at a global scale [1,5–8]. Current monitoring strategies focus on tracking viral mutations by performing molecular analyses, such as rRT-PCR (quantitative real-time reverse-transcription polymerase chain reaction) and the amplicon-based gene sequencing of its surface glycoproteins HA and NA [9]. Additionally, there is a rising demand and expectation for full-length viral genome characterization to comprehend the viral evolution and epidemiology of newly emerging and re-emerging AIV strains. Phylogenetic analysis of all genomic segments of the Eurasian A/goose/Guangdong/1/1996 (GsGd) lineage detected in late 2021 in North America demonstrated the transatlantic spread of the H5N1 strain from Europe, associated with wild bird migration [10,11].

Improved Sanger sequencing and the introduction of second-generation sequencing platforms allow the comprehensive genomic characterization of AIVs from isolates and clinical samples, contributing to a better understanding of human and animal infectious diseases [12–16]. However, these current technologies have limitations, such as a long turn-around time, extensive protocols, high cost per sample, and the need for large bench equipment [17,18]. On the other hand, the advent of the Oxford Nanopore Technology (ONT) platform, a third-generation sequencing platform, circumvents these limitations and further facilitates the use of whole genome sequencing (WGS) in infectious disease diagnostics [19]. ONT has provided cost- and time-effective solutions for sequencing workflows that require a lower cost per sample, fewer initial investments, and less complex library preparation procedures, leading to a shorter time from sample to results. Additionally, the sequencing can be run on a USB-connected sequencer using laptop computers and analyzed with user-friendly data analysis tools [20–22]. ONT's portable devices, such as the MinION, have enabled the remote, real-time analysis of sequencing data outside the laboratory setting [23,24]. However, the technology has several limitations, such as a higher error rate compared to short-read sequencing [25], constant updates of kits and software, and the short shelf life of flow cells and reagents, making selecting the most appropriate workflow more challenging [26].

The features of ONT, particularly the real-time access to the sequence results, make the technology suitable for metagenomic next-generation sequencing (mgNGS), in which AIV nucleic acid can quickly be identified and characterized directly from clinical samples. The success of viral WGS using ONT directly from clinical samples primarily hinges on a multi-step preparation process. This process includes nucleic acid extraction, sequencing library preparation, and the subsequent assembly and analysis of the generated reads, culminating in sequence results [27]. Nucleic acid extraction is the first and critical step to maximize the applicability of ONT in diagnostics settings. There are multiple available nucleic acid extraction protocols, and the selection of the optimal method is complex and depends on the sample type and the desired outcome [28]. Therefore, multiple studies have been conducted to assess the impact of different extraction procedures in nucleic acid recovery from clinical samples using ONT [27,29–31]. Previous work that analyzed complex microbial diversity and the metagenomic use of Nanopore sequencing has shown that the yield and length of DNA extracted by different protocols impacted the microbial abundance from urine and tongue dorsum samples [29,30]. Another study has assessed the impact of different extraction procedures in AIV RNA recovery from nasal samples using the Illumina MiSeq platform. The research compared five extraction protocols, and the protocol MagNA pure compact RNA isolation (automated extraction based on the magnetic isolation of nucleic acids) consistently gave the best results in AIV segment coverage depth at different time points after inoculating the virus in ferrets [32].

Even though similar work has been conducted on comparing different extraction protocols for AIV recovery from clinical samples using Illumina (short-read sequencing), no data are available for a similar evaluation using ONT (long-read sequencing). Therefore, the objective of this study is to compare four commercially available and commonly used RNA extraction protocols (magnetic particle-based, spin column, liquid-phase separation, and the enzymatic method) and evaluate their performance in terms of concentration and purity, followed by metagenomic nanopore sequencing for their comprehensive evaluation.

2. Materials and Methods

2.1. Clinical Samples

The samples used in the study (n = 24) were received at the Iowa State University Veterinary Diagnostic Laboratory (ISU-VDL) in 2022. The samples were confirmed positive at the National Veterinary Services Laboratory (NVSL) in Ames, IA, for Influenza A by (rRT-PCR) targeting Eurasian lineage goose Guangdong H5 clade 2.3.4.4b. As a tier 1 member of the National Animal Health Laboratory Network (NAHLN), the samples received in ISU-VDL were handled and disposed of according to the Guidelines for Avian Influenza viruses established by the U.S. Department of Agriculture and Animal and Plant Health and Inspection Service (USDA-APHIS). A complete list of samples and their details is presented in Table 1. All samples were further flushed and manually homogenized using 3 to 5 mL of phosphate-buffered saline (PBS) to elute the tissues. PBS was selected in our methodology because it is a widely available transport media, it is compatible with ONT downstream applications (no interference in the following steps), non-toxic, presents buffering capability and pH stability, and it has been widely used for AIV transport and storage [33–35]. The liquid from each sample was then collected and aliquoted into 1.5 mL Eppendorf tubes and briefly centrifuged at 12,000 rpm for 30 s. Then, total RNA was extracted from the supernatant obtained from the samples.

Table 1. Description of samples used in the study.

Sample ID	Sample Type	Host	Date of Collection
1	Assorted tissues [a]	Turkey vulture (*Cathartes aura*)	04/28/2022
2	Brain	Red-tailed hawk (*Buteo jamaicensis*)	04/27/2022
3	Respiratory tissues [b]	Red-tailed hawk (*Buteo jamaicensis*)	04/27/2022
4	Respiratory tissues [b]	Great horned owl (*Bubo virginianus*)	04/28/2022
5	Brain	Great horned owl (*Bubo virginianus*)	04/28/2022
6	Brain	Turkey vulture (*Cathartes aura*)	04/28/2022
7	Respiratory tissues [b]	Turkey vulture (*Cathartes aura*)	04/28/2022
8	Brain	Great horned owl (*Bubo virginianus*)	05/12/2022
9	Respiratory tissues [b]	Great horned owl (*Bubo virginianus*)	05/12/2022
10	Intestine	American green-winged teal (*Anas crecca carolinensis*)	04/26/2022
11	Respiratory tissues [b]	American green-winged teal (*Anas crecca carolinensis*)	04/26/2022
12	Intestine	Falcon	04/18/2022
13	Respiratory tissues [b]	Falcon	04/18/2022
14	Trachea	Chicken (*Gallus gallus domesticus*)	04/01/2022
15	Lung	Chicken (*Gallus gallus domesticus*)	04/01/2022
16	Brain	Chicken (*Gallus gallus domesticus*)	04/01/2022
17	Spleen swabs	Chicken (*Gallus gallus domesticus*)	04/01/2022
18	Air sac swabs	Chicken (*Gallus gallus domesticus*)	04/01/2022
19	Liver	Eagle (*Haliaeetus leucocephalus*)	05/01/2022
20	Trachea	Eagle (*Haliaeetus leucocephalus*)	05/01/2022
21	Brain	Eagle (*Haliaeetus leucocephalus*)	05/01/2022
22	Liver	Eagle (*Haliaeetus leucocephalus*)	05/01/2022
23	Intestine	Eagle (*Haliaeetus leucocephalus*)	05/01/2022
24	Lung	Eagle (*Haliaeetus leucocephalus*)	05/01/2022

[a] Assorted tissues = combination of multiple organs, including respiratory (lung, trachea), enteric (intestine), and central nervous system. [b] Respiratory tissues = combination of trachea and lung.

Nucleic acid extraction was carried out twice on each sample using each protocol (two sections), resulting in 48 individual observations per kit. These two sets of experiments were conducted to test the repeatability of the results (Supplementary Figure S1).

2.2. Nucleic Acid Extraction Kits Used in This Study

Four different nucleic acid extraction methods were tested using different commercial extraction kits: magnetic particle-based, silica column, liquid-phase separation, and enzymatic extraction methods (Table 2). Each method is fully described below, and the experimental workflow is shown in Figure 1.

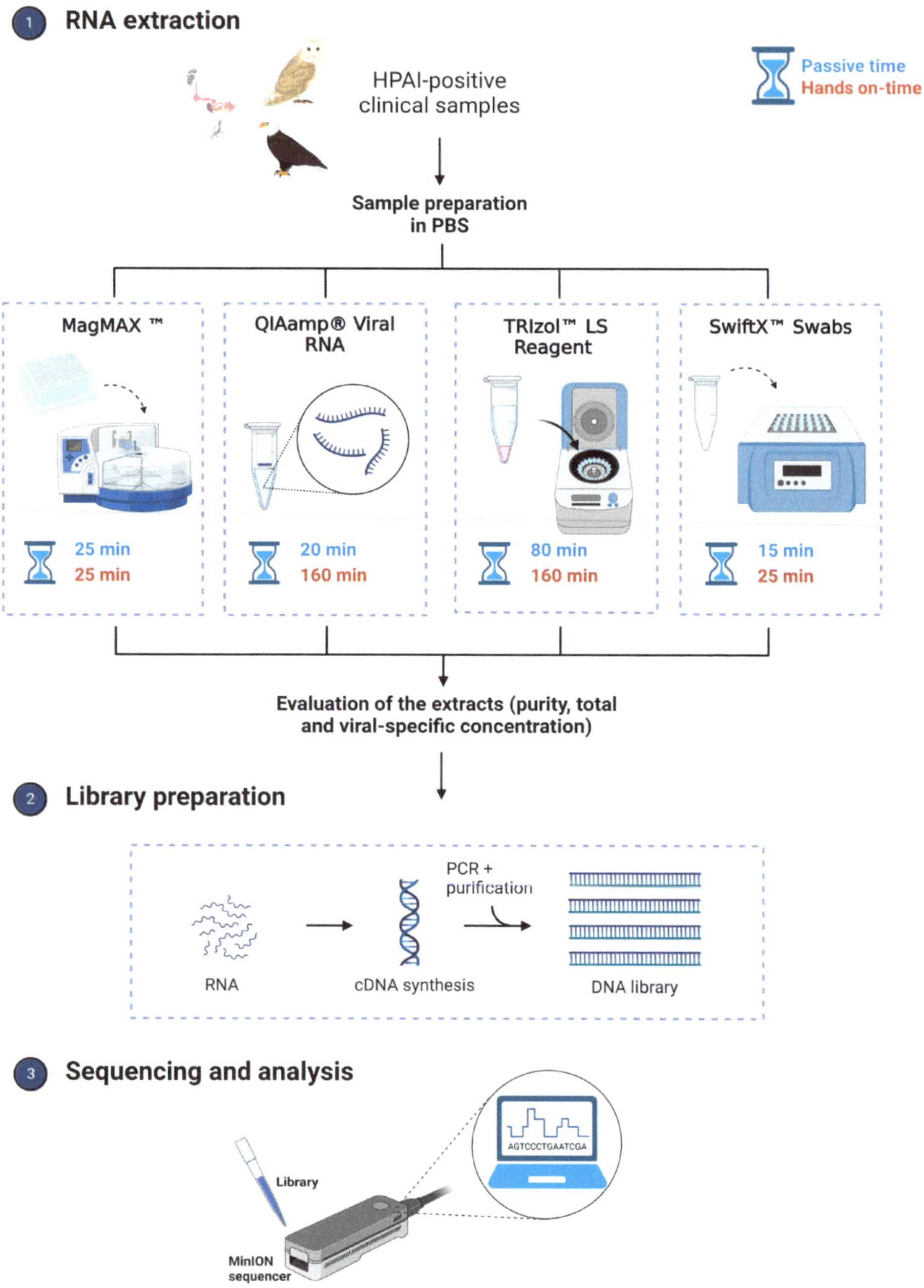

Figure 1. Experimental workflow. The total time (spent extracting 24 samples) was split into passive and hands-on time for each protocol.

Table 2. Description of the four protocols regarding technical (method, cost, equipment required, automation) and functional aspects (starting and elution volume).

Protocol	Extraction Method	Cost Per Sample (US$)	Equipment Requirement	Automation Potential	Starting Volume (μL)	Elution Volume (μL)
MagMAX Pathogen RNA/DNA™	Magnetic particle-based	4.60	Magnetic robot	Yes	100	90
QIAamp® Viral RNA	Silica membrane	5.50	Centrifuge	Available	140	40–60
TRIzol™ LS Reagent (DNA/RNA)	Liquid-phase separation	1.90	Centrifuge	No	250	50
SwiftX™ Swabs (DNA/RNA)	Enzymatic	1.30	Thermal block	No	100	200

(1) Method (A): Magnetic particle-based method using MagMAX™ Pathogen RNA/DNA Kit (Thermo Fisher Scientific, Waltham, MA, USA)

One aliquot of the supernatant from each sample (100 μL) was used to extract the viral RNA following the manufacturer's instructions. Briefly, the steps consisted of the lysis of the samples using 240 μL of the lysis buffer for bead beating, two washing steps, and a final elution step in 90 μL. For the lysis buffer preparation, RNA carrier was not included to avoid sequencing the extraneous RNA. Extraction was performed using the KingFisher™ Flex Purification System (Thermo Fisher Scientific, Waltham, MA, USA).

(2) Method (B): Silica column using QIAamp® Viral RNA (QIAGEN, Hilden, Germany):

A 140 μL aliquot from the supernatant of each sample was used to extract viral RNA following the manufacturer's instructions with a few modifications. First, the carrier RNA was not added to the viral lysis (AVL) buffer to avoid sequencing the extraneous RNA. Additionally, the elution step was modified to increase the RNA elution volume, and it consisted of (1) the addition of 30 μL of the elution buffer, (2) incubation at room temperature for one minute, and (3) centrifuging at 8000 rpm for one minute. These sequential steps were performed twice, resulting in a 60 μL total eluate.

(3) Method (C): Liquid-phase separation using TRIzol™ LS Reagent (Invitrogen, Waltham, MA, USA)

A 250 μL aliquot of the supernatant from each sample was homogenized with 750 μL of TRIzol reagent for cell lysis, followed by chloroform addition and phase separation (a lower red phenol–chloroform phase, white interphase, and a colorless upper aqueous phase containing the RNA). Following this step, the RNA was collected from the aqueous phase, precipitated in 500 μL of isopropanol, and centrifugation was performed for 15 min at 18,400× g at 4 °C for pellet formation. The pellet was resuspended in 1 mL of 75% ethanol and centrifuged for 5 min at 7500× g at 4 °C. The dried pellet was eluted in 50 μL of nuclease-free water.

(4) Method (D) Enzymatic extraction SwiftX™ Swabs (Xpedite Diagnostics GmbH, Hallbergmoos, Germany)

The extraction buffer (component E) was activated by dissolving two enzyme blends (components C and P) following the manufacturer's instructions. Subsequently, extraction was performed from the liquid samples by mixing 100 μL of the activated component E with 100 μL of each sample. The solution was incubated for 15 min at 90 °C and then cooled down and homogenized by vortexing the final elution.

Extracted RNA from all methods was kept at 4 °C till further rRT-PCR testing and evaluation. All analyses were performed within a week to preserve RNA integrity.

2.3. Evaluation of the Extracted RNA

2.3.1. Viral-Specific RNA Quantification

To assess the performance of each method in detecting viral-specific RNA, samples extracted from each method were tested for IAV using rRT-PCR targeting the virus Matrix gene. Testing was performed on the ABI 7500 Fast Real-Time PCR system (Applied Biosystems, Foster City, CA, USA) using a 20 μL total reaction volume containing 8 μL of RNA extract, 0.8 μL of Influenza Virus primers and probe mix (Avian Influenza Virus RNA Test kit—VetMAX™ Gold AIV Detection kit, Thermo Fisher Scientific, Waltham, MA, USA), 5 μL TaqMan Fast Virus 1-Step Master Mix (Life Technologies. Carlsbad, CA, USA), and 6.2 μL of nuclease-free water. The cycling conditions were 50 °C for 5 min and 95 °C for 20 s, followed by 40 cycles of 95 °C for 15 s and 60 °C for 1 min. Samples with C_T (cycle threshold) values equal to or higher than 40 were considered negative. The C_T value was used to approximate the IAV RNA concentration within each sample. The rRT-PCR detection rate was used as an evaluation parameter. This was a binary classification: samples with a C_T value less than 40 were assigned the value 1 (positive), while those with a C_T value of 40 or higher were assigned the value 0 (negative).

2.3.2. Total RNA Quantification and Purity Evaluation

The RNA concentration was assessed using the Qubit 4.0 Fluorometer and Qubit™ RNA HS Assay Kit (Thermo Fisher Scientific, Waltham, MA, USA) according to the manufacturer's protocol. Left-side censoring was established at 0.25 ng/μL for all samples with concentration values below the assay's limit of detection (0.25 ng/μL). The purity of each extract was verified using the NanoDrop Spectrophotometer (Thermo Fisher Scientific, Waltham, MA, USA) based on an A260/A280 ratio, and sample values between 1.9 and 2.2 were considered to have a high RNA purity.

2.3.3. Generation of MinION Nanopore Libraries, Sequencing, and Data Analysis

After extracting and evaluating the extracts, three samples (sample numbers five, fourteen, and sixteen—Table 1) were selected, extracted by the four protocols (n = 12), and used to prepare sequencing libraries. These samples were selected based on their tissue type, with the trachea representing the respiratory tract and the brain representing the neurological system, two systems commonly affected by the highly pathogenic avian influenza. Additionally, the selected samples had a variety of total and viral-specific (rRT-PCR C_T value) RNA concentrations (C_T values from 11.4 to 23; total RNA concentration from 378 to 1975 ng/μL) to evaluate the performance of ONT across a wide range of concentrations in the tested samples.

Two separate sequencing libraries were prepared with ONT's PCR-cDNA sequencing–barcoding protocol (SQK-PCB109) following the manufacturer's instructions. Briefly, the steps included (1) reverse transcription and strand switching, (2) a PCR step and the addition of barcoding to the transcripts, and (3) adapter ligation to the amplified cDNA library. After library preparation, each sequencing library was pooled and loaded onto a separate MinION R9.4.1 (FLO-MIN106D) flow cell (ONT) after priming with the Flow Cell Priming Kit (EXP FLP002) according to the manufacturer's instructions. The library containing sample 14 was run in a flow cell with 1141 pores, with 100 fmol of the library loaded. In contrast, for samples 5 and 16, the flow cell had 1314 pores, and 260 fmol of the library was loaded. The flow cells ran for 14 and 12 h, respectively, using the MinION Mk1B sequencer. MinKNOW software (21.06.0 version) was used to start and monitor the progress of the sequencing run. Guppy (5.0.11 version) within MinKNOW was used for base calling (fast accuracy base calling mode) and demultiplexing. The quality filtering employed a minimum score of seven, whereas length filtering applied to sequences within the range of 50 to 3000 bases. The generated FASTQ files were further analyzed using the WIMP tool within EPI2ME (Agent version 3.6.2) to calculate the total yield (in millions of bases), read length, read quality, and the number of specific AIV reads generated during the runs, to compare the effect of the four extraction methods on the generated sequences. Additionally, the Nanoplot [36] tool provided by Galaxy software v 22.05 (https://usegalaxy.org/) was used to assess the N50 from the generated FASTQ files. This sequencing approach is a mgNGS without prior enrichment. Although mgNGS is known for its poor sensitivity in viral detection, we chose not to apply any enrichment to ensure a fair comparison between methods.

2.3.4. Protocol Applicability and Sample Type Comparison

Establishing an applicable extraction process with the MinION nanopore sequencing platform will create an easy operational protocol for identifying and characterizing AIV from clinical samples. In our study, we assessed the protocol's applicability based on several key factors, including its flexibility (such as the ability to extract from various sample types), reproducibility, susceptibility to personal bias, the balance between hands-on and passive time, cost considerations, and input/output volumes. Our study's primary objective was to identify the most suitable protocol; therefore, we examined the applicability characteristics of the methods to guide our selection. The sample types are another crucial element influencing the extracted RNA and generated reads. As a result, we also compared the performance of the extraction protocols with different tissue types by contrasting the total RNA concentration and rRT-PCR detection rates.

2.4. Statistical Analysis

All statistical analyses were performed on the R statistical software [37]. Tables and figures were used to describe and assess the performance of the extraction protocols; figures were generated using the ggplot2 package [38] in R statistical software. Mixed-effects regression models were used to evaluate statistical differences in the performance of the extraction protocols for each variable assessed.

2.4.1. Statistical Analysis of RNA Quantification and Evaluation of Purity

Tables 3 and S1 and Figures 2–6 illustrate and compare the extraction protocols' performances in quantifying the total and IAV-specific RNA, extract purity, and rRT-PCR detection rates.

Table 3. Description of the selected samples for nanopore sequencing.

Sequencing Sample		1	2	3
	Animal ID	CN	GHO	CN
	Tissue type	Trachea	Brain	Brain
Protocol A (MagMAX™)	Av conc	9.8	32.5	35.7
	C_T	18.8	11.4	23.0
	Purity	1.6	2.1	2.0
	Total number of reads (Mb)	41.3	44.1	54.2
	AIV reads (count)	7	3340	3
	N50 (bases)	177	143	254
Protocol B (QIAamp® Viral RNA)	Av conc	21.8	15.55	66.5
	C_T	19.3	12.9	19.5
	Purity	1.9	2.0	1.9
	Total number of reads (Mb)	8.5	2.3	22.4
	AIV reads (count)	5	157	4
	N50 (bases)	187	139	228
Protocol C (TRIzol™ LS Reagent)	Av conc	368	1975	985
	C_T	17.4	6.9	18.8
	Purity	1.8	2.0	1.9
	Total number of reads (Mb)	26.1	46.4	33.6
	AIV reads (count)	49	5833	6
	N50	213	180	196
Protocol D (SwiftX™ Swabs)	Av conc	9.5	41.5	20.6
	C_T	27.2	13.2	25.3
	Purity	2.1	1.5	1.6
	Total number of reads (Mb)	6.8	19.8	10
	AIV reads (count)	5	778	2
	N50	149	142	204

CN: chicken. GHO: great horned owl.

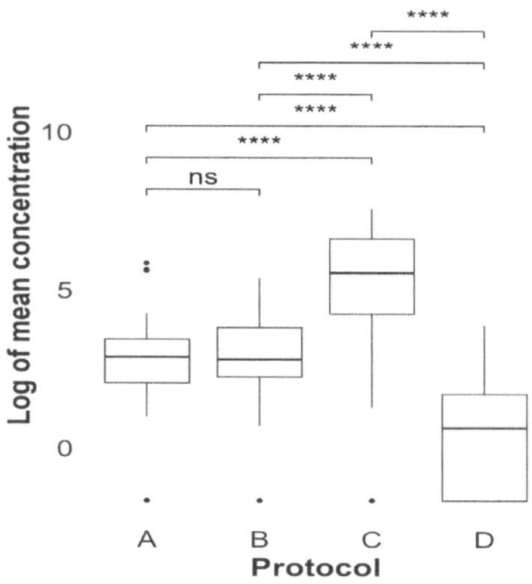

Figure 2. The log mean concentration distribution for each extraction protocol is represented as MagMAX Pathogen RNA/DNA™ (A), QIAamp® Viral RNA (B), TRIzol™ LS Reagent (C), and SwiftX™ Swabs (D). Statistical differences between protocols are indicated atop the boxplots using the results from a mixed-effect regression model (protocol as a fixed effect and tissue type nested within bird as a random effect). No significance "ns"; "****" indicate *p*-values > 0.05 and ≤0.0001, respectively. An alpha value of 0.05 was used, and *p*-values were adjusted using the Sidak method for 6 tests.

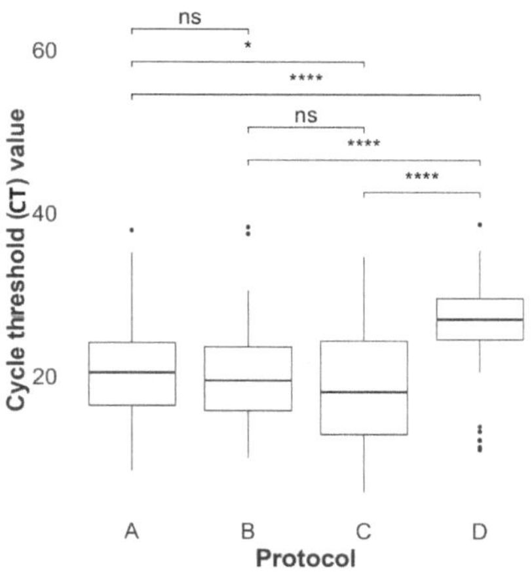

Figure 3. The distribution of cycle threshold values for each extraction protocol is represented as MagMAX Pathogen RNA/DNA™ (A), QIAamp® Viral RNA (B), TRIzol™ LS Reagent (C), and SwiftX™ Swabs (D). Statistical differences between protocols are indicated atop the boxplots using the results from a mixed-effect regression model (C_T as the protocol as a fixed effect and tissue type nested within bird as a random effect). No significance "ns", "*", and "****" indicate *p*-values > 0.05, ≤0.05, and ≤0.0001, respectively. An alpha value of 0.05 was used, and *p*-values were adjusted using the Sidak method for 6 tests.

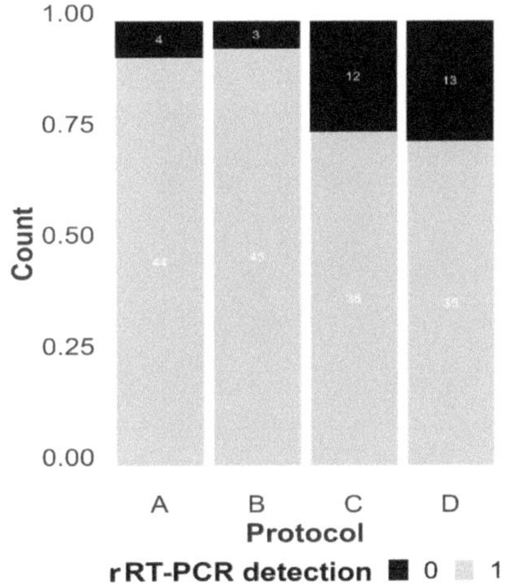

Figure 4. The count of positive samples by rRT-PCR by extraction protocol, represented as MagMAX Pathogen RNA/DNA™ (A), QIAamp® Viral RNA (B), TRIzol™ LS Reagent (C), and SwiftX™ Swabs (D). The total number of evaluated extracts per protocol was 48, considering that we extracted 24 samples in two different sections, resulting in 48 individual results per protocol. An extract has a positive detection (1) when the C_T value is less than (<) 40 and a negative detection (0) when the C_T value is equal to or higher than 40.

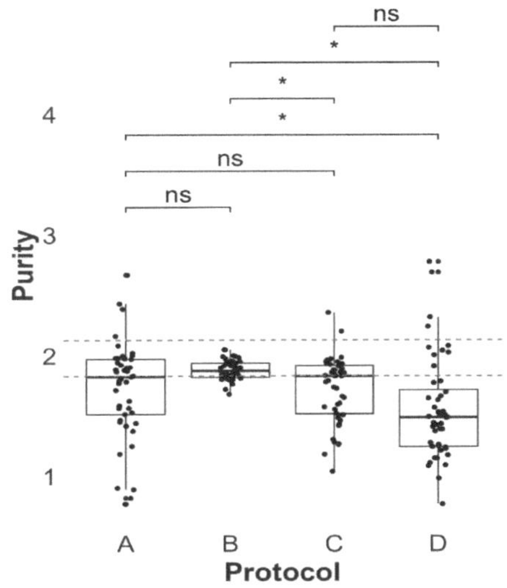

Figure 5. The distribution of purity values for each extraction protocol is represented as MagMAX Pathogen RNA/DNA™ (A), QIAamp® Viral RNA (B), TRIzol™ LS Reagent (C), and SwiftX™ Swabs (D). Statistical differences between protocols are indicated atop the boxplots using the results from a mixed-effect regression model (purity (pure or impure) was the response variable, the extraction protocol was the fixed effect, and tissue type nested within the bird was used as a random effect). "ns" and "*" indicate *p*-values > 0.05 and ≤0.05 respectively. An alpha value of 0.05 was used, and *p*-values were adjusted using the Sidak method for 6 tests. The red dashed lines indicate the range of absorbance ratio values between 1.9 and 2.2 within which an extract is considered pure.

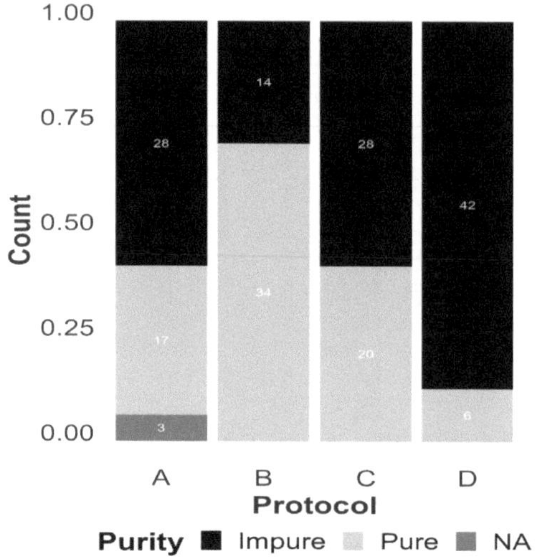

Figure 6. The count (numbers within the bars) of pure and impure extracts by extraction protocol, represented as MagMAX Pathogen RNA/DNA ™ (A), QIAamp® Viral RNA (B), TRIzol™ LS Reagent (C), and SwiftX™ Swabs (D). An extract is considered pure if the absorbance ratio values lie between 1.9 and 2.2. "NA": purity could not be assessed due to insufficient extract volume.

Linear mixed regression models were used to assess the least squares mean differences in the log mean RNA concentration and least squares mean differences in C_T values between protocols. In these models, the listed variables were each used as response variables, the extraction protocol was the fixed effect, and tissue type nested within each animal ID was used as a random effect to account for sample-specific attributes that could influence the performance of the extraction protocols.

The values obtained from the purity assessment were discretized into two categorical groups (pure or impure) based on having an A260/A280 ratio value within the range of 1.9–2.2 (inclusive) or not. Similarly, rRT-PCR C_T values below 40 were considered positive; otherwise, they were negative, hence also discreet. Logistic mixed regression models were thereafter used to assess purity and IAV rRT-PCR detection rates across the extraction protocols.

2.4.2. Statistical Analysis of the Generated Nanopore Sequencing Data

Table 3 and Figure 6 also illustrate and compare the extraction protocols' performances in quantifying the total yield (in a million bases), read length, read quality, and the number of specific IAV reads generated during the runs.

As all the listed variables are continuous, linear mixed regression models assessed the least squares mean differences between the extraction protocols. The total yield, read length, read quality, and the natural log of the IAV reads were each used as the response or dependent variables in the mixed models, the extraction protocols were the fixed effects, and the tissue type nested within each animal ID was used as the random effect.

3. Results

3.1. IAV Detection Rate and RNA Concentration

TRIzol demonstrated statistically significant superiority in terms of the mean log concentration of total RNA compared to all other methods across different samples (with a mean log concentration of 202.74 ng/µL) and a lower AIV-specific C_T value compared to the magnetic particle-based and enzymatic methods (mean C_T of 19.49), as shown in Figures 2 and 3. However, its ability to extract AIV from clinical samples was inconsistent, reflected by its lower detection rate in rRT-PCR results (Figure 4) compared to MagMAX and QIAmp. TRIzol had false negative results in 12 out of 48 extracts, while MagMAX and QIAmp had false negative results in 4 and 3 extracts, respectively. MagMAX and QIAamp performed similarly regarding their total RNA concentration and qPCR results. There was no statistically significant difference between the MagMAX and QIAmp mean log concentration results, with MagMAX showing a mean log concentration of 23.57 ng/μL and QIAmp 21.40 ng/μL. Additionally, there was no statistical difference regarding the MagMAX and QIAmp mean C_T values. It was also noteworthy that viral-specific concentration did not follow the same tendency as total concentration (i.e., some samples with a high total RNA concentration showed low AIV copy numbers, as predicted by high C_T values rather than low C_T values, Supplementary Material, Table S1). Other samples, such as spleen and air sac swabs, had a low total concentration and high AIV copy numbers. This difference may be due to the RNA in clinical samples representing the host rather than viral RNA. SwiftX Swabs consistently performed the worst, showing the lowest mean log concentration and the lowest detection rate by qPCR (with a mean log concentration of 1.8 ng/μL and mean C_T of 26.86), statistically inferior to the other protocols in both the evaluated parameters.

3.2. Purity Analysis

Regarding purity evaluation between the protocols, QIAamp exhibited the best performance across different samples, resulting in higher log odds of observing outcomes within the desirable range of 1.9–2.2 of RNA extracts (a probability of 72.66% of the occurrence of a pure sample in our logistic regression model). On the other hand, there was no significant statistical difference in the mean purity ratio between TRIzol and MagMAX (Figure 5), and both presented a similar number of samples classified as "impure" from our analysis. Finally, the Swift Swabs protocol presented the highest number of samples classified as "impure" and statistically lower log odds for the purity analysis (Figure 6).

3.3. Sequencing Performance

Although there were no statistical differences among the total yields (i.e., total generated bases from the sequencing run presented in million bases (Mb)) between MagMAX, TRIzol, and Swift Swabs, MagMAX had a higher read count than the other methods, resulting in an average of 46.53 million bases. In contrast, QIAmp showed the lowest yield, averaging 11.07 Mb.

Although most reads were from the host genome, there was a correlation between the number of total bases and the number of AIV-specific reads generated. As observed for QIAmp (B) and Swift Swabs (D), they showed fewer total bases and fewer logAIV reads (Figure 7d). The summary of the extraction evaluation and sequencing data is expressed in Table 3.

To assess the fragment length of the sequences, we compared the N50 generated by each protocol using the Nanoplot tool in Galaxy. N50 is a commonly used parameter for assessing the contiguity of ONT-generated sequencing data, and it is defined as the read length that 50% of the reads are equal to or more than. A higher N50 reflects a corresponding increase in the average read length and suggests a greater likelihood of contiguity in the assembly of reads. TRIzol produced longer reads, with a mean N50 of 196 bases, and Swift Swabs, the shortest reads, with a mean N50 of 165 bases. However, the kits had no significant length difference (Figure 7c).

To address the wide range of AIV reads obtained across the samples, we applied a log transformation to the read counts, compressing higher values and increasing the distribution of small values (Figure 7b). TRIzol showed the highest log-transformed AIV read counts (mean log reads of 4.78 and a median of 3.89). QIAmp produced fewer AIV reads, with the lowest mean AIV log reads of 2.68 and a median of 1.61.

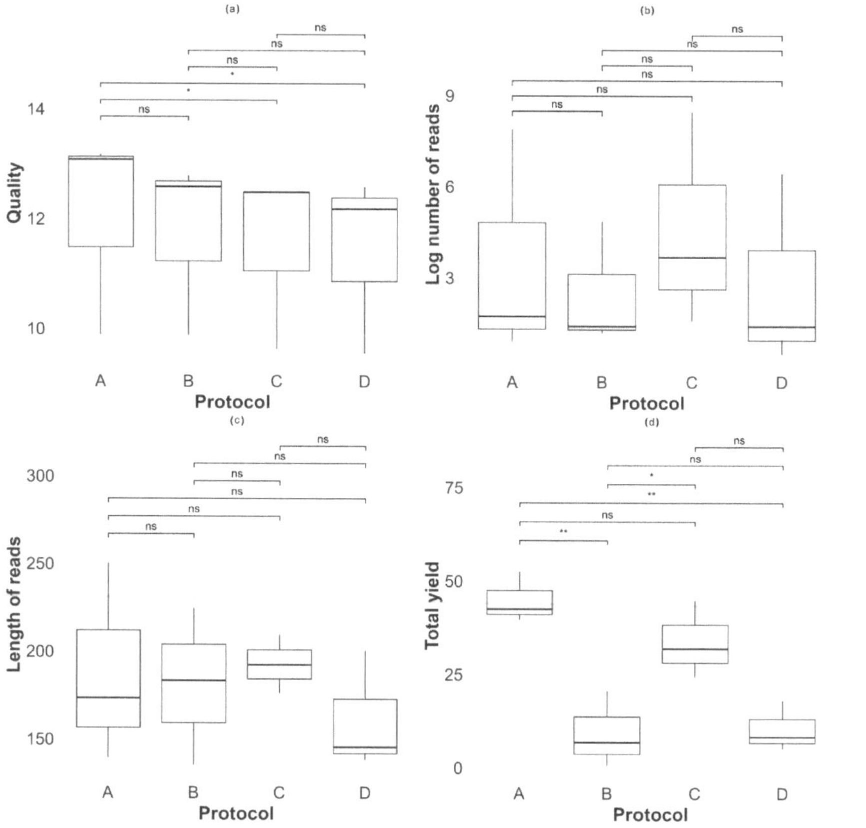

Figure 7. Metagenomic nanopore sequencing results by protocol. A-D plots of the different aspects evaluated to assess the sequence performance of the extraction protocols, represented as MagMAX Pathogen RNA/DNA™ (A), QIAamp® Viral RNA (B), TRIzol™ LS Reagent (C), and SwiftX™ Swabs (D). The boxplots represent the results from the three samples selected for mNGS. (**a**) Quality scores from the generated reads. (**b**) Log-transformed number of Influenza A reads generated. (**c**) Length of the generated reads expressed in bases. (**d**) Total yield (number of total reads) generated by protocol. Statistical differences between protocols are indicated atop the boxplots using the results from a mixed-effect regression model (read quality/log number of reads/read length, yield as the protocol as a fixed effect, and tissue type nested within bird as a random effect). "ns," "*", and "**"indicate p-values > 0.05, ≤0.05, and ≤0.0001 respectively. An alpha value of 0.05 was used, and p-values were adjusted using the Sidak method for six tests.

Finally, to evaluate the accuracy of the generated reads, we assessed the mean read quality score using the WIMP tool. The quality score is based on the Phred score, and across the different samples we evaluated, all four protocols exhibited an average quality score above 12, representing an accuracy higher than 90%. Furthermore, when comparing the mean read quality among the protocols for each sample, there was no statistical difference between their mean quality score, indicating a comparable read quality performance (Figure 7a).

3.4. Applicability of Different Extraction Protocols

The extraction procedure applicability was also established as a comparison parameter, considering that we aimed to combine the MinION's practicality with a suitable extraction workflow for AIV. Applicability in the current study was associated with the simplest, most reproducible method (reducing individual bias while performing the method), cost, flexibility with different tissue types, the equipment needed to execute each protocol, and input/output volumes.

Overall, MagMAX and Swift Swabs were the least time-consuming, with a reduced hands-on time of 25 min. Despite needing specific extraction equipment (Kingfisher Flex) for MagMAX, it would concomitantly allow the extraction of 96 samples, which is convenient for a diagnostic laboratory setting with a high caseload. The SwiftX Swabs method is advantageous overall because it only requires a regular heat block. In contrast, QIAmp and TRIzol were the most time-consuming; they included sequential centrifuging steps and presented less passive time because they required multiple pipetting and mixing steps. It is noteworthy that QIAmp was performed manually during this study. However, automation of the protocol is possible, which would significantly reduce the time, especially for extracting a high number of samples.

Additionally, there were specific limitations associated with some methods. For instance, the TRIzol method is highly error-prone because it depends on personal decisions during aqueous phase pipetting and pellet visualization, leading to inconsistencies and inaccuracies. Meanhile, Swift Swabs presented a limitation considering the final aspect of the extract; some of the extracts solidified and prevented the separation of a clear solution for further application. This condition might have affected the rRT-PCR results and the purity of the samples extracted by Swift Swabs.

3.5. Sample Type Comparison

Considering that different sample types were included in the study, the C_T value and rRT-PCR detection rate were evaluated across these samples to assess the extraction protocols' performance (Table S1 and Figure S2 in the Supplementary Materials). Brain and lung tissues consistently tested positive (detection rate = 1) across different protocols, except for a single brain sample (sample #21) that showed a C_T value greater than 40 (detection rate = 0) when extracted with TRIzol (Method C). Notably, brain tissue exhibited the lowest mean C_T value across all extraction protocols. TRIzol had a lower detection rate for swab samples (air sac and spleen swabs), with three out of four extracts testing negative in the rRT-PCR test. Additionally, the SwiftX Swabs (Method D) showed a lower detection rate in liver and trachea samples, with all six extracts testing negative in the rRT-PCR test.

4. Discussion

As a foreign animal disease (FAD), avian influenza impacts the poultry industry and brings economic and social requirements for its detection and control [1]. The output of a nanopore sequencing run is strongly influenced by all the preceding steps, including the nucleic acid extraction, enrichment, and library preparation steps. Therefore, all the procedures involved in sample preparation for AIV detection and sequencing must be evaluated to establish a reproducible, rapid, and accurate diagnostic workflow using ONT. Extraction is the base step upon which all the other steps for an optimal sequencing run are built, and it is essential for obtaining high-quality nucleic acid. Thus, in this study, we evaluated the extraction step by comparing four commercial extraction kits. The extraction is based on three main steps: the disruption of cells and tissue, denaturation of nucleoprotein complexes, and inactivation of nucleases (DNase and RNase) [39]. After extraction, the target nucleic acid should be in a high concentration and free of contaminants such as proteins, carbohydrates, or lipids [40]. The different principles, reagents, and procedures used by each protocol impact the RNA recovery and purity, interfering with pathogen detection and characterization with NGS. Additionally, input and output sample volume, throughput, automation, and cost differ across the methods, leading to differences in the suitability for diagnostics settings.

4.1. Performance of the Kits—Evaluating the Extracts' Concentration (Total and Viral-Specific) and Purity

We evaluated the RNA concentration obtained from four extraction methods, categorizing our results into total RNA concentration assessed by fluorometry, and AIV-specific concentration by rRT-PCR. As shown in Figure 3 and Table S1 TRIzol LS (Method C) had the highest RNA recovery efficiency across different tissue types. Other studies comparing RNA concentrations between QIAmp (Method B) and acid guanidium thiocyanate–phenol–chloroform extraction (a similar extraction principle as TRIzol) procedures used different sample types (blood, tissues, exhaled breath, and airborne environment) and revealed similar outcomes [41–43]. Although TRIzol had the lowest C_T values in tissue samples, it had a lower rRT-PCR detection rate in swab samples than the other kits (Table S1). Knepp et al. (2003) reported comparable results after examining various nucleic acid extraction methods for Enterovirus RNA recovery from cell culture [44]. This difference in the TRIzol LS recovery rate can be attributed to the method's superior performance with tissue samples but not with relatively cell-free samples such as swabs [45,46]. The inconsistent detection rate of TRIzol LS is a significant limitation of this method in a diagnostic setting, since swabs are the primary sample type for AIV detection and monitoring.

Our investigation showed that SwiftX™ Swabs' efficacy in RNA extraction was lower than the other evaluated kits. This led to a reduced recovery rate indicated by a lower log concentration and higher C_T values. This protocol has been validated as a tool for RNA extraction from fresh swabs and saliva samples. It is intended to work best when swabs are placed directly into the reagent solution without prior dilution in transport media [47]. In our study, we utilized tissue samples with a high cell concentration, and the swabs were subjected to freezing before extraction. To date, no further studies have assessed the potential of this method for AIV extraction. Hence, additional research is needed before recommending incorporating this approach as a standard diagnostic procedure.

Our study found that the magnetic particle-based method (MagMAX) and the silica column (QIAmp) had similar results in total RNA concentration and rRT-PCR performance for different sample types. However, previous studies have reported that the magnetic bead method was more effective in extracting nucleic acids from fecal samples for gut microbiota profiling [28] and yielded lower C_T values for detecting SARS-CoV-2 [48] when compared to the silica method. Nevertheless, in agreement with our PCR detection rates results, the silica column and magnetic particle-based methods presented high agreement between positive and negative results in the previous study, while TRIzol showed an inferior performance in detecting the viral RNA from the cell culture samples tested [48]. Both methods (MagMAX and QIAmp) are widely used in diagnostic settings, and based on our findings, they are effective approaches for RNA recovery from tissue samples.

As measured by the 260/280 ratio, the RNA purity was also evaluated between the different extraction methods. QIAamp (spin column) produced the best results, but that did not directly correlate with better sequence results. Deng et al. (2005) also compared RNA extraction methods regarding purity by assessing A260/A280, and the spin column procedure had the optimal ratio for most of the tested samples when compared to TRIzol LS [41]. However, another study found comparable purity results when assessing the performance of both methods [43]. The differences in purity results between these studies might be related to a higher efficiency achieved during the washing steps for the TRIzol procedure, which increased the purity of the extraction outcome. In addition, avoiding pipetting contaminants accidentally from the interphase would prevent RNA contamination with protein or phenol [49]. Conversely, a decrease in QIAGEN purity might happen due to the silica membrane clogging. This is more frequent when extracting tissue samples with higher amounts of particles/cells, as demonstrated by Muyal et al. 2009, obtaining a lower A260/A280 ratio [43].

4.2. Sequencing Performance Evaluation

This study aimed to select the optimum extraction protocol for AIV recovery from clinical samples that would be applied for mNGS with ONT. We compared the sequencing results of three samples extracted using each protocol to complete the evaluation of the four commercial extraction methods. We assessed the total number of reads generated, the number of specific AIV reads, and the sequences' length and quality to determine the best extraction protocol.

The outcome of ONT sequencing relies on the extracted RNA's quality and quantity. Our study found that TRIzol had the highest viral concentration, as evidenced by a lower C_T value, and resulted in a high number of avian influenza reads. Obtaining a high number of viral reads is crucial, given that the accurate identification and characterization of the pathogen depends on the depth and breadth of coverage, which can be increased with high-throughput sequencing platforms like ONT. Moreover, the higher error rate of ONT compared to Illumina can be overcome by increasing coverage depth, which allows for confident variant calling [32,50]. Therefore, selecting an extraction protocol that yields more AIV reads is necessary. Previous studies have shown the importance of protocol selection to the final AIV genome assembly for NGS outcome, highlighting that the magnetic particle protocol outperformed regarding AIV segments coverage depth [32].

Regarding the quality impact on ONT data, we hypothesized that the purity of the original samples would not have significantly affected our results, given that we used a library preparation kit (SQK-PCB109) incorporating a PCR step. PCR can be used to select successfully barcoded nucleic acids and amplify them, which, in turn, can dilute and decrease impurities in the samples. This process may explain why other low-purity samples extracted with MagMax and TRIzol protocols still outperformed QIAgen, which had better purity results. Therefore, the purity of the samples may have been improved during the library preparation step. However, ONT offers a wide range of library preparation kits, and for the PCR-free protocols, the original purity from the samples may play a role in sequencing data generation.

Although ONT is a long-read NGS platform, the average length of the generated reads was relatively short. This may be due to several factors in our study, including the freezing–thawing process (as the samples were not fresh), the presence of RNases, and multiple pipetting and vortexing steps throughout the process [51,52]. However, given the segmented genome of IAV, fragment length was not a major concern in our study.

The major limitation of our sequencing outcome was the low amount of AIV reads generated from the clinical samples tested. This limitation can be attributed to most nucleic acid in the samples being from the host genome. Furthermore, the lack of target enrichment strategies and host depletion procedures compromised the assay's sensitivity. Previous research has shown that DNase treatment is necessary for successful AIV RNA sequencing from clinical samples [32]. Additionally, other studies have described various protocols for AIV NGS directly from clinical samples. These protocols include amplicon sequencing [19,23,53] or sequence-independent enrichment [54] approaches to increase the number of viral reads and improve genome coverage. Although mgNGS is known for its poor sensitivity in viral detection, we chose not to apply any enrichment to ensure a fair comparison between methods.

4.3. Sample Type Impact

Based on our results, brain samples presented the highest total RNA and specific viral concentration. These findings are explained by the fact that HPAI viral strains have a systemic distribution in chicken visceral organs, and brain neurons are commonly affected [55]. HPAIV had not previously been associated with clinical signs and lesions in wild birds until the H5N1 Eurasian–African lineage altered the pathobiological dynamics of the disease in these species [56]. In our clinical cases, the birds showed neurological signs and microscopic lesions compatible with a systemic viral infection, including brain inflammation. Those findings also support the higher viral load in brain samples.

Respiratory samples, especially oropharyngeal swabs, are the most common sample type used in the AIV diagnostic routine; therefore, evaluating the extraction step impact in these samples would be more beneficial. Given the limitations of our study, where access to oropharyngeal swabs was unavailable, we conducted the extraction using air sac and spleen swabs instead. These two alternatives share similarities, such as having fewer host cells and serving as tissues suitable for viral detection because HPAIV strains can be systemically distributed throughout the infected birds [2]. In our work, the respiratory tissues showed a high total RNA concentration, except for in the case of Swift Swabs (as shown in Table S1). Furthermore, the swabs had the lowest concentration values, which is explained by less cellularity in this sample type, reducing the amount of host RNA. However, even with a lower total RNA concentration, air sac swabs presented a high viral load, reflected by its low mean C_T value obtained with both the MagMAX and QIAmp protocols. TRIzol was unable to detect AIV from air sac swab samples. One possible explanation is that the air sac swab sample type may have a lower cellularity, resulting in less RNA extraction and a smaller pellet forming, which could affect RNA visualization and capture, highlighting a major limitation of TRIzol extraction. Moreover, SwiftX Swabs was less efficient than MagMAX and QIAmp, as evidenced by its higher C_T value.

4.4. The Applicability of the Kits

Further comparison between the four methods was implemented based on the suitability of the workflow, to assess their applicability as a standard diagnostic procedure. The automated MagMAX presented many advantages, such as removing consecutive centrifugation steps, column separation, and using hazardous chemicals [40]. In addition, it allows the simultaneous extraction of up to 96 samples in a 25 min reaction. Conversely, it had a higher cost per sample and required a specific instrument for its performance. TRIzol and QIAmp, on the other hand, were more time-consuming and did not allow high-throughput viral RNA extraction in our conditions. TRIzol specifically presented critical stages during the manual extraction of the samples, such as the phase separation step and the need for visual pellet formation. In addition, it was laborious and prone to personal bias due to multiple steps, which limits its large-scale routine application [57]. We recognize that QIAmp is also compatible with automated extraction, which would benefit its application in diagnostic laboratories.

Finally, we identified SwiftX™ Swabs as a promising procedure due to its cost-effectiveness, decreased hands-on time, and minimal steps and equipment required, making it a good candidate for point-of-care diagnostics. However, due to the sample type (tissue samples) we included in the study, the extraction output was unsuitable for AIV detection, considering that after being heated with the extraction solution, some samples clotted (e.g., became solid instead of an aqueous solution), leading to extracts of worse quality and quantity. In addition, the swabs utilized in the study were frozen, and the kit was intended to be performed on fresh swabs, which could explain its inferior performance with the swabs. Notably, there is a different extraction kit offered by Xpedite Diagnostics, SwiftX™ DNA, which could be utilized to extract DNA or RNA from complex (high cellularity) samples. This protocol has additional lysing steps, and a cellular capture based on adding beads suspension and further heat lysis and releasing the nucleic acids in the sample. Additional analysis should be conducted to evaluate the suitability of SwiftX™ DNA or similar technologies for AIV recovery from tissues.

While our study found that TRIzol yielded superior results in total and viral-specific concentrations, it is important to note that this kit had several drawbacks. These disadvantages included inconsistencies in viral detection when using swab samples (commonly used for routine avian influenza virus diagnostics), a lengthy protocol, and susceptibility to personal bias. In contrast, the QIAmp kit excelled in purity but underperformed in various sequencing parameters across different samples. Lastly, although MagMAX did not outperform the other methods in our evaluation, it offers several advantages. It is an automated protocol, allowing for the simultaneous processing of up to 96 samples in the KingFisher. MagMAX demonstrated consistency and reproducibility, with a viral concentration and purity comparable to other methods. Furthermore, MagMAX performed well with the MinION sequencing platform, yielding a high number of total and specific AIV reads.

5. Limitations

This study had some limitations. Firstly, the different extraction methods used in this study had varying input and output volumes, which could affect the final RNA concentration. Our primary aim was to evaluate commercially available methods based on the routine protocols established by their manufacturers. Future studies can be performed to compare different input and output volumes to optimize each method further. Secondly, although nasal and cloacal swabs are the most common sample types for AIV diagnosis, they were not the majority of samples tested in this study. This is due to the study's circumstances (e.g., a veterinary diagnostic laboratory receiving birds for necropsy and submitting swabs for NVSL Laboratory AIV confirmation tests). However, since AIV causes systemic disease in various bird species, testing different tissue types remains valuable for diagnosing this virus and other systemic diseases affecting poultry. Regarding the comparison between the automated MagMAX extraction protocol and other manual procedures, we acknowledge that an automated option is available for the Qiagen protocol, which could enhance both the speed and consistency of the results. However, we included only the automated MagMAX protocol in our study because it was readily available in our laboratory, as well as in other veterinary diagnostic laboratories across the U.S. Lastly, we did not pursue additional host depletion strategies to enhance the sensitivity of the metagenomic NGS (e.g., a higher centrifugation speed and time, DNase and RNase depletion). Consequently, the number of AIV reads from clinical samples using ONT was limited. Therefore, it was not possible to properly compare the final mapping or assembly results obtained from each RNA sample. It is possible that extending the sequencing run could have improved the recovery of the avian influenza virus genome from the samples; however, this was not performed in the current study. Further testing with host depletion approaches is necessary to improve mNGS for more effective virus identification and characterization.

6. Conclusions

None of the protocols evaluated was superior for all the aspects assessed in this study. Different choices regarding the suitability of each method in different situations could be made based on the data presented in this manuscript, which highlights the advantages and disadvantages for each method. However, in our hands, the MagMAX™ Pathogen RNA/DNA Kit overall had many advantages in its applicability (speed and scalability) and consistent sequencing performance (yield, compatible number of AIV-specific reads, and segment length) that would allow it to be routinely used for the first step of an NGS workflow. TRIzol™ LS Reagent performed better regarding the RNA and viral concentration, while the best purity ratios were obtained with QIAamp® Viral RNA, but both kits encountered issues regarding their ease of use and speed. Finally, although SwiftX™ Swabs had promising performance features related to its simplified processing steps and time, the performance was not comparable to the other protocols. We recognize the limitation of not using swabs as the primary sample type in our study, given the significance of this sample type for AIV diagnosis, and the fact that SwiftX™ swabs were specifically designed for use with such samples. We emphasize that our findings were related specifically to AIV samples, and these methods could perform differently when used for different pathogens that are not segmented or have longer genome sizes; therefore, they should be evaluated based on the intended target.

Supplementary Materials: The following supporting information can be downloaded at: https://www.mdpi.com/article/10.3390/v16091429/s1, Table S1: Mean total RNA concentration, expressed in nanograms per microliters, and C_T value from each sample by protocol. Samples are ordered according to the animal species, and number IDs are added corresponding to the numbering described in Table 1; Figure S1: Mean cycle threshold (C_T values, log concentration, and purity for each protocol in the two experimental sessions (1 and 2); Figure S2: The count of positive samples by rRT-PCR by sample type and by extraction protocol, represented as MagMAX Pathogen RNA/DNA™ (A), QIAamp® Viral RNA (B), TRIzol™ LS Reagent (C), and SwiftX™ Swabs (D). An extract has a positive detection (1) when the C_T value is less than (<) 40 and a negative detection (0) when the C_T value is equal to or higher than 40. AGT: American green-winged teal. CN: chicken. EE: eagle. FN: falcon. GHO: great horned owl. HK: hawk. TV: turkey vulture.

Author Contributions: Conceptualization, M.C., A.H., Y.S., D.L.S. and M.E.-G.; methodology, A.H.; software, M.C. and A.H.; validation, M.C., A.H., Y.S. and M.E.-G.; formal analysis, M.C., A.H., Y.S. and M.E.-G.; investigation, M.C., A.H., Y.S., D.L.S. and M.E.-G.; resources, Y.S., D.L.S. and M.E.-G.; data curation, O.O.; writing—original draft preparation, M.C.; writing—review and editing, M.C., A.H., O.O., Y.S., D.L.S. and M.E.-G.; supervision, M.E.-G.; project administration, M.E.-G.; funding acquisition, A.H., Y.S., D.L.S. and M.E.-G. All authors have read and agreed to the published version of the manuscript.

Funding: This research was funded by the US Department of Agriculture (USDA) Animal and Plant Health Inspection Service, grant number AP22VSD&B000C010.

Institutional Review Board Statement: Not applicable.

Informed Consent Statement: Not applicable.

Data Availability Statement: The raw data presented in this study are openly available in the SRA under the accession numbers SRR27468981, SRR27468980, SRR27468979, SRR27468978, SRR27468977, SRR27468976, SRR27468975, SRR27468974, SRR27468973, SRR27468972, SRR27468971, SRR27468970, and the BioProject accession number PRJNA1062777.

Acknowledgments: We thank the Veterinary Diagnostic Laboratory at Iowa State University and Mostafa Shelkamy for excellent technical assistance.

Conflicts of Interest: The authors declare no conflicts of interest.

References

1. Available online: https://www.woah.org/en/disease/avian-influenza/ (accessed on 23 April 2023).
2. McMullin, P.F. *Diseases of Poultry*, 14th ed.; Swayne, D.E., Boulianne, M., Logue, C.M., McDougald, L.R., Nair, V., Suarez, D.L., de Wit, S., Grimes, T., Johnson, D., Kromm, M., et al., Eds.; John Wiley & Sons: Hoboken, NJ, USA, 2020; Volume I.
3. USDA Animal and Plant Health Inspection Service Veterinary Services. *Final Report for the 2014–2015 Outbreak of Highly Pathogenic Avian Influenza (HPAI) in the United States*; USDA: Riverdale, MD, USA, 2016.
4. USDA Animal and Plant Health Inspection Service. 2022–2023 Confirmations of Highly Pathogenic Avian Influenza in Commercial and Backyard Flocks. Available online: https://www.aphis.usda.gov/aphis/ourfocus/animalhealth/animal-disease-information/avian/avian-influenza/hpai-2022/2022-hpai-commercial-backyard-flocks (accessed on 22 November 2023).
5. Sajeer P, M. Disruptive technology: Exploring the ethical, legal, political, and societal implications of nanopore sequencing technology. *EMBO Rep.* **2023**, *24*, e56619. [CrossRef] [PubMed]
6. Quick, J.; Ashton, P.; Calus, S.; Chatt, C.; Gossain, S.; Hawker, J.; Nair, S.; Neal, K.; Nye, K.; Peters, T. Rapid draft sequencing and real-time nanopore sequencing in a hospital outbreak of Salmonella. *Genome Biol.* **2015**, *16*, 114. [CrossRef] [PubMed]
7. Quick, J.; Loman, N.J.; Duraffour, S.; Simpson, J.T.; Severi, E.; Cowley, L.; Bore, J.A.; Koundouno, R.; Dudas, G.; Mikhail, A. Real-time, portable genome sequencing for Ebola surveillance. *Nature* **2016**, *530*, 228–232. [CrossRef] [PubMed]
8. Quick, J.; Grubaugh, N.D.; Pullan, S.T.; Claro, I.M.; Smith, A.D.; Gangavarapu, K.; Oliveira, G.; Robles-Sikisaka, R.; Rogers, T.F.; Beutler, N.A. Multiplex PCR method for MinION and Illumina sequencing of Zika and other virus genomes directly from clinical samples. *Nat. Protoc.* **2017**, *12*, 1261–1276. [CrossRef]
9. World Organisation for Animal Health. Avian Influenza (Including infections with High Pathogenicity Avian Influenza Viruses). In *WOAH Terrestrial Manual*; World Organisation for Animal Health: Paris, France, 2021; Chapter 3.3.4.
10. Bevins, S.N.; Shriner, S.A.; Cumbee Jr, J.C.; Dilione, K.E.; Douglass, K.E.; Ellis, J.W.; Killian, M.L.; Torchetti, M.K.; Lenoch, J.B. Intercontinental movement of highly pathogenic avian influenza A (H5N1) clade 2.3. 4.4 virus to the United States, 2021. *Emerg. Infect. Dis.* **2022**, *28*, 1006. [CrossRef]

11. Caliendo, V.; Lewis, N.; Pohlmann, A.; Baillie, S.; Banyard, A.; Beer, M.; Brown, I.; Fouchier, R.; Hansen, R.; Lameris, T. Transatlantic spread of highly pathogenic avian influenza H5N1 by wild birds from Europe to North America in 2021. *Sci. Rep.* **2022**, *12*, 11729. [CrossRef]
12. Wan, X.-F.; Dong, L.; Lan, Y.; Long, L.-P.; Xu, C.; Zou, S.; Li, Z.; Wen, L.; Cai, Z.; Wang, W. Indications that live poultry markets are a major source of human H5N1 influenza virus infection in China. *J. Virol.* **2011**, *85*, 13432–13438. [CrossRef]
13. Pasick, J. Advances in the molecular based techniques for the diagnosis and characterization of avian influenza virus infections. *Transbound. Emerg. Dis.* **2008**, *55*, 329–338. [CrossRef]
14. Wei, S.-H.; Yang, J.-R.; Wu, H.-S.; Chang, M.-C.; Lin, J.-S.; Lin, C.-Y.; Liu, Y.-L.; Lo, Y.-C.; Yang, C.-H.; Chuang, J.-H. Human infection with avian influenza A H6N1 virus: An epidemiological analysis. *Lancet Respir. Med.* **2013**, *1*, 771–778. [CrossRef]
15. Hoffmann, E.; Stech, J.; Guan, Y.; Webster, R.; Perez, D. Universal primer set for the full-length amplification of all influenza A viruses. *Arch. Virol.* **2001**, *146*, 2275–2289. [CrossRef]
16. Deng, Y.-M.; Spirason, N.; Iannello, P.; Jelley, L.; Lau, H.; Barr, I.G. A simplified Sanger sequencing method for full genome sequencing of multiple subtypes of human influenza A viruses. *J. Clin. Virol.* **2015**, *68*, 43–48. [CrossRef] [PubMed]
17. Díaz-Sánchez, S.; Hanning, I.; Pendleton, S.; D'Souza, D. Next-generation sequencing: The future of molecular genetics in poultry production and food safety. *Poult. Sci.* **2013**, *92*, 562–572. [CrossRef] [PubMed]
18. Rang, F.J.; Kloosterman, W.P.; de Ridder, J. From squiggle to basepair: Computational approaches for improving nanopore sequencing read accuracy. *Genome Biol.* **2018**, *19*, 90. [CrossRef] [PubMed]
19. Crossley, B.M.; Rejmanek, D.; Baroch, J.; Stanton, J.B.; Young, K.T.; Killian, M.L.; Torchetti, M.K.; Hietala, S.K. Nanopore sequencing as a rapid tool for identification and pathotyping of avian influenza A viruses. *J. Vet. Diagn. Investig.* **2021**, *33*, 253–260. [CrossRef]
20. Jain, M.; Olsen, H.E.; Paten, B.; Akeson, M. The Oxford Nanopore MinION: Delivery of nanopore sequencing to the genomics community. *Genome Biol.* **2016**, *17*, 239.
21. Petersen, L.M.; Martin, I.W.; Moschetti, W.E.; Kershaw, C.M.; Tsongalis, G.J. Third-generation sequencing in the clinical laboratory: Exploring the advantages and challenges of nanopore sequencing. *J. Clin. Microbiol.* **2019**, *58*, e01315–e01319. [CrossRef]
22. Kono, N.; Arakawa, K. Nanopore sequencing: Review of potential applications in functional genomics. *Dev. Growth Differ.* **2019**, *61*, 316–326. [CrossRef]
23. de Vries, E.M.; Cogan, N.O.; Gubala, A.J.; Mee, P.T.; O'Riley, K.J.; Rodoni, B.C.; Lynch, S.E. Rapid, in-field deployable, avian influenza virus haemagglutinin characterisation tool using MinION technology. *Sci. Rep.* **2022**, *12*, 11886. [CrossRef]
24. Runtuwene, L.R.; Tuda, J.S.; Mongan, A.E.; Suzuki, Y. On-site MinION sequencing. In *Single Molecule and Single Cell Sequencing*; Advances in Experimental Medicine and Biology; Springer: Singapore, 2019; Volume 1129, pp. 143–150. [CrossRef]
25. Wang, Y.; Zhao, Y.; Bollas, A.; Wang, Y.; Au, K.F. Nanopore sequencing technology, bioinformatics and applications. *Nat. Biotechnol.* **2021**, *39*, 1348–1365. [CrossRef]
26. Sauvage, T.; Cormier, A.; Delphine, P. A comparison of Oxford nanopore library strategies for bacterial genomics. *BMC Genom.* **2023**, *24*, 627. [CrossRef]
27. Eagle, S.H.; Robertson, J.; Bastedo, D.P.; Liu, K.; Nash, J.H. Evaluation of five commercial DNA extraction kits using Salmonella as a model for implementation of rapid Nanopore sequencing in routine diagnostic laboratories. *Access Microbiol.* **2023**, *5*, 000468.v3. [CrossRef] [PubMed]
28. Panek, M.; Čipčić Paljetak, H.; Barešić, A.; Perić, M.; Matijašić, M.; Lojkić, I.; Vranešić Bender, D.; Krznarić, Ž.; Verbanac, D. Methodology challenges in studying human gut microbiota–effects of collection, storage, DNA extraction and next generation sequencing technologies. *Sci. Rep.* **2018**, *8*, 5143. [CrossRef] [PubMed]
29. Zhang, L.; Chen, T.; Wang, Y.; Zhang, S.; Lv, Q.; Kong, D.; Jiang, H.; Zheng, Y.; Ren, Y.; Huang, W. Comparison Analysis of Different DNA Extraction Methods on Suitability for Long-Read Metagenomic Nanopore Sequencing. *Front. Cell. Infect. Microbiol.* **2022**, *12*, 919903. [CrossRef] [PubMed]
30. Trigodet, F.; Lolans, K.; Fogarty, E.; Shaiber, A.; Morrison, H.G.; Barreiro, L.; Jabri, B.; Eren, A.M. High molecular weight DNA extraction strategies for long-read sequencing of complex metagenomes. *Mol. Ecol. Resour.* **2022**, *22*, 1786–1802. [CrossRef]
31. Petersen, C.; Sørensen, T.; Westphal, K.R.; Fechete, L.I.; Sondergaard, T.E.; Sørensen, J.L.; Nielsen, K.L. High molecular weight DNA extraction methods lead to high quality filamentous ascomycete fungal genome assemblies using Oxford Nanopore sequencing. *Microb. Genom.* **2022**, *8*, 000816. [CrossRef]
32. Di, H.; Thor, S.W.; Trujillo, A.A.; Stark, T.J.; Marinova-Petkova, A.; Jones, J.; Wentworth, D.E.; Barnes, J.R.; Davis, C.T. Comparison of nucleic acid extraction methods for next-generation sequencing of avian influenza A virus from ferret respiratory samples. *J. Virol. Methods* **2019**, *270*, 95–105. [CrossRef]
33. Dixit, B.; Murugkar, H.; Nagarajan, S.; Dixit, M.; Shrivastav, A.; Kumar, A.; Jha, A.; Mishra, A.; Singh, R.; Kumar, M. Evaluation of different transport media for survival of H5N1 highly pathogenic avian influenza virus. *Preprint* **2024**. [CrossRef]
34. Killian, M.L. Avian influenza virus sample types, collection, and handling. In *Animal Influenza Virus: Methods and Protocols*; Humana: New York, NY, USA, 2020; pp. 113–121.
35. Zhang, X.-C.; Liu, S.; Hou, G.-Y.; Zhuang, Q.-Y.; Wang, K.-C.; Jiang, W.-M.; Wang, S.-C.; Li, J.-P.; Yu, J.-M.; Du, X. Comparison of three media for transport and storage of the samples collected for detection of avian influenza virus. *J. Virol. Methods* **2015**, *222*, 202–205. [CrossRef]

36. De Coster, W.; Rademakers, R. NanoPack2: Population-scale evaluation of long-read sequencing data. *Bioinformatics* **2023**, *39*, btad311. [CrossRef]
37. *R Core Team: A Language and Environment for Statistical Computing*; R Foundation for Statistical Computing: Vienna, Austria, 2019; Available online: https://www.R-project.org (accessed on 27 April 2023).
38. Wickham, H. ggplot2. *Wiley Interdiscip. Rev. Comput. Stat.* **2011**, *3*, 180–185. [CrossRef]
39. Buckingham, L. *Molecular Diagnostics: Fundamentals, Methods and Clinical Applications*; FA Davis: Philadelphia, PA, USA, 2019.
40. Tan, S.C.; Yiap, B.C. DNA, RNA, and protein extraction: The past and the present. *J. Biomed. Biotechnol.* **2009**, *2009*, 574398. [CrossRef]
41. Deng, M.Y.; Wang, H.; Ward, G.B.; Beckham, T.R.; McKenna, T.S. Comparison of six RNA extraction methods for the detection of classical swine fever virus by real-time and conventional reverse transcription–PCR. *J. Vet. Diagn. Investig.* **2005**, *17*, 574–578. [CrossRef]
42. Fabian, P.; McDevitt, J.J.; Lee, W.-M.; Houseman, E.A.; Milton, D.K. An optimized method to detect influenza virus and human rhinovirus from exhaled breath and the airborne environment. *J. Environ. Monit.* **2009**, *11*, 314–317. [CrossRef] [PubMed]
43. Muyal, J.P.; Muyal, V.; Kaistha, B.P.; Seifart, C.; Fehrenbach, H. Systematic comparison of RNA extraction techniques from frozen and fresh lung tissues: Checkpoint towards gene expression studies. *Diagn. Pathol.* **2009**, *4*, 9. [CrossRef] [PubMed]
44. Knepp, J.H.; Geahr, M.A.; Forman, M.S.; Valsamakis, A. Comparison of automated and manual nucleic acid extraction methods for detection of enterovirus RNA. *J. Clin. Microbiol.* **2003**, *41*, 3532–3536. [CrossRef] [PubMed]
45. Torii, S.; Furumai, H.; Katayama, H. Applicability of polyethylene glycol precipitation followed by acid guanidinium thiocyanate-phenol-chloroform extraction for the detection of SARS-CoV-2 RNA from municipal wastewater. *Sci. Total Environ.* **2021**, *756*, 143067. [CrossRef]
46. Zheng, X.; Deng, Y.; Xu, X.; Li, S.; Zhang, Y.; Ding, J.; On, H.Y.; Lai, J.C.; Yau, C.I.; Chin, A.W. Comparison of virus concentration methods and RNA extraction methods for SARS-CoV-2 wastewater surveillance. *Sci. Total Environ.* **2022**, *824*, 153687. [CrossRef]
47. Available online: https://www.xpedite-dx.com/products/swiftx-swabs/ (accessed on 27 April 2023).
48. Eisen, A.K.A.; Demoliner, M.; Gularte, J.S.; Hansen, A.W.; Schallenberger, K.; Mallmann, L.; Hermann, B.S.; Heldt, F.H.; de Almeida, P.R.; Fleck, J.D. Comparison of different kits for SARS-CoV-2 RNA extraction marketed in Brazil. *bioRxiv* **2020**. [CrossRef]
49. Toni, L.S.; Garcia, A.M.; Jeffrey, D.A.; Jiang, X.; Stauffer, B.L.; Miyamoto, S.D.; Sucharov, C.C. Optimization of phenol-chloroform RNA extraction. *MethodsX* **2018**, *5*, 599–608. [CrossRef]
50. Wilker, P.R.; Dinis, J.M.; Starrett, G.; Imai, M.; Hatta, M.; Nelson, C.W.; O'Connor, D.H.; Hughes, A.L.; Neumann, G.; Kawaoka, Y.; et al. Selection on haemagglutinin imposes a bottleneck during mammalian transmission of reassortant H5N1 influenza viruses. *Nat. Commun.* **2013**, *4*, 2636. [CrossRef]
51. Gallego Romero, I.; Pai, A.A.; Tung, J.; Gilad, Y. RNA-seq: Impact of RNA degradation on transcript quantification. *BMC Biol.* **2014**, *12*, 42. [CrossRef] [PubMed]
52. Lu, W.; Zhou, Q.; Chen, Y. Impact of RNA degradation on next-generation sequencing transcriptome data. *Genomics* **2022**, *114*, 110429. [CrossRef] [PubMed]
53. King, J.; Harder, T.; Beer, M.; Pohlmann, A. Rapid multiplex MinION nanopore sequencing workflow for Influenza A viruses. *BMC Infect. Dis.* **2020**, *20*, 648. [CrossRef] [PubMed]
54. Chrzastek, K.; Lee, D.-h.; Smith, D.; Sharma, P.; Suarez, D.L.; Pantin-Jackwood, M.; Kapczynski, D.R. Use of Sequence-Independent, Single-Primer-Amplification (SISPA) for rapid detection, identification, and characterization of avian RNA viruses. *Virology* **2017**, *509*, 159–166. [CrossRef] [PubMed]
55. Pantin-Jackwood, M.J.; Swayne, D. Pathogenesis and pathobiology of avian influenza virus infection in birds. *Rev. Sci. Tech. l'OIE* **2009**, *28*, 113–136. [CrossRef]
56. Pantin-Jackwood, M.J. Pathobiology of avian influenza in domestic ducks. In *Animal Influenza*; John Wiley & Sons, Inc.: Ames, IA, USA, 2016; pp. 337–362.
57. Fanson, B.G.; Osmack, P.; Di Bisceglie, A.M. A comparison between the phenol–chloroform method of RNA extraction and the QIAamp viral RNA kit in the extraction of hepatitis C and GB virus-C/hepatitis G viral RNA from serum. *J. Virol. Methods* **2000**, *89*, 23–27. [CrossRef]

viruses

MDPI

Article

Specific and Sensitive Visual Proviral DNA Detection of Major Pathogenic Avian Leukosis Virus Subgroups Using CRISPR-Associated Nuclease Cas13a

Qingqing Xu [1,2,3], Yaoyao Zhang [1], Yashar Sadigh [1], Na Tang [2,3], Jiaqian Chai [4], Ziqiang Cheng [4], Yulong Gao [5], Aijian Qin [6], Zhiqiang Shen [2,3], Yongxiu Yao [1,*] and Venugopal Nair [1,7,8,*]

1 The Pirbright Institute and UK-China Centre of Excellence for Research on Avian Diseases, Pirbright, Guildford, Surrey GU24 ONF, UK; zjzlxqq@126.com (Q.X.); yaoyao.zhang@pirbright.ac.uk (Y.Z.); Yashar.sadigh@coventry.ac.uk (Y.S.)

2 UK-China Centre of Excellence for Research on Avian Diseases, Shandong Binzhou Animal Science and Veterinary Medicine Academy, Binzhou 256600, China; tangna0543@163.com (N.T.); bzshenzq@163.com (Z.S.)

3 Sino-UK Laboratory for Poultry Disease Research, Shandong Binzhou Animal Science and Veterinary Medicine Academy, Binzhou 256600, China

4 College of Veterinary Medicine, Shandong Agricultural University, Tai'an 271018, China; jqchai@sdau.edu.cn (J.C.); czqsd@126.com (Z.C.)

5 State Key Laboratory of Veterinary Biotechnology, Division of Avian Infectious Diseases, Harbin Veterinary Research Institute, The Chinese Academy of Agricultural Sciences, Harbin 150008, China; gaoyulong@caas.cn

6 Ministry of Education Key Lab for Avian Preventive Medicine, Yangzhou University, Yangzhou 225109, China; aijian@yzu.edu.cn

7 The Jenner Institute Laboratories, University of Oxford, Oxford OX3 7DQ, UK

8 Department of Biology, University of Oxford, Oxford OX1 3RB, UK

* Correspondence: yongxiu.yao@pirbright.ac.uk (Y.Y.); venugopal.nair@pirbright.ac.uk (V.N.)

Abstract: Avian leukosis viruses (ALVs) include a group of avian retroviruses primarily associated with neoplastic diseases in poultry, commonly referred to as avian leukosis. Belonging to different subgroups based on their envelope properties, ALV subgroups A, B, and J (ALV-A, ALV-B, and ALV-J) are the most widespread in poultry populations. Early identification and removal of virus-shedding birds from infected flocks are essential for the ALVs' eradication. Therefore, the development of rapid, accurate, simple-to-use, and cost effective on-site diagnostic methods for the detection of ALV subgroups is very important. Cas13a, an RNA-guided RNA endonuclease that cleaves target single-stranded RNA, also exhibits non-specific endonuclease activity on any bystander RNA in close proximity. The distinct trans-cleavage activity of Cas13 has been exploited in the molecular diagnosis of multiple pathogens including several viruses. Here, we describe the development and application of a highly sensitive Cas13a-based molecular test for the specific detection of proviral DNA of ALV-A, B, and J subgroups. Prokaryotically expressed LwaCas13a, purified through ion exchange and size-exclusion chromatography, was combined with recombinase polymerase amplification (RPA) and T7 transcription to establish the SHERLOCK (specific high-sensitivity enzymatic reporter unlocking) molecular detection system for the detection of proviral DNA of ALV-A/B/J subgroups. This novel method that needs less sample input with a short turnaround time is based on isothermal detection at 37 °C with a color-based lateral flow readout. The detection limit of the assay for ALV-A/B/J subgroups was 50 copies with no cross reactivity with ALV-C/D/E subgroups and other avian oncogenic viruses such as reticuloendotheliosis virus (REV) and Marek's disease virus (MDV). The development and evaluation of a highly sensitive and specific visual method of detection of ALV-A/B/J nucleic acids using CRISPR-Cas13a described here will help in ALV detection in eradication programs.

Keywords: avian leukosis viruses; CRISPR-Cas13a diagnosis; RPA; Lateral flow detection; ALV detection

Citation: Xu, Q.; Zhang, Y.; Sadigh, Y.; Tang, N.; Chai, J.; Cheng, Z.; Gao, Y.; Qin, A.; Shen, Z.; Yao, Y.; et al. Specific and Sensitive Visual Proviral DNA Detection of Major Pathogenic Avian Leukosis Virus Subgroups Using CRISPR-Associated Nuclease Cas13a. *Viruses* **2024**, *16*, 1168. https://doi.org/10.3390/v16071168

Academic Editor: Chi-Young Wang

Received: 10 May 2024
Revised: 4 July 2024
Accepted: 9 July 2024
Published: 20 July 2024

1. Introduction

Avian leukosis virus (ALV) is a major group of avian pathogens associated with severe neoplastic disease affecting multiple cell types commonly referred to as avian leukosis. The prevalence of multiple ALV envelope subgroups together with widespread diversity and recombination make the detection of ALV very challenging [1]. Among the commercial poultry populations, ALV subgroups A, B, and J (ALV-A, ALV-B, and ALV-J) are the most common ALVs. Viruses belonging to ALV-A and ALV-B, widespread in some countries, are primarily associated with lymphoid leukosis (LL) and sarcomas. While diseases caused by ALV-C and ALV-D are less commonly reported, ALV-E is the ubiquitous endogenous retrovirus of low pathogenicity [1]. ALV-J was first isolated from meat-type chickens in 1988, primarily causing myeloid leukosis in chickens [2]. Although ALV-J has been eradicated from most countries, it continues to induce diseases in poultry populations in China. Co-infections of ALV-A, ALV-B, and ALV-J can occur in the same chicken, including commercial laying hens [3,4]. Such co-infections provide a potential opportunity for recombination between different subgroups of ALVs [5,6]. As a pathogen that is predominantly transmitted vertically through the eggs, the control of ALV in poultry populations is mainly achieved through eradication programs where the efficient and accurate detection and removal of carrier birds are crucial to prevent ALV transmission in the flocks. Successful ALV eradication is thus very much dependent on the efficacy of specific, sensitive, and reliable diagnostic methods for detecting ALV-positive carrier birds.

In the past two decades, a number of routine ALV detection methods including enzyme-linked immunosorbent assay (ELISA), immunofluorescence assay (IFA), and different types of PCR together with virus isolation protocols have been widely used in ALV eradication programs. However, these methods have advantages as well as drawbacks. For example, the widely used group-specific antigen detection ELISA cannot differentiate between exogenous and endogenous ALV as it detects the conserved p27 antigen [7]. While PCR and IFA can be used to detect and differentiate between endogenous and exogenous ALV, both techniques are not used widely in the field due to the requirement of sophisticated instrumentation [8,9]. Virus isolation in cell culture is used and considered as the gold standard diagnostic test. However, virus isolation is time-consuming, requiring at least 6 days to obtain the results, with additional time required for the identification of the ALV subgroups. Current PCR-related assays and isothermal methods such as RPA (recombinase polymerase amplification) and LAMP (loop-mediated isothermal amplification) also suffer from limitations including low specificity and the requirement of complex instrumentation [10,11].

Recently, orthologs of CRISPR-associated enzymes such as Cas13a nuclease have shown great promise in nucleic acid detection assays in different biological systems, including many viruses [12,13]. Cas13a is an RNA-guided RNA nuclease that targets and cleaves the RNA. After Cas13a cleaves its target RNA, it adopts an enzymatically "active" state and binds and cleaves neighboring non-targeted RNA regardless of homology, which is referred to as "collateral cleavage". It is this property of Cas13a that led to the establishment of SHERLOCK (specific high-sensitivity enzymatic reporter unlocking), a Cas13a-based molecular detection platform. SHERLOCK combines RPA (recombinase polymerase amplification) with the T7 transcription of amplified DNA to RNA and the collateral effect of CRISPR-Cas13a. The assay starts with pre-amplification of either a DNA (RPA) or RNA (RT-RPA) target input, followed by the conversion of amplified DNA to RNA via T7 transcription and then detection by Cas13−crRNA complexes, which activate and cleave RNA reporters that are used to create a signal after being cleaved if the target sequence is present in the pool of amplified nucleotides. Detection can be performed as a colorimetric lateral flow reaction with the RNA reporter flanked by a fluorescein and biotin on separate ends or a fluorescence-based reaction with the reporter sequence coupled to a fluorophore on one end and a quencher on the other end [14]. While the performance of RPA-based assays is variable and influenced by multiple factors including primers, template sequence, and amplicon length, SHERLOCK is fairly robust. In combination with lateral flow RNA reporters or quenched fluorescent RNAs, SHERLOCK can generate a colorimetric lateral flow or fluorescent readout, respectively, upon Cas13a recognition of target nucleic acid species with high specificity at single-nucleotide level discrimination and single-molecule sensitivity. SHERLOCK has been successfully applied for the detection of multiple viruses including Avian influenza A (H7N9) virus, Dengue virus (DENV), Zika virus (ZIKV), Ebola virus, SARS-CoV-2, Feline calicivirus (FCV), Porcine reproductive, and respiratory syndrome virus (PRRSV), as well as other molecules such as N1-methyladenosine and miRNA [15–21]. In the present study, the Cas13a detection using the purified Leptotrichia wadei Cas13a (LwaCas13a), a custom FAM-Biotin reporter and in vitro transcribed target RNA corresponding to the viral glycoprotein gp85 gene with a lateral flow readout, was developed for the visual detection of proviral DNA extracted from ALV-A-, ALV-B-, and ALV-J-infected DF-1 cells (Figure 1). The assay has proved to be sensitive and specific.

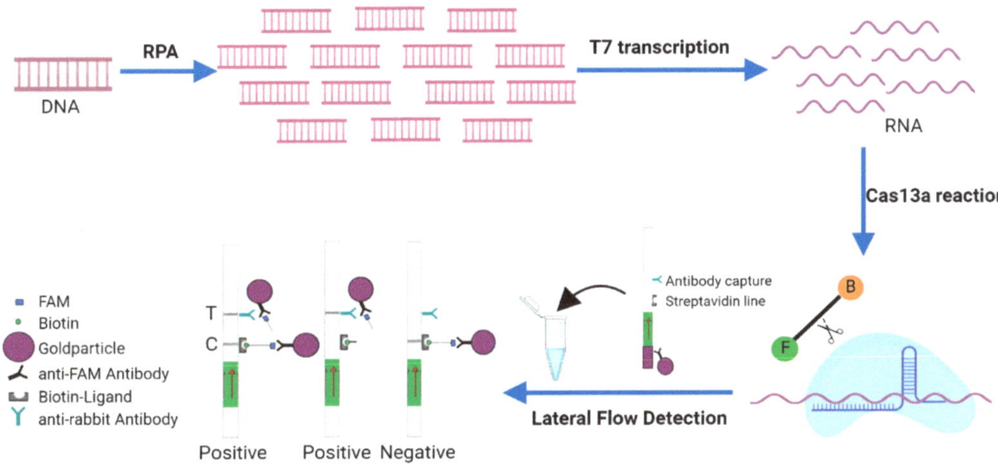

Figure 1. SHERLOCK detection of DNA from ALV-infected DF-1 cells. The region of interest is isothermally amplified by the RPA assay from DNA extracted from ALV-infected DF-1, then converted to RNA by T7 transcription. Cognate binding of the Cas13a–crRNA complex to amplified RNA targets triggers the collateral activity of Cas13a, which cleaves RNA reporters tagged with a fluorescein (F) and biotin (B) at each end. Detection is then performed as a colorimetric lateral flow reaction by placing the lateral flow strip into the reaction tube. The result can be visualized by the accumulation of the FAM/Biotin ssRNA reporter that conjugates to anti-FAM gold nanoparticles at the control or test lines depending on whether the reporter is intact. In the absence of reporter RNA cleavage, the RNA reporter is absorbed at the streptavidin line and captures anti-FAM antibodies. If the RNA reporter is destroyed by the collateral effect, then antibodies will flow through to a second capture line.

2. Materials and Methods

2.1. Viruses and Nucleic Acid Extraction

Virus stocks of prototype ALV subgroups ALV-A (RAV-1), ALV-B (RAV-2), ALV-C (RAV-49), ALV-D (RAV-50), ALV-E (RAV-0), and ALV-J (HPRS-103) maintained in the Viral Oncogenesis group at the Pirbright Institute were used in the experiments. ALV stocks were inoculated into DF-1 cells cultured in T25 flasks with Dulbecco's modified Eagle's medium (DMEM) (Invitrogen, Waltham, MA, USA) supplemented with 10% fetal bovine serum (FBS) at 38.5 °C in a 5% CO_2 incubator. Passaging of the infected DF-1 cells was carried out two times in DMEM containing 2% FBS at 38.5 °C in a 5% CO_2 incubator for 5 days. The harvested cells were lysed in 1× Proteinase K-based DNA extraction buffer (10 mM Tris-HCl, pH 8, 1 mM EDTA, 25 mM NaCl, and 200 µg/mL Proteinase K) at 65 °C for 30 min for the extraction of ALV subgroup-specific proviral DNA for RPA amplifications. DNA extracted from REV- and MDV-transformed cell lines was used as controls to determine the specificity of the assay.

2.2. RPA Primer Design and crRNA Preparation

For designing the RPA primer sets (between 30 and 35 nt), the previously published ALV sequences from NCBI were first aligned using DNASTAR. Based on the results of the sequence comparison, specific primers mainly targeting the gp85 gene were designed for discrimination of the three subgroups with amplicon sizes between 100 and 200 nt. The T7 promoter sequence was appended to the 5′end of the RPA forward primers. Primers were synthesized by Integrated DNA Technologies (IDT). To generate a complete crRNA template, the 28 nt spacer sequence was joined with a 5′direct repeat (DR) sequence with an additional upstream T7 RNA polymerase promoter sequence (T7-3G) to allow for T7 transcription [14]. The entire sequence was synthesized as the DNA reverse complement and the crRNAs were generated through in vitro transcription (IVT) according to the instructions of the HiScribe T7 Quick High Yield RNA Synthesis Kit (New England Biolabs, Ipswich, MA, USA). Briefly, the crRNA templates and T7-3G oligonucleotides were annealed after a 5 min denaturation at 95 °C in a PCR thermocycler and slow cooling to 4 °C. Double-stranded DNA was then transcribed to crRNA by incubation for 4 h at 37 °C and purified using Agencourt RNA Clean XP Kit (Beckman Coulter, Brea, CA, USA) according to the manufacturer's instructions.

2.3. Expression and Purification of LwaCas13a

LwaCas13a protein expression and purification were carried out as previously reported with modifications [14]. Rosetta (DE3) competent cells transformed with the pC013-TwinStrep-SUMO-huLwaCas13a plasmid (https://www.addgene.org/90097/, accessed on 5 October 2019) were grown up and 20 mL of overnight culture was added into two liters of Luria Broth (LB) medium and incubated in a shaking incubator at 37 °C. When the OD600 value of the culture reached 0.6, protein expression was induced using IPTG to a final concentration of 500 µM and the cells were grown at 25 °C for 16 h. Cell pellets obtained after centrifugation at 3000× *g* for 20 min at 4 °C were crushed and resuspended in lysis buffer (250 mM NaCl, 20 mM Tris-HCl, 1 mM DTT, and pH 8.0). The suspension was sonicated on ice followed by centrifugation. The supernatant containing the protein was incubated with 5 mL of Strep-Tactin Sepharose (GE Healthcare, Chicago, IL, USA) for 2 h at 4 °C by gentle shaking and protein-bound Strep-Tactin resin was washed three times with cold lysis buffer. The resin was then resuspended in SUMO digest buffer (30 mM Tris-HCl, 500 mM NaCl, 1 mM DTT, 0.15% NP-40, and pH 8.0), along with 250 U of SUMO protease to cleave overnight at 4 °C with gentle rotation. To maximize protein elution, the resin was washed twice with one column volume of lysis buffer following the separation of the resin from the suspension by gravity flow. For cation exchange and gel filtration purification, 250 mM of elute diluted in cation exchange buffer (5% glycerol, 1 mM DTT, 20 mM HEPES, and pH 7.0) was loaded into a 5 mL HiTrap SP HP cation exchange column (GE Healthcare) via fast protein liquid chromatography (FPLC; AKTA PURE, GE Healthcare). The protein was then eluted over a salt gradient with 250 mM to 2 M NaCl in the elution buffer/cation exchange buffer. The presence of recombinant protein in the resulting fractions was tested by SDS-PAGE. The protein-containing fractions were pooled and concentrated to 1 mL in S200 size-exclusion buffer (1 M NaCl, 10 mM HEPES, 2 mM DTT, 5 mM MgCl2, and pH 7.0) using a centrifugal filter unit (Millipore, Burlington, MA, USA). The concentrated protein was then loaded onto a gel filtration column (Superdex 200 Increase 10/300 GL; GE Healthcare) for FPLC. Fractions containing protein were pooled and the buffer was exchanged with storage buffer (50 mM Tris-HCl, 600 mM NaCl, 5% glycerol, and 2 mM DTT) and stored at −80 °C.

2.4. LwaCas13a Detection Assay

Detection reactions, consisting of RPA pre-amplification and T7 transcription for the detection of Cas13a function, were performed as described in Max et al. [14] with a few modifications. An amount of 3 μL of 10 μM forward primer, 3 μL of 10 μM reverse primer, 30 μL TwistAmp Rehydration Buffer, and 6 μL nuclease-free water were added to the RPA strips containing a dried enzyme pellet to prepare four individual RPA reactions that can be scaled up according to the reactions needed, followed by adding 1 μL of DNA template extracted from infected DF-1 cells to each reaction. Reactions were allowed to proceed for between 10 min and 40 min at 37 °C according to the instructions of the TwistAmp® Basic kit (TwistDx, Maidenhead, UK). To establish the Cas13a lateral flow detection with a visual readout, 10 μL of LwaCas13a assay reaction consisting of 1.0 μL RPA product, 0.25 μL HEPES (1M, pH 6.8), 0.1 μL $MgCl_2$ (1M), 0.4 μL rNTP solution mix (25 mM each), 1.0 μL LwaCas13a (63.3 μg/mL), 0.5 μL Murine RNase inhibitor (40 U/μL), 0.25 μL T7 RNA polymerase (5 U/μL), 0.5 μL crRNA (10 ng/μL), 0.1 μL LF-RNA reporter 1 (100 μM), and 6.25 μL nuclease-free water was first prepared. Following the addition of 50 μL HybriDetect assay buffer, the HybriDetect 1 lateral flow strip (TwistDx) was dipped into the solution and incubated for 3 min for the readout. After incubation, the images were taken using a smartphone.

2.5. Specificity and Sensitivity of the Assay

DNA samples containing the proviral DNA of the different ALV subgroups extracted from DF-1 cells infected with the prototype strains, together with REV and MDV as negative controls, were used to determine the specificity of the assay.

In order to determine the sensitivity of the assay, gel-extracted PCR amplicons of ALV-A/B/J amplified by specific primers targeting the *gp85* region (Table 1) were used for cloning into a plasmid as standard references. Concentrations of all three standard references were determined by UV spectrophotometry. DNA copy numbers (copies/μL) were calculated using the formula $(6.02 \times 10^{23}) \times (\text{ng}/\mu\text{L} \times 10^{-9})/(\text{DNA length} \times 660)$. An amount of 1 μL of each serial dilution containing 10^4 to 10^1 copies/μL DNA was used as the input DNA template to detect the sensitivity of this method.

Table 1. Specific primers for ALV-A/B/J identification.

Targets	Sequences (5′-3′)	Product Sizes (bp)
ALV-A	H5: GGATGAGGTGACTAAGAAAG envA: AGAGAAAGAGGGGCGTCTAAGGAGA	694
ALV-B	H5: GGATGAGGTGACTAAGAAAG envB: ATGGACCAATTCTGACTCATT	846
ALV-J	H5: GGATGAGGTGACTAAGAAAG H7: CGAACCAAAGGTAACACACG	545

2.6. Application of the Assay on Field Samples

In order to verify the application of the LwaCas13a assay for diagnostic purposes on field samples, 23 validated ALV-A/B/J-positive hepatic tissue samples collected from different chicken farms were used for the extraction of DNA and RNA by using a AxyPrep™ Body Fluid Viral DNA/RNA Miniprep Kit (AXYGEN, 20019KC5, New York, USA). An amount of 1 μL of DNA extracted from each specimen was used as a template in the PCR and RPA reactions, respectively. The presence of ALV-A/B/J proviral DNA was confirmed with subgroup-specific primers targeting the *gp85* gene (Table 1) using the following cycle conditions: pre-denaturation at 95 °C for 5 min; 30 cycles of denaturation at 95 °C for 20 s, annealing at 58 °C for 30 s, extending at 72 °C for 1 min. Samples were assayed and analyzed following the previously described Cas13a detection and lateral flow methods. The images were taken using a smartphone.

3. Results

3.1. Design of Primers and crRNAs and crRNA Preparation

As described above, the assay starts with pre-amplification of either a DNA (RPA) or RNA (RT-RPA) target input. For RPA, primers are typically designed with NCBI Primer-BLAST to be 30~35 nt and the amplicon sizes are 100~200 bp. In order to target a broad range of ALV strains in the same subgroup, the conserved crRNA sequences were identified by the alignment of multiple *gp85* gene sequences within each ALV subgroup retrieved from the NCBI. To identify the best primers and crRNA, we designed one crRNA with six pairs of RPA primers for ALV-A, one crRNA with three pairs of RPA primers for ALV-B, and two crRNAs for ALV-J, one with three pairs and the other one with two pairs of RPA primers, respectively. The sequences of the designed RPA primers and crRNA IVT templates are listed in Table 2. Each of the ALV subgroup-specific crRNAs were generated by IVT from DNA templates, and 5 μL per aliquot (300 ng/μL concentration in nuclease-free water) was stored at −80 °C.

Table 2. The sequences of primers and crRNAs designed for Cas13a detection in this study.

Primer	Sequence (5′-3′)	Sizes
ALV-A1-F	GAAATTAATACGACTCACTATAGGGACTGGCGGTCCTGACAACAGCACCACCCTCACT	143 bp
ALV-A1-R	GTAATATTAGTAATGTTAGGGAGAGACTGGGAAC	
ALV-A2-F	GAAATTAATACGACTCACTATAGGGGATATGTCTCTGATACAAATTGCGCCACCT	170 bp
ALV-A2-R	CAGCTGTAGTTCAGGTGGCTCATCCCACATAG	
ALV-A3-F	GAAATTAATACGACTCACTATAGGGCGGAAACTGACCGGTTAGTCTCGTCAGCTGACT	147 bp
ALV-A3-R	AACCTAACAGCTGTAGTTCAGGTGGCTCATCC	
ALV-A4-F	GAAATTAATACGACTCACTATAGGGATATGTCTCTGATACAAATTGCGCCACCTCGGA	176 bp
ALV-A4-R	AACCTAACAGCTGTAGTTCAGGTGGCTCATCCCA	
ALV-A5-F	GAAATTAATACGACTCACTATAGGGCTGATACAAATTGCGCCACCTCGGAAACTGAC	165 bp
ALV-A5-R	CTAACAGCTGTAGTTCAGGTGGCTCATCCCA	
ALV-A6-F	GAAATTAATACGACTCACTATAGGGAAACTGACCGGTTAGTCTCGTCAGCTGACT	165 bp
ALV-A6-R	TAATGTTAGGGAGAGACTGGGAACCTAACAG	
crRNA IVT template for A1-A6	CTGACAACAGCACCACCCTCACTTATCGGTTTTAGTCCCCTTCGTTTTT GGGGTAGTCTAAATCCCCTATAGTGAGTCGTATTAATTTC	
ALV-B1-F	GAAATTAATACGACTCACTATAGGGCTAATATTACTCAGATCCCTAGTGTGGCTGG	134 bp
ALV-B1-R	AGGATTGCTCCCTGGGTCAGTCAAGAGGATG	
ALV-B2-F	GAAATTAATACGACTCACTATAGGGTGGACCGGAGACAAGTTACACACATCCTCTTG	157 bp
ALV-B2-R	TGTAGCCATATGCACCGCAATATTCACTTCCCAT	
ALV-B3-F	GAAATTAATACGACTCACTATAGGGCTCTTGACTGACCCAGGGAGCAATCCTTTC	155 bp
ALV-B3-R	GAGCAATTGTACATCTCCCAAAATCTGTAG	
crRNA IVT template for B1-B3	TCTAACTCCTCGAAACCGTTTACAGTAGGTTTTAGTCCCCTTCGTTTTTGGGGTAGTCTAAA TCCCCTATAGTGAGTCGTATTAATTTC	
ALV-J1-F	GAAATTAATACGACTCACTATAGGGGATATTTTAGGGTCTCAGATGATCAAGAACGGAAC	142 bp
ALV-J1-R	CTTCCACCCCACCAGTCCCATTAAAATTCCCATCA	
ALV-J2-F	GAAATTAATACGACTCACTATAGGGCTTGATAAAGGCTCTTAACACAAACCTCCCTTG	191 bp
ALV-J2-R	CTTCCACCCCACCAGTCCCATTAAAATTCCCATCA	
ALV-J3-F	GAAATTAATACGACTCACTATAGGGGTACGTGTGTTACCTTTGGTTCGATGTGCT	172 bp
ALV-J3-R	GATTGGTTGACATAGGGTCTTATACGAGGGTC	
crRNA IVT template for J1-J3	GCTATAAAGAGAACAATCACAGCAGAGTGTTTTAGTCCCCTTCGTTTTTGGGGTAGTCTAAATCC CCTATAGTGAGTCGTATTAATTC	
ALV-J4-F	GAAATTAATACGACTCACTATAGGGCATTTCTGACTGGGCACCCTGGGAAGGTGAGC	147 bp
ALV-J4-R	TAACCACGCACACAAGTATCATTTGAAAGAAG	
ALV-J5-F	GAAATTAATACGACTCACTATAGGGGGATGAGGTGACTAAGAAAGATGAGGCGAGC	183 bp
ALV-J5-R	ACACAAGTATCATTTGAAAGAAGAAGTAACC	
crRNA IVT template for J4-J5	CAAGAAAGACCCGGAGAAGACACCCTTGGTTTTAGTCCCCTTCGTTTTTGGGGTAGTCTAAAT CCCCTATAGTGAGTCGTATTAATTTC	

3.2. Expression and Purification of LwaCas13a

Rosetta *E. coli* cells transformed with TwinStrep-SUMO-LwaCas13a protein expression plasmid were induced with 500 μM IPTG and grown for 16 h at 25 °C. The harvested cells were resuspended, sonicated, and centrifuged to remove the debris. After IPTG induction, the LwaCas13a protein was expressed (Figure 2A), and the target protein was mainly in the supernatant. The recombinant protein was enriched from the total cell protein by affinity Strep-Tactin purification. The native LwaCas13a was obtained following removal of the SUMO tag after digestion with SUMO protease and further purified using ion-exchange

(IEC) and size-exclusion chromatography (SEC) on an FPLC system. The expression and purification of the LwaCas13a protein was determined by SDS-PAGE and Coomassie blue staining as shown in Figure 2. The purified 138.5 kD LwaCas13a was then diluted to a final concentration of 2 mg/mL in protein storage buffer and stored as 5 μL aliquots at −80 °C.

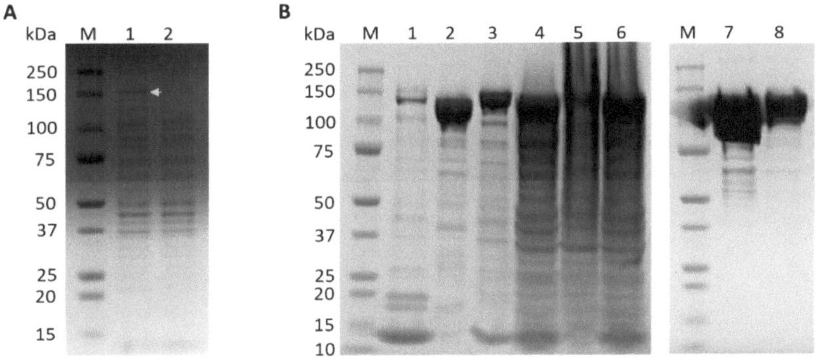

Figure 2. Expression and purification of LwaCas13a. (**A**) LwaCas13a expression detection. Lane M, protein marker; lane 1, IPTG-induced bacterial sample (the LwaCas13a band is indicated by the arrow); lane 2, uninduced bacterial sample. (**B**) LwaCas13a purification. Lane M, protein marker; lane 1, Strep-Tactin resin post SUMO cleavage; lane 2, eluted fraction post SUMO protease cleavage; lane 3, Strep-Tactin resin before SUMO protease cleavage; lane 4, flow-through following Strep-Tactin batch binding; lane 5, cell pellet after clearing of lysate; lane 6, cleared cell lysate; lane 7, final product after SEC; lane 8, concentrated sample post IEC.

3.3. Validation of the LwaCas13a Lateral Flow Detection

Lateral flow strips from TwistDx are designed to detect biotin and FAM-labeled RNA reporter. As shown in Figure 1, the first line (control line) with streptavidin will bind to biotin, capturing all the intact probes. Anti-fluorescein antibodies labeled with gold nanoparticles (NPs) will bind the fluorescein end of the reporter and form a dark purple color at this first line. When RNA reporters are cleaved because of target presence and collateral activity, gold NP–labeled antibodies will flow over to a second line of anti-rabbit secondary antibody (test line), capturing all the antibodies and forming a dark purple color at the second line that indicates the presence of the target. As a result, the negative sample only forms one band at the control line as all reporter molecules are intact and captured at this line. As shown and described by others, a faint band may appear at the test line for the non-target control or the negative strips are allowed to sit at room temperature for over 10 min, but this signal is much fainter than a true positive signal [22–24]. For the positive samples, there could be one test line present when the RNA reporter is fully cleaved or both a control and test line present if the RNA reporter is partially cleaved.

Optimal RPA was performed for different amplification durations ranging from 20 to 60 min. Each reaction includes 9 μL of the reconstituted RPA mixture and 1 μL of tested sample in a PCR strip tube. In RPA pre-amplification, the negative control with the target molecule known to be absent was also included. The assay using the DNA extracted from prototype strains of ALV-A-, B-, and J- (RAV-1, RAV-2, and HPRS-103, respectively)-infected DF-1 cells showed that A6F/A3R, B3F/B3R, and J4F/J4R primer sets were efficient and capable of specific amplification producing the expected test bands (Figure 3A, top panel). The binding sites of these RPA primers and crRNAs which are used in the subsequent LwaCas13a lateral flow detection are shown in Figure 4. To optimize the reaction conditions, different temperatures and incubation times were examined. While the test bands that correlated to 10 min of RPA were weak, extending the amplification time to 30 min and longer increased the intensity of the test band. Based on the optimization data, the amplification duration was set at 40 min for ALV-A and 30 min for ALV-B/J RPA reactions. Since the RPA amplification reaction is initiated following MgOAc addition, we also want to know if the nucleic acid amplification was initiated during sample preparation at room temperature. We prepared two pairs of RPA reactions consisting of one positive and one negative for each pair and allowed one pair to be at room temperature and the other pair to be at 37 °C for 30 min. The crude RPA products were examined on a 2% agarose gel. As shown in Figure 3B, no significant changes between positive and negative samples of ALV-A and J were observed on the gel at room temperature amplification. However, the detection of the amplicons at 37 °C indicated apparent differences.

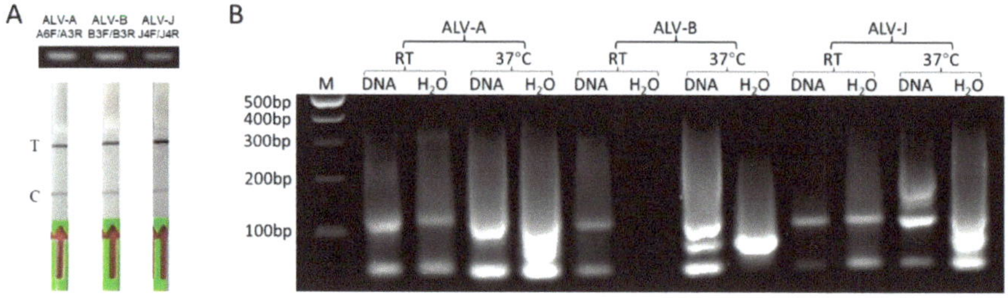

Figure 3. Validation of the LwaCas13a lateral flow detection. (**A**) Top panel: agarose gel electrophoresis of RPA products using specific primers A6F/A3R for ALV-A, B3F/B3R for ALV-B, and J4F/J4R for ALV-J. Bottom panel: the corresponding Cas13a assay result of ALV/A/B/J by imaging of the lateral flow dipstick is displayed. T: test line, C: control line. (**B**) RPA pre-amplifications optimization. RPA reactions were run for ALV-A/B/J at room temperature (RT) or 37 °C with proviral DNA and water control with primer pairs A6F/A3R, B3F/B3R, and J4F/J4R for subgroups ALV-A/B/J, respectively. Proviral DNAs of RAV-1, RAV-2, and HPRS-103 extracted from infected DF-1 were used as templates for ALV-A, ALV-B, and ALV-J, respectively.

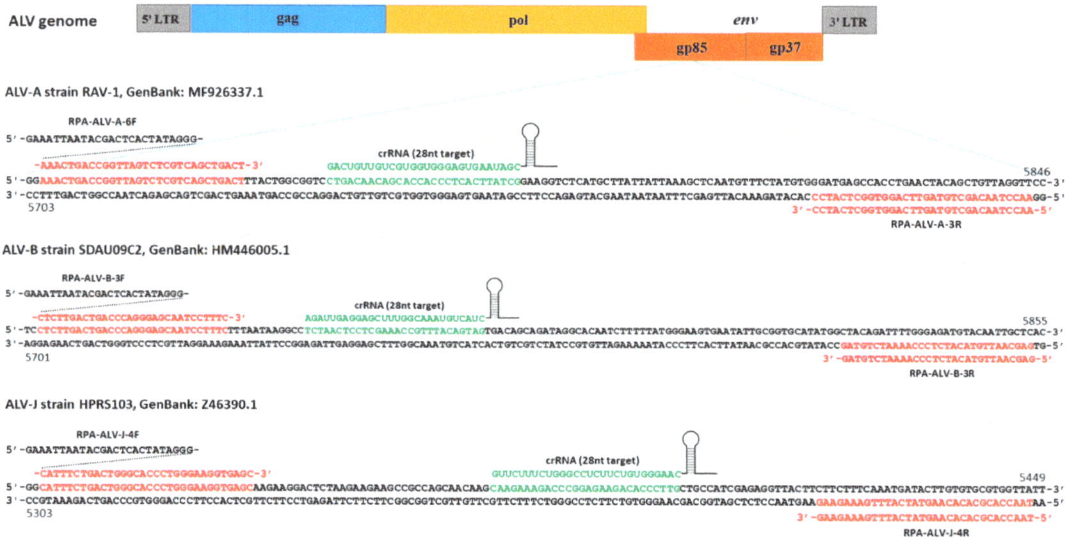

Figure 4. Binding sites of RPA primers and crRNAs. The RPA primers and crRNA sequences targeting *gp85* of the ALV-A/B/J genome selected through experimental optimization are shown. The nucleotide sequences and the numbering showing the genomic location at both ends of the selected sequences are based on RAV-1 (GenBank accession number: MF926337.1), SDAU09C2 (GenBank accession number: HM446005.1), and HPRS103 (GenBank accession number: Z46390.1) for ALV-A, ALV-B, and ALV-J, respectively.

Having obtained the specific RPA bands for the ALV-A, B, and J subgroups, the Cas13a assay was performed in a total volume of 10 µL. For this, Cas13a-SHERLOCK master mix was prepared by adding the components as described in Section 2. Subsequently, 50 µL HybriDetect assay buffer was added to the 10 µL Cas13a detection products followed by placing a HybriDetect 1 lateral flow strip (TwistDx) into the solution and incubation in an upright position. After 3 min incubation, the images of dipsticks were taken using a smartphone. As shown in Figure 3A, bottom panel, a strong band appeared in the test line region for all three samples tested, demonstrating the successful establishment of the Cas13a lateral flow detection of proviral DNA for the ALV-A/B/J subgroups.

3.4. Specificity and Sensitivity of the Cas13a Lateral Flow Detection

The specificity of the assay for the detection of ALV-A, B, and J subgroups was determined by examining the signals for ALV subgroups C, D, and E and other avian oncogenic viruses REV and MDV. Results of the specificity test clearly demonstrated that the assay was ALV A, B, and J subgroup-specific with no cross reactivity (Figure 5). In order to determine the sensitivity of the assay, 10-fold serial dilutions containing 10^4 to 10^2 copies/µL followed by two 2-fold dilutions to make 50 and 25 copies/µL (an additional dilution to 10 copies/uL was made to ALV-J). Each of the individual DNA templates were tested as shown in Figure 6. Results of the sensitivity test demonstrated that each assay could reliably detect a minimum of approximately 50 copies of the respective DNA targets in each reaction.

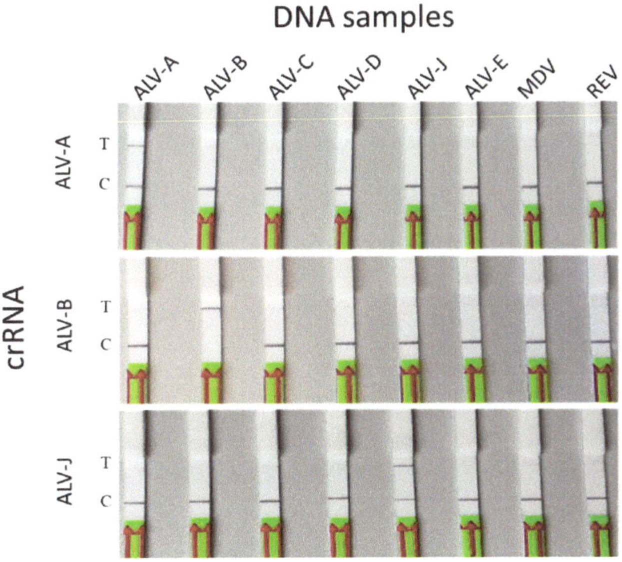

Figure 5. Specificity of ALV-A/B/J-LwaCas13a detection. Specificity detections of ALV-A/B/J with RPA at 37 °C for 30 min and Cas13a reaction at 37 °C for 40 min. DNA samples include proviral DNAs of RAV-1, RAV-2, RAV-49, RAV-50, HPRS-103, and RAV-60 for ALV-A, ALV-B, ALV-C, ALV-D, ALV-J, and ALV-E, respectively, and genomic DNAs of MDV (vaccine strain CVI-988) and REV infection cells. T: test line; C: control line.

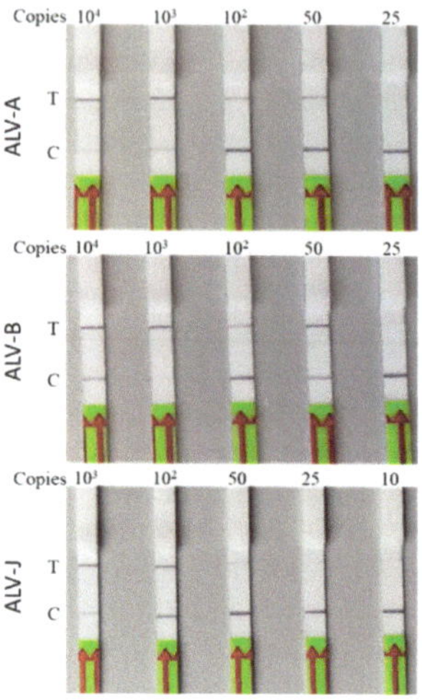

Figure 6. Sensitivity testing of ALV-A/B/J-LwaCas13a detection. Sensitivity detection results of ALV-A/B/J-Cas13a with RPA at 37 °C for 30 min and LwaCas13a reaction at 37 °C for 40 min. Gradient-diluted cloning vector of ALV-A/B/J plasmid DNAs were detected using ALV-A/B/J-LwaCas13a assays. The detection limit of ALV-A/B/J is 50 copies/reaction for all three. T, test line; C, control line.

3.5. Assay Performance on Field Samples

Finally, the assay was evaluated for its efficacy for the detection of ALV-A-, B-, and J-specific DNA in field samples of naturally infected cases. For this, we used 5 ALV-A-positive, 6 ALV-B-positive, and 12 ALV-J-positive field samples to determine the efficacy of detection of specific DNA, in comparison to PCR tests. As shown in Figure 7, lateral flow detection strips of ALV-A, B, and J subgroups demonstrated clear positive bands, correlating with the PCR tests carried out on these field samples, confirming the use of the Cas13a lateral flow assay for the specific proviral DNA detection of ALV-A, B, and J subgroups from field samples.

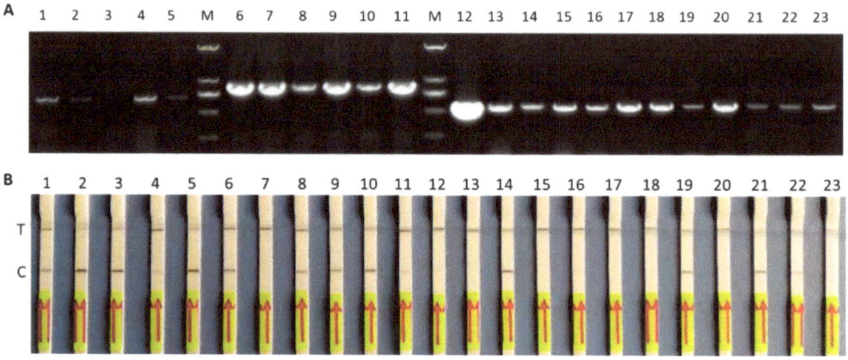

Figure 7. LwaCas13a detection on field samples. (**A**) Agarose gel electrophoresis of PCR products using specific primers. Lane M, DNA Marker 2000; lanes 1 to 5 are ALV-A-positive samples, lanes 6 to 11 are ALV-B-positive samples, and lanes 12 to 23 are ALV-J-positive samples. (**B**) ALV/A/B/J-LwaCas13a assay results with primer pair A6F/A3R for ALV-A samples (lanes 1–5), B3F/B3R for ALV-B samples (lanes 6–11), and J4F/J4R for ALV-J samples (lanes 12–23). T: test line, C: control line.

4. Discussion

Avian leukosis viruses, the common naturally occurring avian retrovirus pathogens, are associated with neoplastic diseases and other production problems in chickens [1]. With no effective vaccine or medication available, control of ALV infection is achieved mainly through systematic eradication program consisting of the early detection and removal of virus-shedding birds to break the chain of transmission that occurs through the congenital route and contact infections [25]. Several methods for ALV detection have been established. While antigen–antibody reaction-based detection can be used in the field with minimal equipment, the method has relatively low sensitivity [7,26]. PCR and RT-qPCR, the highly sensitive nucleic acid-based detection assays, are not suitable for poorly equipped laboratories or field diagnosis due to the requirement of expensive equipment [8,9,26]. Considering the importance of the accurate and sensitive detection of virus-infected birds for successful eradication, the availability of rapid, accurate ALV diagnostic tools is key for the success of the eradication.

In this study, a LwaCas13a detection assay was developed and optimized to detect viruses belonging to the common pathogenic subgroups ALV-A, ALV-B, and ALV-J. Primer sets and crRNAs specific for these subgroups were designed based on the consensus from the alignment of the nucleotide sequences of the viral *gp85* gene published in GenBank. Only the most distinct region that differed between different subgroups, but was highly conserved within *gp85* sequences of the same subgroup, was used to design the specific RPA primers. While the sequences of ALV-J *gp85* differed greatly from those of the other ALV subgroups, it has close sequence identity to env-like sequences of the EAV family of endogenous avian retroviruses [27,28]. As the ancient EAV-HP retroviral elements are present in all gallus species, these could interfere with the specific amplification of the ALV-J *gp85* gene. Thus, the chosen primers need to selectively amplify only the region specific to the exogenous ALV-J sequences. The H5/H7 primer set has been used successfully for detection of ALV-J [29]. The forward primer H5, located on the 3′ region of the pol gene, was conserved across several ALV subgroups. The reverse primer H7, located on a well-conserved region of the ALV-J *gp85* gene, could distinguish ALV-J from other subgroups. In our study, the primer pairs J1, J2, and J3 were first designed mainly focusing on the region around the H7 primer binding sequences. Although the experiments generated RPA amplification products, the Cas13a detection assay could not distinguish ALV-J from other exogenous ALV proviral DNA, probably due to the interference with the EAV-HP sequences. Hence, for the ALV-J detection, we modified the assay using another forward (JF4) and reverse (JR4) primer pair located at the 3′end of the pol and at the 5′end of the *gp85*, respectively. Tests using this new primer pair showed a good specificity to ALV-J amplification. Thus, the primer sets A6F/A3R, B3F/B3R, and J4F/J4R for RPA with the corresponding crRNAs for LwaCas13a detection performed accurately for the detection of the respective ALV subgroups.

In order to evaluate the specificity of the LwaCas13a detection method, we extracted proviral DNA from DF-1 cells infected with prototypes of ALV subgroups A, B, C, D, E, and J. In addition, DNAs from cells infected with Marek's disease virus and reticuloendotheliosis virus were extracted for use as controls. As expected, only the ALV-A/B/J subgroup-infected DNA samples could be detected with the corresponding RPA primers and crRNAs by this method, demonstrating the specificity of the test (Figure 5). The LwaCas13a detection assay also showed a detection limit of 50 copies per reaction for each of the subgroups. Perhaps due to this limited sensitivity of the assay, no significant difference in intensity was observed between the T and C lines in the lateral flow strip-based readout of the assay, when a number of reporter RNAs were cleaved. Despite this, we have demonstrated that the LwaCas13a lateral flow can be used for specific and sensitive proviral DNA detection of the major ALV subgroups A, B, and J. When the turnaround time was considered, the described method in this study requires 1.5 h of average assay time including 30 min of rapid DNA extraction, 30 min of RPA for DNA amplification, and 40 min of LwaCas13a detection.

Unlike PCR-based DNA amplification assays, there are no rules for the design of RPA primers other than the suggestion from the TwistDx website (www.twistdx.co.uk/rpa/). Besides genuine amplifications, RPA also allows for undesired primer interactions such as hairpins and primer dimer formation. Some of such artefacts will serve as templates for further recombination/extension events and enter an exponential amplification. Then, the detectable low-molecular-weight DNA consisting of a primer-derived sequence ("prime noise") will be generated (Figure 3B). The sensitivity of amplification and speed of RPA are directly affected by the amplicon size due to the effects of primer noise. An amplicon length ideally is between 100 and 200 bp, which tends to have an improved product/noise ratio. At low temperatures, amplicon doubling times lengthen more rapidly than energy consumption rates, which can result in fuel "burn-out". The observations of our study are consistent with the information given by the manufacturer that RPA amplification occurs over a broad range of temperatures (25 to 42 °C), making the assay robust against inadvertent temperature changes. It has also been reported that RPA is quite robust to mismatches even with 5~9 base pair mismatches in the primers [30]. However, this is not the case with the mismatches in the crRNA:target duplex, where even two or more mismatches can prevent the activation of Cas13a. As a result, SHERLOCK can easily distinguish the sequences of similar viruses. Furthermore, due to the additional specificity of the crRNA, it is not necessary to evaluate primer sets for specific amplicons using gel electrophoresis.

Although the efficiency of RPA is variable and influenced by factors such as primer and template sequence, the collateral cleavage activity of Cas13a can compensate for the low efficiency of RPA, making this assay achieve satisfactory results [31]. Moreover, as both reactions can occur at 37 °C, the method only demands simple heat source systems such as chemical heaters, water baths, or even body heat, and the results can be visualized with naked eye [16,20]. Furthermore, the method is not dependent on the cold chain as all the critical RPA reagents can be provided as a single lyophilized pellet. The entire procedure can be completed within 1.5 h and requires only a small sample volume of 10 μL for both RPA and SHERLOCK. Requiring only a basic heat source for incubation and a simple lateral flow readout, the LwaCas13a assay developed in this study can be considered as a rapid, efficient, and accurate field test for the diagnosis of ALV in low-resource settings.

5. Conclusions

A visual nucleic acid detection method based on CRISPR-LwaCas13a was established for the common pathogenic ALV subgroups A, B, and J. The method which combines RPA pre-amplification with the identification of a specific crRNA sequence makes the LwaCas13a lateral flow detection more accurate. The current study presented for the first time an alternative tool for the rapid, sensitive, and specific detection of ALV, particularly in resource-poor settings.

Author Contributions: Conceptualization, Q.X., Z.S., Y.Y. and V.N.; Data curation, Q.X.; Formal analysis, Q.X., Y.Y. and V.N.; Funding acquisition, N.T., A.Q., Z.S., Y.Y. and V.N.; Investigation, Q.X., Y.Z., Y.S., N.T., J.C., Z.C., Y.G., A.Q. and Z.S.; Methodology, Q.X., Y.Z., Y.Y. and V.N.; Resources, Y.Z.; Supervision, Y.Y. and V.N.; Validation, Q.X.; Writing—original draft, Q.X.; Writing—review and editing, Y.Y. and V.N. All authors have read and agreed to the published version of the manuscript.

Funding: This work was supported by the National Key Research and Development Program of China [grant number 2023YFE0106100], the National Natural Science Foundation of China [grant number 31761133002], the Natural Science Foundation of Shandong Province [grant number ZR2020KC006], the Biotechnology and Biological Sciences Research Council (BBSRC) [grant numbers BB/P016472/1, BB/L014262/1, BBS/E/PI/23NB0003, BBS/E/I/00007032 and BB/R012865/1], and the BBSRC Newton Fund Joint Centre Awards on "UK-China Centre of Excellence for Research on Avian Diseases" [grant number BBS/OS/NW/000007].

Institutional Review Board Statement: Not applicable.

Informed Consent Statement: Not applicable.

Data Availability Statement: All datasets generated for this study are included in the article.

Conflicts of Interest: The authors report no conflicts of interest.

References

1. Payne, L.N.; Nair, V. The long view: 40 years of avian leukosis research. *Avian Pathol. J. World Vet. Poult. Assoc.* **2012**, *41*, 11–19. [CrossRef] [PubMed]
2. Venugopal, K. Avian leukosis virus subgroup J: A rapidly evolving group of oncogenic retroviruses. *Res. Vet. Sci.* **1999**, *67*, 113–119. [CrossRef] [PubMed]
3. Fenton, S.P.; Reddy, M.R.; Bagust, T.J. Single and concurrent avian leukosis virus infections with avian leukosis virus-J and avian leukosis virus-A in australian meat-type chickens. *Avian Pathol. J. World Vet. Poult. Assoc.* **2005**, *34*, 48–54. [CrossRef] [PubMed]
4. Spencer, J.L.; Benkel, B.; Chan, M.; Nadin-Davis, S. Evidence for virus closely related to avian myeloblastosis-associated virus type 1 in a commercial stock of chickens. *Avian Pathol. J. World Vet. Poult. Assoc.* **2003**, *32*, 383–390. [CrossRef] [PubMed]
5. Li, T.; Xie, J.; Liang, G.; Ren, D.; Sun, S.; Lv, L.; Xie, Q.; Shao, H.; Gao, W.; Qin, A.; et al. Co-infection of vvMDV with multiple subgroups of avian leukosis viruses in indigenous chicken flocks in China. *BMC Vet. Res.* **2019**, *15*, 288. [CrossRef] [PubMed]
6. Liu, H.; Ma, K.; Liu, M.; Yang, C.; Huang, X.; Zhao, Y.; Qi, K. Histologic findings and viral antigen distribution in natural coinfection of layer hens with subgroup J avian leukosis virus, marek's disease virus, and reticuloendotheliosis virus. *J. Vet. Diagn. Investig.* **2019**, *31*, 761–765. [CrossRef] [PubMed]
7. Yun, B.; Li, D.; Zhu, H.; Liu, W.; Qin, L.; Liu, Z.; Wu, G.; Wang, Y.; Qi, X.; Gao, H.; et al. Development of an antigen-capture Elisa for the detection of avian leukosis virus p27 antigen. *J. Virol. Methods* **2013**, *187*, 278–283. [CrossRef] [PubMed]
8. Dai, M.; Feng, M.; Liu, D.; Cao, W.; Liao, M. Development and application of SYBR Green I real-time PCR assay for the separate detection of subgroup J Avian leukosis virus and multiplex detection of avian leukosis virus subgroups A and B. *Virol. J.* **2015**, *12*, 52. [CrossRef] [PubMed]
9. Qin, L.; Gao, Y.; Ni, W.; Sun, M.; Wang, Y.; Yin, C.; Qi, X.; Gao, H.; Wang, X. Development and application of real-time PCR for detection of subgroup j avian leukosis virus. *J. Clin. Microbiol.* **2013**, *51*, 149–154. [CrossRef]
10. Wang, Y.; Kang, Z.; Gao, Y.; Qin, L.; Chen, L.; Wang, Q.; Li, J.; Gao, H.; Qi, X.; Lin, H.; et al. Development of loop-mediated isothermal amplification for rapid detection of avian leukosis virus subgroup A. *J. Virol. Methods* **2011**, *173*, 31–36. [CrossRef]
11. Zhang, X.; Liao, M.; Jiao, P.; Luo, K.; Zhang, H.; Ren, T.; Zhang, G.; Xu, C.; Xin, C.; Cao, W. Development of a loop-mediated isothermal amplification assay for rapid detection of subgroup J avian leukosis virus. *J. Clin. Microbiol.* **2010**, *48*, 2116–2121. [CrossRef] [PubMed]
12. Gootenberg, J.S.; Abudayyeh, O.O.; Lee, J.W.; Essletzbichler, P.; Dy, A.J.; Joung, J.; Verdine, V.; Donghia, N.; Daringer, N.M.; Freije, C.A.; et al. Nucleic acid detection with CRISPR-Cas13a/C2c2. *Science* **2017**, *356*, 438–442. [CrossRef] [PubMed]
13. Zhao, L.; Qiu, M.; Li, X.; Yang, J.; Li, J. Crispr-cas13a system: A novel tool for molecular diagnostics. *Front. Microbiol.* **2022**, *13*, 1060947. [CrossRef] [PubMed]
14. Kellner, M.J.; Koob, J.G.; Gootenberg, J.S.; Abudayyeh, O.O.; Zhang, F. Sherlock: Nucleic acid detection with CRISPR nucleases. *Nat. Protoc.* **2019**, *14*, 2986–3012. [CrossRef] [PubMed]
15. Abbott, T.R.; Dhamdhere, G.; Liu, Y.; Lin, X.; Goudy, L.; Zeng, L.; Chemparathy, A.; Chmura, S.; Heaton, N.S.; Debs, R.; et al. Development of CRISPR as an antiviral strategy to combat SARS-CoV-2 and influenza. *Cell* **2020**, *181*, 865–876.e12. [CrossRef] [PubMed]
16. Chang, Y.; Deng, Y.; Li, T.; Wang, J.; Wang, T.; Tan, F.; Li, X.; Tian, K. Visual detection of porcine reproductive and respiratory syndrome virus using CRISPR-Cas13a. *Transbound. Emerg. Dis.* **2020**, *67*, 564–571. [CrossRef] [PubMed]
17. Chen, Y.; Yang, S.; Peng, S.; Li, W.; Wu, F.; Yao, Q.; Wang, F.; Weng, X.; Zhou, X. N1-methyladenosine detection with CRISPR-Cas13a/C2c2. *Chem. Sci.* **2019**, *10*, 2975–2979. [CrossRef] [PubMed]
18. Huang, J.; Liu, Y.; He, Y.; Yang, X.; Li, Y. CRISPR-Cas13a based visual detection assays for feline calicivirus circulating in Southwest China. *Front. Vet. Sci.* **2022**, *9*, 913780. [CrossRef]
19. Liu, Y.; Xu, H.; Liu, C.; Peng, L.; Khan, H.; Cui, L.; Huang, R.; Wu, C.; Shen, S.; Wang, S.; et al. CRISPR-cas13a nanomachine based simple technology for avian influenza a (H7N9) virus on-site detection. *J. Biomed. Nanotechnol.* **2019**, *15*, 790–798. [CrossRef]
20. Myhrvold, C.; Freije, C.A.; Gootenberg, J.S.; Abudayyeh, O.O.; Metsky, H.C.; Durbin, A.F.; Kellner, M.J.; Tan, A.L.; Paul, L.M.; Parham, L.A.; et al. Field-deployable viral diagnostics using CRISPR-Cas13. *Science* **2018**, *360*, 444–448. [CrossRef]
21. Qin, P.; Park, M.; Alfson, K.J.; Tamhankar, M.; Carrion, R.; Patterson, J.L.; Griffiths, A.; He, Q.; Yildiz, A.; Mathies, R.; et al. Rapid and fully microfluidic Ebola virus detection with CRISPR-Cas13a. *ACS Sens.* **2019**, *4*, 1048–1054. [CrossRef]
22. Broughton, J.P.; Deng, X.; Yu, G.; Fasching, C.L.; Servellita, V.; Singh, J.; Miao, X.; Streithorst, J.A.; Granados, A.; Sotomayor-Gonzalez, A.; et al. CRISPR-Cas12-based detection of SARS-CoV-2. *Nat. Biotechnol.* **2020**, *38*, 870–874. [CrossRef] [PubMed]
23. Arizti-Sanz, J.; Freije, C.A.; Stanton, A.C.; Petros, B.A.; Boehm, C.K.; Siddiqui, S.; Shaw, B.M.; Adams, G.; Kosoko-Thoroddsen, T.F.; Kemball, M.E.; et al. Streamlined inactivation, amplification, and Cas13-based detection of SARS-CoV-2. *Nat. Commun.* **2020**, *11*, 5921. [CrossRef] [PubMed]
24. Patchsung, M.; Jantarug, K.; Pattama, A.; Aphicho, K.; Suraritdechachai, S.; Meesawat, P.; Sappakhaw, K.; Leelahakorn, N.; Ruenkam, T.; Wongsatit, T.; et al. Clinical validation of a Cas13-based assay for the detection of SARS-CoV-2 RNA. *Nat. Biomed. Eng.* **2020**, *4*, 1140–1149. [CrossRef] [PubMed]

25. Gao, Q.; Yun, B.; Wang, Q.; Jiang, L.; Zhu, H.; Gao, Y.; Qin, L.; Wang, Y.; Qi, X.; Gao, H.; et al. Development and application of a multiplex PCR method for rapid differential detection of subgroup A, B, and J Avian leukosis viruses. *J. Clin. Microbiol.* **2014**, *52*, 37–44. [CrossRef] [PubMed]
26. Payne, L.N.; Gillespie, A.M.; Howes, K. Unsuitability of chicken sera for detection of exogenous ALV by the group-specific antigen Elisa. *Vet. Rec.* **1993**, *132*, 555–557. [CrossRef] [PubMed]
27. Sacco, M.A.; Howes, K.; Smith, L.P.; Nair, V.K. Assessing the roles of endogenous retrovirus EAV-hp in avian leukosis virus subgroup J emergence and tolerance. *J. Virol.* **2004**, *78*, 10525–10535. [CrossRef] [PubMed]
28. Venugopal, K.; Smith, L.M.; Howes, K.; Payne, L.N. Antigenic variants of J subgroup avian leukosis virus: Sequence analysis reveals multiple changes in the ENV gene. *J. Gen. Virol.* **1998**, *79 Pt 4*, 757–766. [CrossRef] [PubMed]
29. Smith, L.M.; Brown, S.R.; Howes, K.; McLeod, S.; Arshad, S.S.; Barron, G.S.; Venugopal, K.; McKay, J.C.; Payne, L.N. Development and application of polymerase chain reaction (PCR) tests for the detection of subgroup J avian leukosis virus. *Virus Res.* **1998**, *54*, 87–98. [CrossRef]
30. Boyle, D.S.; Lehman, D.A.; Lillis, L.; Peterson, D.; Singhal, M.; Armes, N.; Parker, M.; Piepenburg, O.; Overbaugh, J. Rapid detection of HIV-1 proviral DNA for early infant diagnosis using recombinase polymerase amplification. *mBio* **2013**, *4*, e00135-13. [CrossRef]
31. Wessels, H.H.; Mendez-Mancilla, A.; Guo, X.; Legut, M.; Daniloski, Z.; Sanjana, N.E. Massively parallel Cas13 screens reveal principles for guide RNA design. *Nat. Biotechnol.* **2020**, *38*, 722–727. [CrossRef] [PubMed]

viruses

MDPI

Article

The Oncolytic Avian Reovirus p17 Protein Inhibits Invadopodia Formation in Murine Melanoma Cancer Cells by Suppressing the FAK/Src Pathway and the Formation of theTKs5/NCK1 Complex

Chao-Yu Hsu [1,2,†], Jyun-Yi Li [3,†], En-Ying Yang [3], Tsai-Ling Liao [2,4], Hsiao-Wei Wen [5], Pei-Chien Tsai [2,6], Tz-Chuen Ju [3], Lon-Fye Lye [7], Brent L. Nielsen [8] and Hung-Jen Liu [2,3,6,9,10,*]

1. Division of Urology, Department of Surgery, Tungs' Taichung MetroHarbor Hospital, Taichung 435, Taiwan; t4361@ms.sltung.com.tw
2. Ph.D. Program in Translational Medicine, National Chung Hsing University, Taichung 402, Taiwan; tlliao1972@gmail.com (T.-L.L.); ptsai@dragon.nchu.edu.tw (P.-C.T.)
3. Institute of Molecular Biology, National Chung Hsing University, Taichung 402, Taiwan; tcju@dragon.nchu.edu.tw (T.-C.J.)
4. Department of Medical Research, Taichung Veterans General Hospital, Taichung 407, Taiwan
5. Department of Food Science and Biotechnology, National Chung Hsing University, Taichung 402, Taiwan; hwwen@nchu.edu.tw
6. Department of Life Sciences, National Chung Hsing University, Taichung 402, Taiwan
7. Department of Medical Research, Tungs' Taichung MetroHarbor Hospital, Taichung 435, Taiwan; lonfyelye@gmail.com
8. Department of Microbiology and Molecular Biology, Brigham Young University, Provo, UT 84602, USA; bnielsen28@gmail.com
9. The iEGG and Animal Biotechnology Center, National Chung Hsing University, Taichung 402, Taiwan
10. Rong Hsing Research Center for Translational Medicine, National Chung Hsing University, Taichung 402, Taiwan

* Correspondence: hjliu5257@nchu.edu.tw; Tel.: +886-4-22840485 (ext. 243); Fax: +886-4-22874879

† These authors contributed equally to this work.

Citation: Hsu, C.-Y.; Li, J.-Y.; Yang, E.-Y.; Liao, T.-L.; Wen, H.-W.; Tsai, P.-C.; Ju, T.-C.; Lye, L.-F.; Nielsen, B.L.; Liu, H.-J. The Oncolytic Avian Reovirus p17 Protein Inhibits Invadopodia Formation in Murine Melanoma Cancer Cells by Suppressing the FAK/Src Pathway and the Formation of theTKs5/NCK1 Complex. *Viruses* **2024**, *16*, 1153. https://doi.org/10.3390/v16071153

Academic Editor: Craig Meyers

Received: 9 June 2024
Revised: 5 July 2024
Accepted: 13 July 2024
Published: 17 July 2024

Abstract: To explore whether the p17 protein of oncolytic avian reovirus (ARV) mediates cell migration and invadopodia formation, we applied several molecular biological approaches for studying the involved cellular factors and signal pathways. We found that ARV p17 activates the p53/phosphatase and tensin homolog (PTEN) pathway to suppress the focal adhesion kinase (FAK)/Src signaling and downstream signal molecules, thus inhibiting cell migration and the formation of invadopodia in murine melanoma cancer cell line (B16-F10). Importantly, p17-induced formation of invadopodia could be reversed in cells transfected with the mutant $PTEN_{C124A}$. p17 protein was found to significantly reduce the expression levels of tyrosine kinase substrate 5 (TKs5), Rab40b, non-catalytic region of tyrosine kinase adaptor protein 1 (NCK1), and matrix metalloproteinases (MMP9), suggesting that TKs5 and Rab40b were transcriptionally downregulated by p17. Furthermore, we found that p17 suppresses the formation of the TKs5/NCK1 complex. Coexpression of TKs5 and Rab40b in B16-F10 cancer cells reversed p17-modulated suppression of the formation of invadopodia. This work provides new insights into p17-modulated suppression of invadopodia formation by activating the p53/PTEN pathway, suppressing the FAK/Src pathway, and inhibiting the formation of the TKs5/NCK1 complex.

Keywords: avian reoviruses; p17; p53/PTEN; FAK/Src; TKs5/NCK1 complex; Rab40b; MMP9; invadopodia

1. Introduction

Invadopodia are actin-rich protrusions of the plasma membrane that are associated with sites of proteolytic degradation of the extracellular matrix (ECM) in cancer invasiveness and metastasis [1,2]. Invadopodia are found in invasive cancer cells and are important for their ability to invade through the ECM [3]. Invadopodia are generally visualized by the holes they create in ECM-coated plates, in combination with immunohistochemistry for the invadopodia localizing proteins including actin, cortactin, and tyrosine kinase substrate 5 (Tks5) [1,2,4]. The large scaffolding protein TKs5 is phosphorylated by Src kinase and is important for invadopodia maturation and formation [5,6]. Tks5 functions as a tether mediating the targeting of transport vesicles containing matrix metalloproteinases (MMPs; MMP2 and MMP9) and Tks5 to the extending invadopodia [7]. A previous study suggested that the small GTPase Rab40b levels are increased in metastatic breast cancers and are required for MMP2 and MMP9 secretion from the invadopodia in breast cancer cells [8]. It is also crucial for breast tumor growth and metastasis in vivo [8]. Furthermore, a recent study revealed that the Rab40b-TKs5-dependent transport pathway mediates invadopodia extension [7]. MMPs are able to degrade many components of ECM and are important for normal processes, including tissue remodeling and wound healing. The matrix degradation activity of invadopodia is attributed to the targeted secretion of matrix-degrading enzymes such as MMPs. MMP2, MMP9, and MMP14 have been shown to enhance cancer progression due to their ability to degrade basement membrane components. These MMPs are enriched at the invadopodia and are necessary for cancer metastasis [9–15]. It was reported that MMP2 and MMP9 are not transported to invadopodia by endosomes, but instead are targeted directly from the Golgi [8] through microtubule motors (kinesin) and by actin regulators (cortactin), suggesting that these MMPs are targeted to invadopodia through at least two different membrane transport pathways.

Avian reovirus (ARV) is nonenveloped and belongs to the family Reoviridae. Several reports have demonstrated that ARV is an oncolytic virus which induces apoptosis of cancer cells, regulates cell immune response, and exposes tumor-associated antigens to the immune system [16–22]. ARV has 10 double-stranded RNA genome segments. It can replicate in the cytoplasm of infected cells. The S1 genome segment of ARV has three open reading frames that are translated into proteins σC, p10, and p17, respectively. It was found that p17 is a nucleocytoplasmic shuttling protein [23] that has been demonstrated to regulate several cellular signal pathways to modulate cell cycle retardation, the formation of autophagy, angiogenesis, viral protein synthesis, and virus replication [23–28]. To date, although recent studies have suggested that p17 retards the cell cycle of several cancer cell lines [17,25], reduces tumor size in vivo [17], and suppresses angiogenesis by promoting DPP4 secretion [21], it is unclear whether p17 protein modulates cell migration and the formation of invadopodia. The aim of this work was to perform a comprehensive study to investigate whether p17 protein modulates cell migration and the formation of invadopodia and its involved mechanisms. This work reveals, for the first time, that p17 suppresses the formation of invadopodia in B16-F10 cancer cells by activation of the p53/PTEN pathway, inhibition of the FAK/Src pathway, and enhancement of the formation of the TKs5/ non-catalytic region of tyrosine kinase adaptor protein 1 (NCK1) complex.

2. Materials and Methods

2.1. Virus and Cells

In the present study, the S1133 strain of ARV was used. Murine melanoma cancer cell line (B16-F10) [19] was cultured in Dulbecco's modified Eagle's Medium (DMEM) with 5–10% heat-inactivated fetal bovine serum (Hyclone, Logan, UT, USA) and 1% penicillin (100 IU/mL)/streptomycin (100 g/mL) (Gibco, Grand Island, NY, USA). B16-F10 cells were propagated in a 37 °C, 5% CO_2 humidified incubator. Cells were seeded in 10 cm culture dishes one day before each experiment until they reached about 75% confluence.

2.2. Reagents and Antibodies

The Akt III inhibitor, specific for Akt, was purchased from Enzo Life Science (New York, NY, USA). To examine whether p17-modulated decreased levels of TKS5 are regulated by the ubiquitin-proteasome-mediated degradation pathway, cells were transfected with the pCI-neo-p17 plasmid DNA for 6 h followed by treatment with MG132 (1 mM). MG132 was from Calbiochem Co. (San Diego, CA, USA). Gelatin and Alexa-Fluor-gelatin were from Cell Signaling (Danvers, MA, USA). The catalog numbers and dilution factors of the primary and secondary antibodies used in this study are shown in Supplementary Table S1. Antibodies against ARV p17 protein were our laboratory stocks [17].

2.3. Reverse Transcription (RT), Polymerase Chain Reaction (PCR) and Plasmid Construction

Total RNA was extracted from B16-F10 cells using TRIzol kit (Thermo Fisher Scientific Inc. Waltham, MA, USA) based on the manufacturer's procedures. The primer pairs used in this work are shown in Supplementary Table S2. The PCR products were subcloned into the corresponding sites of the pcDNA3.1 vector. In the present study, RT was performed at 42 °C for 15 min and 72 °C for 15 min. PCR was performed with 1 μL of cDNA, 1 μL of each primer, 2 μL of PCR mix, and 15 μL of ddH_2O, in a total volume of 20 μL. The PCR conditions for amplification were 95 °C for 5 min, 35 cycles of 95 °C for 30 s, 55 °C for 60 s or 90 s, and extension at 72 °C for 1 min, followed by 72 °C for 10 min for a final extension. To investigate whether p17-modulated expression of TKs5 and Rab40b is regulated transcriptionally, total RNA was isolated from p17-transfected cells using TRIzol kit. Quantitative real time RT-PCR with iQTM SYBR® Green Supermix kit (Bio-Rad, Hercules, FL, USA) was described previously [16]. The glyceraldehyde-3-phosphate dehydrogenase (GAPDH) gene was used as an internal control.

In order to understand how p17 regulate the formation of invadopodia in B16-F10 cancer cells, pcDNA3.1-$PTEN_{C124A}$ (a dominant-negative), pcDNA3.1-Rab40b, and pcDNA3.1-TKs5 were constructed. If this position is mutated, PTEN will lose its function of removing phosphate groups. The pCI-neo-p17 and pcDNA3.1-p17 plasmids have been described previously [17,26]. PCR products were purified and subcloned into the respective sites of the pcDNA3.1 vector.

2.4. shRNAs

The shRNAs were obtained from the RNAi core facility (Academia Sinica, Taipei, Taiwan). shRNA sequences are shown in Supplementary Table S3. In this work, B16-F10 cancer cells were seeded into 6 cm cell culture dishes. At about 75% confluence, cells were transfected with respective plasmids or shRNAs using Lipofectamine reagent according to the manufacturer's protocol (Invitrogen, Carlsbad, CA, USA).

2.5. Transient Transfection

In this work, cells were transfected or cotransfected with the respective shRNAs or plasmids for 24 h. The scramble plasmid was used as a negative control. Cell viability measurements with the MTT assay were conducted following transfections with the respective shRNAs or plasmids. The transfection efficiency was confirmed either by Western blot or immunofluorescence staining to ensure that the transfection efficiency reached 80–90%. The inhibitory effects of Tpr, p53, PTEN, Rak, and ROCK shRNAs were tested in cells. After transfecting different shRNAs into cells, samples were collected at 0, 6, 12, 18, and 24 h, respectively. The inhibitory effect was confirmed by Western blotting. Additionally, the GFP of pGFP-V-RS vector was expressed, and the transfection efficiency can be confirmed by fluorescence.

2.6. Wound Healing Assays, Invadopodia Detection and Gelatin Degradation Assay

To investigate whether p17 inhibits the migration of B16-F10 cancer cells, the wound healing assay was performed using the pipette tip scratching method. Then, 24 h after transfection with pcDNA3.1-p17, scratch lines were recorded and cells were photographed and recorded. B16-F10 cells were cotransfected with the pcDNA3.1-p17 or shRNAs (Tpr, p53, PTEN, Rak, or ROCK) for 24 h. Since p53, Rak, and ROCK have been suggested to be positive regulators of PTEN, knockdown of these molecules with shRNAs was carried out [26]. The scratch test was used to test and record the migration distances of B16-F10 at 12 and 24 h post transfection. Scratch lines were recorded and cells were photographed and recorded at 0, 12, and 24 h, respectively.

To explore how p17 protein modulates signaling pathways to affect the formation of invadopodia, colocalization of cortactin and β-actin by immunofluorescence staining and gelatin degradation assays were carried out as described previously [29]. B16-F10 cells were cultured on 18 by 18 mm coverslips, followed by transfection with the respective plasmids. Cells were washed twice with 1× PBS and then fixed at the indicated times with 4% paraformaldehyde (Alfa Aesar, Haverhill, MA, USA) for 20 min at room temperature. Next, fixed cells were incubated in PBS with 0.1% Triton X-100 for 10 min. The cells were washed twice with 1× PBS and blocked with Superblock T20 solution (Thermo Scientific, Bellefonte, PA, USA) at room temperature for 1 h. After two washes with 1× PBS, cells were incubated with the cortactin primary antibodies at 4 °C overnight. The solution was removed, and cells were washed three times in PBS, 5 min for each wash. Next, the cells were incubated with β-actin primary antibody (DyLight 554 Phalloidin) and the secondary antibodies overnight at 4 °C overnight (in the dark). Cell nuclei were stained with 49,6-diamidino-2-phenylindole (DAPI) for 10 min. The cells were washed three times with 1× PBS and observed under the confocal microscope (Olympus FV1000, Tokyo, Japan). The gelatin degradation assay makes it possible to assess and quantify cellular protrusions and is crucial in the study of cell invasion. In the process of this assay, fluorophore-conjugated gelatin coated coverslips were prepared and the gelatin coating was carried out as homogeneously as possible. Briefly, the coverslips were washed with 1N hydrochloric acid for 12–16 h, washed with water and sterilized with 70% ethanol. The coverslips were then incubated with 50 μg/mL poly-L-lysine (Merck Ltd. Taipei, Taiwan) for 20 min at room temperature. The coverslips were washed twice with PBS and fixed with ice-cold 0.5% glutaraldehyde (Alfa Aesar) for 15 min, followed by washing with PBS. The coverslips were placed upside down on 80 μL of fluorescent gelatin matrix (0.2% gelatin and Alexa-Fluor-gelatin; 8:1) and incubated at room temperature for 15 min. The coverslips were washed twice with PBS and incubated with the remaining reaction matrix with PBS containing 5 mg/mL sodium borohydride for 10 min followed by two rounds of washing with PBS. B16-F10 cells were then seeded in coverslips containing gelatin matrix until cell confluence reached about 70%. Cells were cotransfected with p17 and the respective plasmids and shRNAs for 24 h. The cells on the coverslip were washed twice with PBS and fixed with 4% formaldehyde at room temperature for 20 min. Next, the fixed cells were washed twice with PBS and blocked in commercially available blocking buffer with final concentration (0.1–0.3%) of Triton X-100 at room temperature for 10–20 min. The cells were washed twice with 1× PBS to remove the remaining Triton X-100 and were immunostained with β-actin primary antibody (DyLight 554 Phalloidin) overnight. Finally, cells were observed under a confocal microscope (Olympus FV1000, Tokyo, Japan) for β-actin, to determine whether the fluorescent matrix was decomposed by invadopodia (no fluorescence produced) and to record and measure regions where the cells degraded the matrix, leaving behind areas that lacked fluorescence.

2.7. Coimmunoprecipitation (Co-IP) Assay

Coimmunoprecipitation assays were performed using a Catch and Release Reversible Immunoprecipitation System (Millipore, Merck Ltd., Taipei, Taiwan), as described previously [17]. Briefly, 6-well plates were seeded with 5×10^5 B16-F10V cancer cells. The cells were cultured in DMEM containing 10% FBS overnight. Cells were transfected with the respective plasmids. Cell lysates were collected 24 h post transfection and washed twice with 1× PBS and scraped in 200 μL of CHAPS lysis buffer (40 mM HEPES (pH 7.5), 120 mM NaCl, 1 mM EDTA, 10 mM pyrophosphate, 10 mM glycerophosphate, 50 mM

NaF, and 0.3% CHAPS). Then, 1000µg of cellular proteins were incubated with 4 ug of the respective antibodies at 4 °C overnight. The immunoprecipitated proteins were analyzed by SDS-PAGE and Western blot assay with the respective antibodies.

2.8. Cell Lysate Preparation and Western Blot Analysis

The B16-F10 cancer cell line was cultured in 6-well culture plates one day before infection with ARV or transfection with the respective constructs, as described above. Cells were collected and washed twice with 1× PBS with lysis buffer (Cell signaling). The concentration of proteins in cell lysates was determined by Bio-Rad Protein assay (Bio-Rad, USA). The sample was mixed with 2.5× sample buffer dye, boiled in the water bath for 15 min, and electrophoresed in 10–15% sodium dodecyl sulphate (SDS)-polyacrylamide gel. Western blot assay was performed with the respective primary antibody and horseradish peroxidase secondary antibody conjugate to analyze expression levels of each individual protein. After membrane incubation with enhanced chemiluminescence (ECL plus) regent (Amersham Biosciences, Little Chalfont, UK, the Western blot bands were detected on X-ray film (Kodak, Rochester, NY, USA).

2.9. Statistical Analysis

Data obtained from three independent experiments are expressed as mean ± standard errors (SE). The results were analyzed for statistical significance using Duncan's multiple range test (MDRT) using Prism 8 software (GraphPad, San Diego, CA, USA). Similar letters (a, b, c) denote no significance.

3. Results

3.1. The ARV p17 Protein Downregulates Nucleoporin Tpr and Activates the p53/PTEN Pathway in B16-F10 Cancer Cells

Our previous study confirmed that p17 inhibits nucleoporin Tpr, thereby promoting the accumulation of p53 in the nucleus and further activating p53, PTEN, and p21 [26]. In order to confirm whether p17 has similar functions in murine melanoma cancer cells, Western blotting was used to analyze the signal changes of p17-transfected or Tpr shRNA cotransfected cells. Our results show that p17 reduces the level of nucleoporin Tpr, and the PTEN expression level and phosphorylated form of p53 are significantly increased (Figure 1A,B). If Tpr shRNA is cotransfected with pCI-neo-p17, the increased levels of PTEN p-p53(S15) are even greater (Figure 1A,B).

3.2. p17 Inhibits Cell Migration of B16-F10 Cancer Cells

To explore whether p17 can inhibit the cell migration of B16-F10 cancer cells, wound healing assays were used. The scratch test was used to test and record the migration distances of B16-F10 at 12 and 24 h post transfection. Our results show, that compared with the control group, p17 can inhibit the migration of B16-F10 cells. Since we demonstrated previously that p17 positively regulates p53 and Rak and drives β-arrestin-mediated PTEN translocation from the cytoplasm to the plasma membrane via a ROCK-1 rependent manner [26], depletion of p53, PTEN, Rak, and ROCk-1 by the use of shRNAs was carried out. Our findings reveal that depletion of p53, PTEN, Rak, and ROCK-1 reversed p17-modulated inhibition of cell migration (Figure 2), suggesting that p17 modulated suppression of cell migration via the p53/PTEN-dependent pathway. Conversely, depletion of Tpr did not affect the p17-modulated inhibition of cell migration (Figure 2).

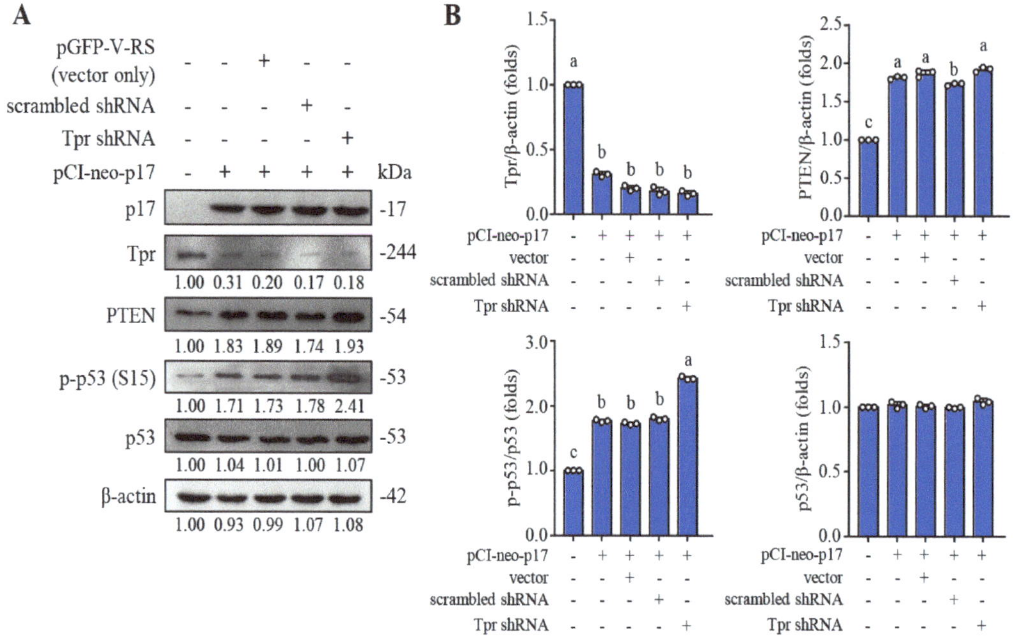

Figure 1. The ARV p17 protein upregulates the p53/PTEN pathway in B16-F10 cancer cells. (**A**) The expression levels of Tpr, PTEN, and p-p53 in p17-transfected cells were analyzed by Western blot. Cells were transfected with shRNAs for 6 h followed by transfection with the pCI-neo-p17 plasmid for 24 h. β-actin was included as a loading control. The image shown is from a single experiment that is representative of at least three separate experiments. Immunoblots were quantitated by densitometric analysis using ImageJ software version 1.53e and normalized to β-actin. Numbers below each lane are relative fold of the control level of a specific protein in mock-treated cells. (**B**) Densitometry analysis results for Western blotting are shown in panel A. Each value represents mean ± SE from three independent experiments, determined using Duncan's multiple range test. Similar letters (a, b, c) denote no significance at $p < 0.05$.

3.3. p17 Inhibits the FAK/Src Pathway and Reduces the MMP9 Level in a PTEN-Dependent Manner

As shown in Figure 3, an increase in the PTEN level and a decreased level of p-FAK (Y397) in B16-F10 cancer cells were observed in pCI-neo-p17 transfected cells (Figure 3A,B). We next wanted to examine whether dephosphorylation of FAK by p17 occurs through a PTEN-dependent manner. Previous reports suggested that FAK is cis- or trans-phosphorylated at Tyr-397, which provides a critical binding site for Src family kinases [30], the p85 regulatory subunit of phosphatidylinositol 3-kinase [31], and phospholipase Cγ [32]. Especially, Src binding to Tyr-397 is required for phosphorylation of Y576/Y577, which is important for full FAK activation. Subsequently, an activated FAK/Src complex mediates the phosphorylation of multiple adhesion components involved in the dynamic regulation of cell motility and invadopodia formation [8,33,34]. In this study, we found that p17 reduces levels of p-FAK(Y379), p-Src (Y416), and MMP9 (Figure 4A,B) and can be reversed in PTEN knockdown cells (Figure 4A,B), suggesting that p17 inhibits the FAK/Src pathway and reduces the MMP9 level in a PTEN-dependent manner.

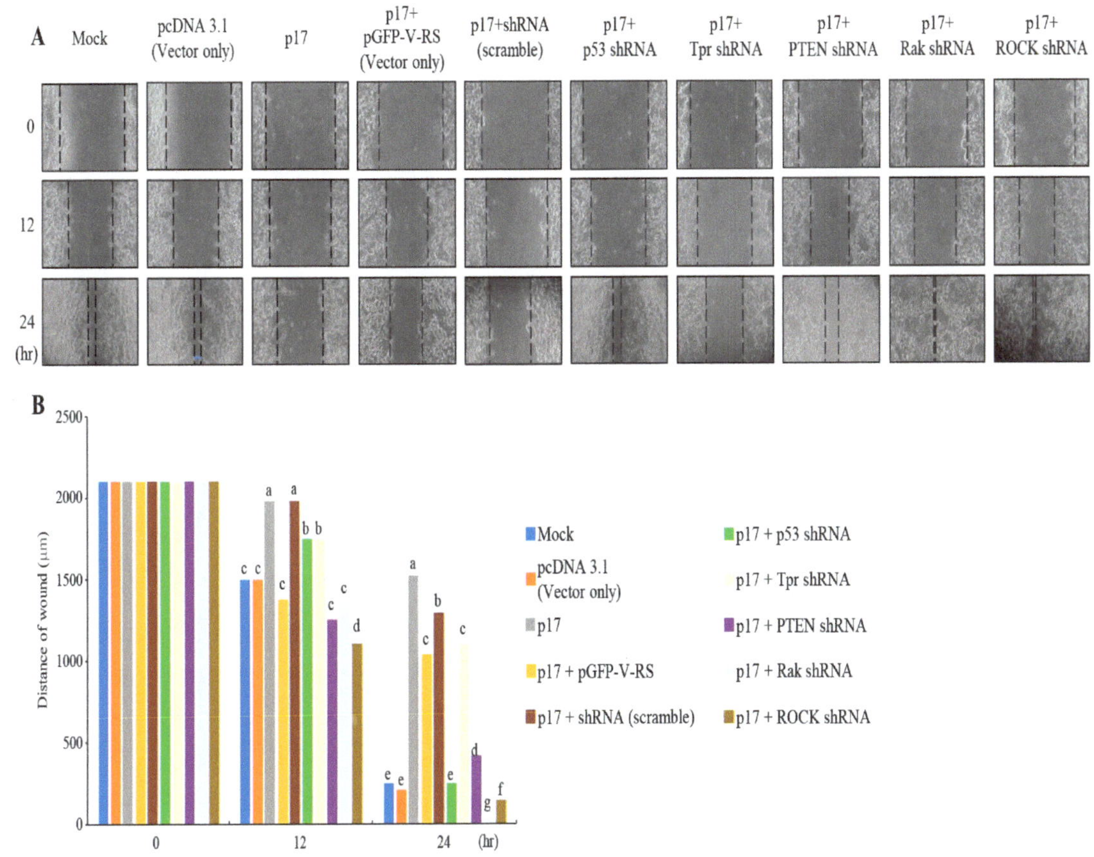

Figure 2. p17 inhibits cell migration of B16-F10 cancer cells. (**A**) To explore whether p17 inhibits cell migration of B16-F10 cancer cells, wound healing assays were used. Cells were transfected with the pcDNA3.1-p17 or cotransfected with shRNAs (p53, Tpr, PTEN, Rak, or ROCK-1) for 24 h. Scratch lines were recorded at 0, 12, and 24 h, respectively. The inhibitory effects of Tpr, p53, PTEN, Rak, and ROCK shRNAs were tested in cells, as shown in Supplementary Figure S1. (**B**)The scratch test was used to analyze the migration distances of B16-F10 at 0, 12, and 24 h post transfection. Scratch lines were recorded at 0, 12, and 24 h, respectively. Each value represents mean ± SE from three independent experiments, determined using Duncan's multiple range test. Similar letters denote no significance at $p < 0.05$.

3.4. *p17 Inhibits the Formation of the FAK/Src Complex*

A previous report indicated that the major autophosphorylation site of FAK (Y397) is responsible for the initial in vivo association of PTEN with FAK, a prerequisite for FAK dephosphorylation by PTEN [35]. PTEN interacts with FAK and reduces its tyrosine phosphorylation at Tyr 397 [36], thereby impeding Src binding to FAK. Thus, we next investigated the molecular interaction of FAK and Src in B16-F10 cancer cells. As shown in Figure 4A, p17 significantly reduces the phosphorylation of FAK and Src, but it has not yet been confirmed whether the formation of the FAK/Src complex is inhibited. Therefore, a coimmunoprecipitation assay was used to analyze the effect of coexpression of PTEN and $PTEN_{C124A}$ mutant in p17-transfected cells. Our coimmunoprecipitation results confirmed that p17 reduces the formation of the FAK/Src complex (Figure 5, left panel). The results show that, compared with the mock group, overexpression of p17 significantly reduced

FAK tyrosine phosphorylation and reduced the amount of FAK/Src complex, while co-overexpression of PTEN can make the inhibitory effect more significant (Figure 5, left and right panels). This inhibitory effect was not altered in cells coexpressing $PTEN_{C124A}$ mutant and p17 (Figure 5, left and right panels). Taking all findings together, p17 activates the p53/PTEN pathway to reduce levels of p-FAK(Y379), thereby reducing Src binding to Tyr-397 and the amount of the FAK/Src complex.

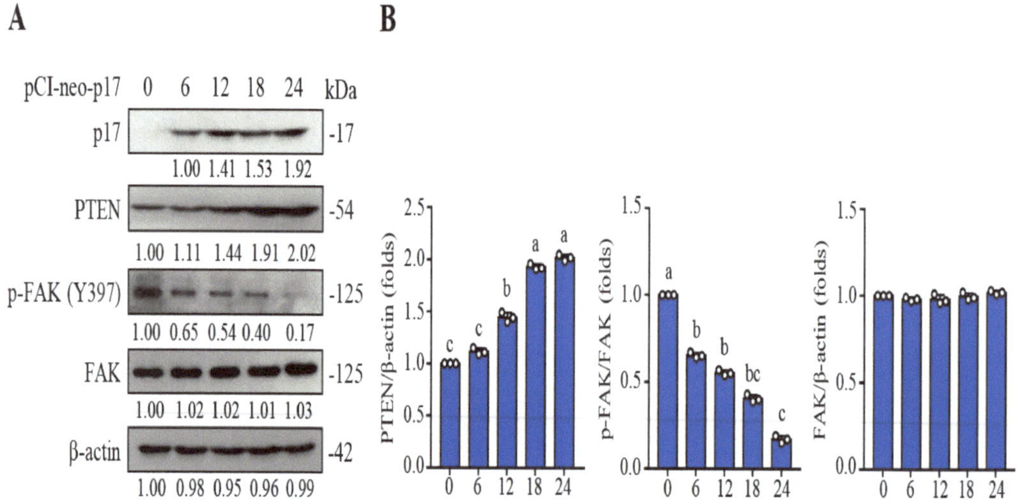

Figure 3. ARV p17 increases the levels of PTEN and reduces the phosphorylated form of FAK in B16-F10 cancer cells in a time-dependent manner. (**A**) The expression levels of PTEN and p-FAK in pCI-neo-p17-transfected cancer cells were analyzed. Whole cell lysates were collected at 0, 6, 12, 18, and 24 h post transfection for Western blot assays. β-actin was included as a loading control. The fold activation and inactivation indicated below each lane were normalized against the 0 h sample. The levels of indicated proteins at 0 h were considered to be 1-fold. Immunoblots were quantitated by densitometric analysis using ImageJ software and normalized to β-actin. (**B**) Densitometry analysis results for Western blots are shown in panel A. Each value represents mean ± SE from three independent experiments, determined using Duncan's multiple range test. Similar letters (a, b, c) denote no significance at $p < 0.05$.

3.5. p17 Reduces the Expression Levels of TKs5, Rab40b, NCK1, and MMP9 and Suppresses the Formation of the TKs5/NCK1 Complex

Previous reports have shown that Src can phosphorylate TKs5 at Y557 to promote cell migration and invadopodia formation [4,34]. TKs4 and TKs5 are Src substrates. They have been identified as invadopodia organizers [34]. The initiation of invadopodia assembly has been related to the PI3K activity. Cells treated with PI3K inhibitors or PI3K-specific siRNA reduced ECM degradation and invadopodia formation [37,38]. Class I PI3K can phosphorylate phosphatidylinositol 4,5-bisphosphate [PIP $(3.4)_2$] to create phosphatidylinositol (3,4,5)-trisphosphate (PIP3) [39] which will recruit kinases involved in invadopodia regulation, such as Akt [38,40]. A previous study suggested that PIP 3 can function as a precursor lipid for PIP $(3.4)_2$, which localizes to invadopodia in Src-transformed fibroblasts [41]. As shown in Figure 6A (left and right panels), the levels of p-PI3K, p-Akt, TKs5, Rab40b, NCK1, and MMP9 all showed a downward trend compared with the control group after transfection with the pCI-neo-p17 construct. These findings reveal that p17 downregulates PI3K, Akt, TKs5, Rab40b, NCK1, and MMP9. Moreover, coexpressing the Rab40b protein in p17-transfected cells reversed the p17-modulated suppression of TKs5 and MMP9, while the decrease in the p-PI3K and p-Akt levels were slightly reversed (Figure 6A, left panel). The decreased level of TKs5 by p17 was not altered. Furthermore, by coexpressing the TKs5 protein, p17-modulated downregulation of MMP9 could be reversed, while the decreased level of NCK1 by p17 was not altered (Figure 6A, right panel). Interestingly, the decreased levels of TKs5 and MMP9 were also seen in Akt III-treated cells (Figure 6B), suggesting that the PI3K/Akt pathway may upregulate TKs5 and MMP9. These findings are consistent with the previous report suggesting that PTEN dephosphorylates PIP3 and FAK, and it can inhibit cell growth, invasion, migration, and focal adhesions [35]. To further study whether depletion of TKS5 and Rab40b affects the downstream MMP9, TKS5 and Rab40b shRNAs were used. The results showed that p17 reduces the levels of MMP9 and this inhibitory effect could be further elevated in TKS5 and Rab40b knockdown cells (Figure 6C).

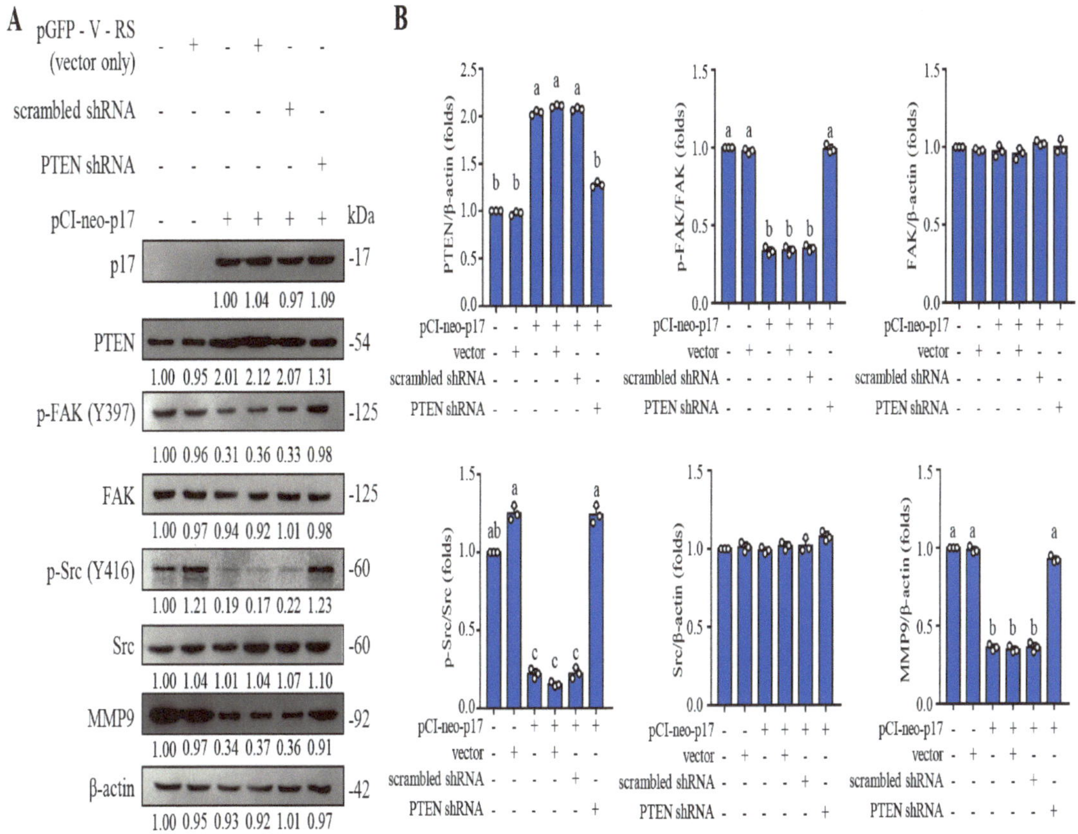

Figure 4. ARV p17 protein upregulates PTEN to inhibit the FAK/Src/MMP9 pathway in B16-F10 cancer cells. (**A**) The expression levels of PTEN, p-FAK, FAK, p-Src, Src, and MMP9 in pCI-neo-p17-transfected cells were analyzed by Western blots. Whole cell lysates were collected at 24 h post transfection. β-actin was used as a loading control. The fold activation and inactivation indicated below each lane were normalized against the mock control. The levels of the indicated proteins in mock treated cells were considered to be 1-fold. (**B**) Immunoblots from panel A were quantitated by densitometric analysis using ImageJ software and normalized to β-actin. Each value represents mean ± SE from three independent experiments, determined using Duncan's multiple range test. Similar letters (a, b, c) denote no significance at $p < 0.05$.

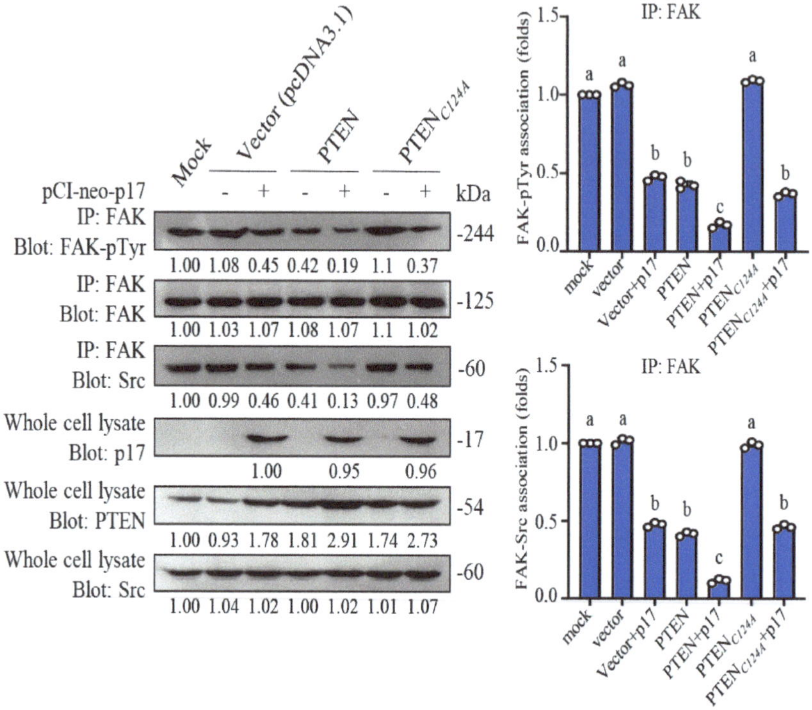

Figure 5. The ARV p17 activates PTEN, leading to inhibition of the FAK/Src complex formation in B16-F10 cancer cells. Coimmunoprecipitation experiments of FAK, FAK-pTyr, and Src were performed. The levels of indicated proteins in cell alone or mock transfection were considered to be 1-fold. Immunoblots from the left panel- were quantitated by densitometric analysis using ImageJ software. Each value represents mean ± SE from three independent experiments, determined using Duncan's multiple range test. Similar letters (a, b, c) denote no significance at $p < 0.05$.

A previous study suggested that PIP(3.4)$_2$ may recruit the scaffold protein Tks5 by binding its PX domain, which will target it for localization with cortactin to the cell membrane [42]. After localization, it is thought that Tks5 regulates invadopodia formation by binding to key actin regulators such as Nck1, Nck2, NWASP, and Grb2, via its third SH3 domain [4,41]. To investigate whether p17 modulates the formation of the TKs5/NCK1 complex, a coimmunoprecipitation assay was carried out. Our data reveal that p17 reduces the amounts of the TKs5/NCK1 complex, and the inhibitory effect could be moderately reversed in cells coexpressing p17 and NCK1 (Figure 6D). The results indicate that p17 suppresses the formation of the TKs5/NCK1 complex. Having shown that the p17 protein downregulates TKs5, Rab40b, and NCK1, we next explored whether p17-modulated decreased levels of TKS5 and Rab40b are regulated by the ubiquitin-proteasome-mediated degradation pathway. Thus, the protease inhibitor MG132 was used to analyze the effect of MG132 on TKS5 expression levels. The results showed that in the presence of MG132, the expression levels of TKs5 were not altered in p17-transfected and MG132-treated cells compared with the p17 transfection group (Figure 6E). To further study whether p17 transcriptionally downregulates the TKs5 and Rab40b genes, the mRNA levels of these genes in p17-transfected B16-F10 cancer cells were quantified by qRT-PCR. As shown in Figure 6F, the mRNA levels of TKs5 and Rab40b genes were significantly reduced in p17-transfected cells, suggesting that p17 transcriptionally downregulates these genes.

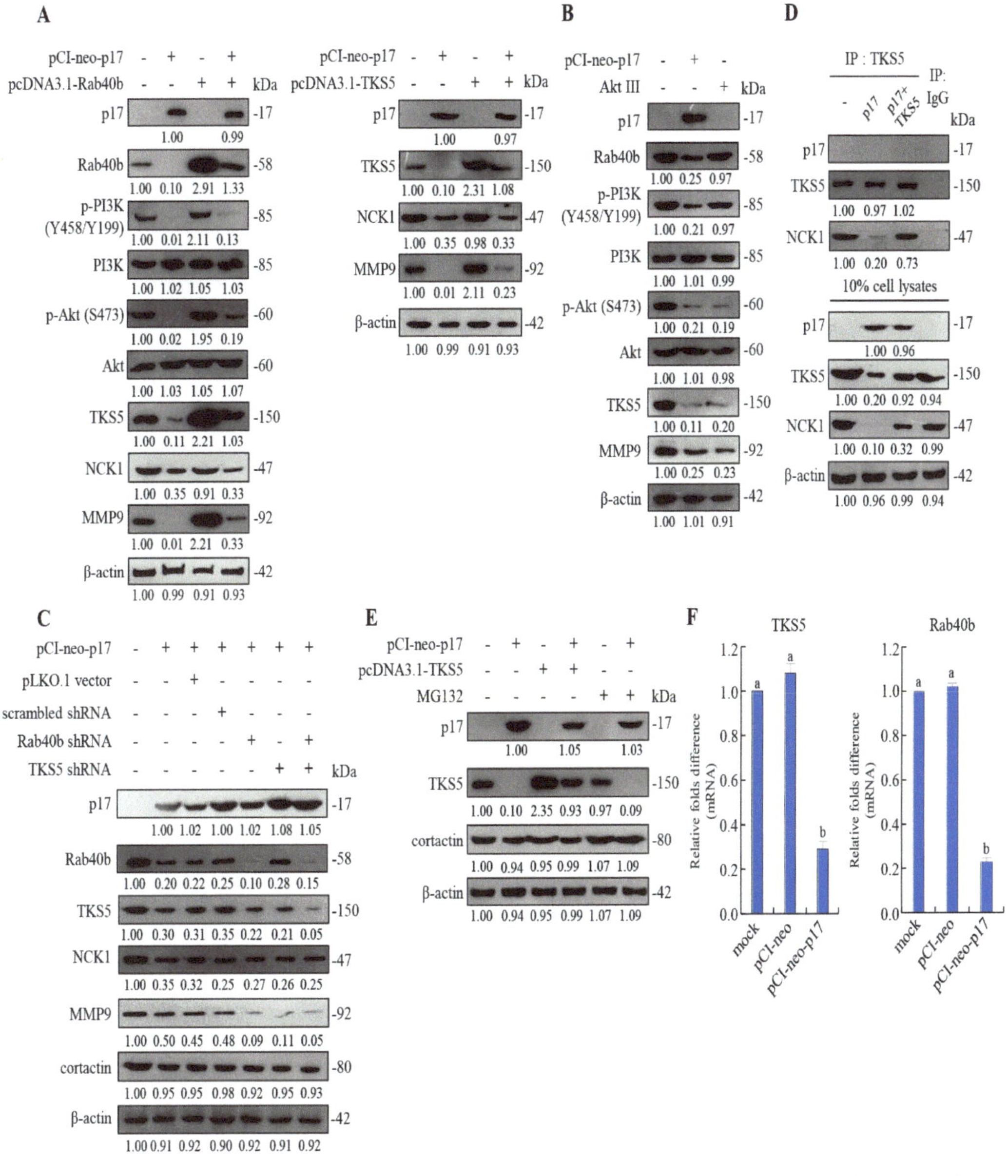

Figure 6. p17 reduces the expression levels of TKs5, Rab40b, NCK1, and MMP9 and suppresses the formation of the TKs5/NCK1 complex in B16-F10 cancer cells. (**A**) The levels of p-PI3K, p-Akt, TKs5, Rab40b, NCK1, and the downstream MMP9 were analyzed by Western blot assays in p17-transfected or p17/Rab40b and p17/TKs5 cotransfected cells, respectively. The level of indicated proteins in cell alone was considered to be 1-fold. The fold activation and inactivation indicated below each lane were normalized against the cell alone group. Immunoblots were quantitated by densitometric analysis using ImageJ software and normalized to β-actin. (**B**) The levels of TKs5 and MMP9 were analyzed in p17-transfected and Akt III-treated cells. (**C**) The levels of Rab40b, TKs5,

NCK1, and MMP9 were analyzed by Western blot assays in p17-transfected or p17/Rab40b shRNA and p17/TKs5 shRNA cotransfected cells, respectively. (**D**) To examine whether p17 modulates the formation of the TKs5/NCK1 complex, coimmunoprecipitation assay was performed in p17-transfected or p17/Tks5-cotransfected cells. (**E**) To examine whether p17-modulated decreased levels of TKS5 are regulated by the ubiquitin-proteasome-mediated degradation pathway, the protease inhibitor MG132 (1 mM) was used to analyze the effect of MG132 on the TKS5 expression level. The levels of TKs5 were analyzed by Western blot. Cells were transfected with the pCI-neo-p17 plasmid DNA for 6 h, followed by treatment with MG132 (1 mM). (**F**) The mRNA levels of TKs5 and Rab40b genes in mock, vector, and p17-transfected cells were analyzed by qRT-PCR. The levels of the mock group in cell alone were considered to be 1-fold. Each value represents mean ± SE from three independent experiments, determined using Duncan's multiple range test. Similar letters (a, b, c) denote no significance at $p < 0.05$. Immunoblots from panels (**A**–**E**) were quantitated by densitometric analysis using ImageJ software. The results are shown in Supplementary Figure S2.

3.6. p17 Inhibits the Formation of Invadopodia in B16-F10 Cancer Cells

Even though it has been demonstrated that p17 modulates suppression of TKs5, NCK1, Rab40b, and MMP9 and reduces complex formation of FAK/Src and TKs5/NCK1 in B16-F10 cancer cells, the impact of p17 on the formation of invadopodia is not yet clear. Thus, we next wanted to examine whether p17 inhibits the formation of invadopodia. Colocalization of cortactin and β-actin by immunofluorescence staining and gelatin degradation assays were performed to analyze whether p17 inhibits the formation of invadopodia, as described in the Methods section. The results of colocalization of cortactin and β-actin by immunofluorescence staining reveal that the amount of invadopodia formation was significantly reduced in the pcDNA3.1-p17-transfected cells compared with the mock control group (Figure 7A). Coexpression of PTEN in p17-transfected cells significantly reduced the formation of invadopodia compared with the mock control group (Figure 7A). Overexpression of PTENC124A, TKs5, and Rab40b significantly increased the formation of invadopodia (Figure 7A), while coexpression of p17 showed a reversion to invadopodia production (Figure 7A). These findings further confirmed the impact of p17 on the formation of invadopodia. In gelatin degradation assays, we found that the fluorescent matrix was decomposed by invadopodia (no fluorescence produced) in cells overexpressing PTENC124A, TKs5, and Rab40b (Figure 7B). The formation of invadopodia could be reversed in cells coexpressing the p17 protein. p17-modulated suppression of invadopodia formation was reversed in Csk-knockdown cells. Taken together, our results reveal that the p17 protein inhibits invadopodia formation by activating the p53/PTEN pathway, suppressing the FAK/Src pathway, and downregulatingTKs5, Rab40b, NCK1, and MMP9.

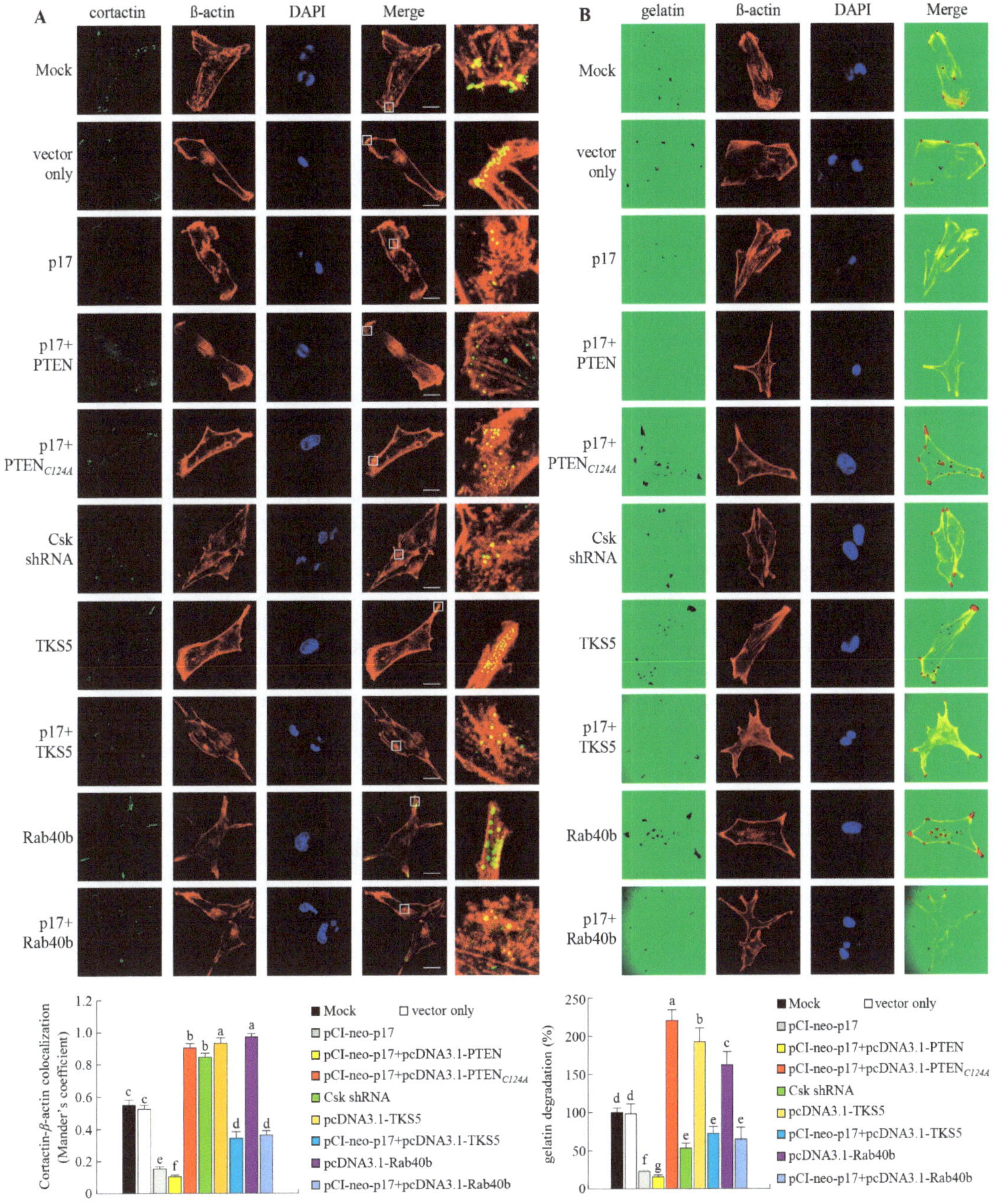

Figure 7. The ARV p17 protein inhibits invadopodia formation in B16-F10 cancer cells. The role of PTEN or PTEN$_{C124A}$ mutant protein in p17-transfected cells was examined. (**A**) Cells were then fixed and processed for immunofluorescence staining of DAPI. β-actin staining (red), cortactin (green), and nuclei (blue) were observed under a confocal microscope. The invadopodia are composed of cortactin

and β-actin. The yellow dots in the merged panels show invadopodia underneath the cells. The square shows the further enlargement area (100×). For quantifying the colocalization of cortactin and β-actin, at least 10 fields of 1 to 2 cells per field were taken for each sample per experiment. Each experiment was performed at least three times, while the exposure settings were unchanged during acquisition of various samples. (**B**) Images showing fluorescent gelatin (green) are from a gelatin degradation assay performed in B16-F10 cells. To quantify invadopodia activity, black areas of gelatin degradation were analyzed using ImageJ. The percent of area corresponds to degradation on a given image and normalized to β-actin. At least 10 fields of 1 to 2 cells per field were taken for each sample per experiment. Quantification of the degradation area was performed with ImageJ software. Each value represents mean ± SE from three independent experiments, determined using Duncan's multiple range test. Similar letters (a, b, c) denote no significance at $p < 0.05$. In this study, all original images are shown in Supplementary Figure S3.

4. Discussion

We previously demonstrated that the ARV p17 protein functions as a nucleoporin Tpr suppressor resulting in p53 accumulation in the nucleus, thereby activating the downstream molecules p21 and PTEN [26]. p17-modulated suppression of cell cycle CDK–cyclin complexes results in cell cycle retardation [17,25]. An in vivo tumorigenesis assay also showed that p17 causes a significant reduction in tumor size [17]. It was also found that p17 suppresses angiogenesis by promoting DPP4 secretion [21]. This work provides novel insights into the mechanisms underlying p17-modulated regulation of related signal pathways to suppress invadopodia formation.

Our findings reveal that p17-modulated inhibition of the formation of invadopodia in B16-F10 cancer cells relies on several different mechanisms. First, p17 activates the p53/PTEN pathway to dephosphorylate FAK at Y397 to inhibit Src binding to FAK at Y397, which prevents Src phosphorylation of TKs5 at Y557 to promote cell migration and invadopodia formation [34,37]. It was demonstrated that Tks5 functions as a tether mediating the targeting of transport vesicles containing MMP2 and MMP9 [7]. TKs5 depletion inhibited secretion of MMP2 and MMP9, suggesting that it directly mediates MMP2 and MMP9 secretion [7]. The upstream FAK signaling is involved in functions such as adhesion to the matrix and cell migration [43]. An earlier report confirmed that PTEN can compete with other signals at the FAK Y397 phosphorylation site and remove FAK phosphorylation [35], inhibiting downstream signals. In PTEN-mutated cells, regardless of whether the cells are in contact with the matrix, FAK will continue to activate Src and other pathways. If a large amount of exogenous PTEN is expressed, it can inhibit the continued activation of FAK. Clinical medicine has confirmed that in many malignant tumors, FAK mRNA transcript levels are 25% to 37% higher than those in normal cells [44]. Since FAK is involved in many cancers, in recent years, there has been a focus on developing anticancer drugs that inhibit FAK [45]. The scaffoldings protein TKs5 is essential for the assembly and function of invadopodia, and it has been confirmed that the TKs5 protein is not required for the structural composition of invadopodia, but is a key protein for stabilizing invadopodia; deletion of TKs5 in Src3T3 cells inhibits the stability of podosomes/invadopodia [6,46–48]. It was found that TKs5/FGD1 forms a complex, and activated CDC42 affects cell migration. If the function of these proteins is lost, MT1-MMP will be unable to function normally. Therefore, the assembly and matrix degradation of collagenolytic pseudopodia are inhibited, and the directionality and speed of tumor cell invasion through the ECM are reduced [49]. Furthermore, several studies have confirmed that reducing TKs5 protein in cancer cells in vitro or in vivo results in reduced cell invasion ability [50,51]. A decrease in Tks4 or Tks5 in cancer cells leads to reduced cell metastasis, suggesting that inhibition of pseudopodia has an additional antimetastatic effect, leading to further reduction in metastasis efficiency [52].

Second, p17 transcriptionally downregulates TKs5, Rab40b, and NCK1 to reduce the formation of TKs5/NCK1 or TKs5/Rab41b complexes, thereby suppressing the formation of invadopodia. It was found that TKs5 forms a complex with Rab40b or NCK1 to regulate invadopodia production and maturation [37]. A previous study suggested that NCK1 activity is important for invadopodia formation and degradation of the external matrix in metastatic breast cancer cells and melanoma cells [53]. TKs5 regulates invadopodia formation by binding to key actin regulators such NCK1 [4,34]. Third, in addition to the p53/PTEN and FAK/Src/Tsk5 signaling axis, our results suggest a mechanism whereby p17 exerts a negative effect on the PI3K/Akt pathway. PI3K can phosphorylate PIP $(3.4)_2$ to generate phosPIP3 [39], which will recruit kinases involved in invadopodia regulation, such as Akt [38,40]. A recent study suggested that Rab40b can recognize and bind to TKs5 located at the end of invadopodia, and will carry MMPs to vesicles to guide the release of invadopodia [7]. TKs5 prompts Rab40b to intervene in the transport of MMP2/MMP9 in the formation of invadopodia [7].

Previous studies have confirmed that highly invasive cancer cells form protruding structures called invadopodia that aggregate actin and degrade ECM [54]. The structure of invadopodia is mainly composed of two different types of actin, β-actin, and cortactin, surrounded by a ring structure rich in actin-binding proteins, N-WASP, and cofilin [3,55]. The resulting invadopodia penetrates deep into the ECM and breaks it down to assist cell migration. In this work, wound healing assays, invadopodia detection by ß-actin and cortactin immunofluorescence staining, and gelatin degradation assays clearly demonstrated that p17 inhibits cell migration and the formation of invadopodia. It was suggested that after cofilin and Arp2/3 conjugates polymerize downstream proteins and actin, cortactin is dephosphorylated, which is necessary to stabilize the invadopodium precursor. In turn, stabilization is required to enable invadopodium [56]. Future studies can further explore whether p17 protein is a cofilin and Arp2/3 complex.

Supplementary Materials: The following supporting information can be down loaded at: https://www.mdpi.com/article/10.3390/v16071153/s1, Figure S1: Inhibitory effects of Tpr, p53, PTEN, Rak and ROCK shRNAs were tested in cells; Figure S2: Immunoblots from Figure 6 (panels A-E) were quantitated by densitometric analysis using ImageJ software; Figure S3: All original blots and images; Supplementary Table S1: The catalog numbers and dilution factor of the respective antibodies used in this study; Supplementary Table S2: Primers used in this study; Supplementary Table S3: shRNAs used in this study.

Author Contributions: H.-J.L. conceived the study and generated the original hypothesis, and supervised the project; C.-Y.H. and J.-Y.L. performed most of the experiments. C.-Y.H., J.-Y.L., E.-Y.Y., T.-L.L., H.-W.W., P.-C.T., T.-C.J., L.-F.L. and B.L.N. analyzed data and statistics; H.-J.L. and B.L.N. revised and edited the manuscript. All authors have read and agreed to the published version of the manuscript.

Funding: This work was financially supported by Ministry of Science and Technology of Taiwan (109-2313-B-005-006-MY3 & 111-2622-B-005-001), The iEGG and Animal Biotechnology Center from The Feature Areas Research Center Program within the framework of the Higher Education Sprout Project by the Ministry of Education (MOE) in Taiwan (112S0023A), National Chung Hsing University, and Taichung Veterans General Hospital (TCVGH-NCHU1117608).

Institutional Review Board Statement: Not applicable.

Informed Consent Statement: Not applicable.

Data Availability Statement: Data are contained within the article and Supplementary Materials.

Conflicts of Interest: The authors declare no conflicts of interest.

References

1. Murphy, D.A.; Courtneidge, S.A. The 'ins' and 'outs' of podosomes and invadopodia: Characteristics, formation and function. *Nat. Rev. Mole. Cell Biol.* **2011**, *12*, 413–426. [CrossRef]
2. Eddy, R.J.; Weidmann, M.D.; Sharma, V.P.; Condeelis, J.S. Tumor Cell Invado podia: Invasive Protrusions that Orchestrate Metastasis. *Trends Cell Biol.* **2017**, *27*, 595–607. [CrossRef] [PubMed]
3. Seano, G.; Primo, L. Podosomes and invadopodia: Tools to breach vascular basement membrane. *Cell Cycle* **2015**, *14*, 1370–1374. [CrossRef]

4. Stylli, S.S.; Stacey, T.T.; Verhagen, A.M.; Xu, S.S.; Pass, I.; Courtneidge, S.A.; Lock, P. Nck adaptor proteins link Tks5 to in va dopodia actin regulation and ECM degradation. *J. Cell Sci.* **2009**, *122 Pt 15*, 2727–2740. [CrossRef] [PubMed]
5. Courtneidge, S.A.; Azucena, E.F.; Pass, I.; Seals, D.F.; Tesfay, L. The Src substrate Tks5, podosomes (invadopodia), and cancer cell invasion. *Cold Spring Harb. Symp. Quant. Biol.* **2005**, *70*, 167–171. [CrossRef]
6. Sharma, V.P.; Eddy, R.; Entenberg, D.; Kai, M.; Gertler, F.B.; Condeelis, J. Tks5 and SHIP2 regulate invadopodium maturation, but not initiation, in breast carcinoma cells. *Curr. Biol.* **2013**, *23*, 2079–2089. [CrossRef]
7. Jacob, A.; Linklater, E.; Bayless, B.A.; Lyons, T.; Prekeris, R. The role and regulation of Rab40b–Tks5 complex during invadopodia formation and cancer cell invasion. *J. Cell Sci.* **2016**, *129*, 4341–4353. [CrossRef]
8. Jacob, A.; Jing, J.; Lee, J.; Schedin, P.; Gilbert, S.M.; Peden, A.A.; Junutula, J.R.; Prekeris, R. Rab40b regulates trafficking of MMP2 and MMP9 during invadopodia formation and invasion of breast cancer cells. *J. Cell Sci.* **2013**, *126*, 4647–4658. [CrossRef] [PubMed]
9. Ala-aho, R.; Kahari, V.M. Collagenases in cancer. *Biochimie* **2005**, *87*, 273–286. [CrossRef] [PubMed]
10. Bjorklund, M.; Koivunen, E. Gelatinase-mediated migration and invasion of cancer cells. *Biochim. Biophys. Acta* **2005**, *1755*, 37–69. [CrossRef] [PubMed]
11. Hofmann, U.B.; Houben, R.; Brocker, E.B.; Becker, J.C. Role of matrix metallopro teinases in melanoma cell invasion. *Biochimie* **2005**, *87*, 307–314. [CrossRef] [PubMed]
12. Kerkela, E.; Saarialho-Kere, U. Matrix metalloproteinases in tumor progression: Focus on basal and squamous cell skin cancer. *Exp. Dermatol.* **2003**, *12*, 109–125. [CrossRef] [PubMed]
13. Lochter, A.; Sternlicht, M.D.; Werb, Z.; Bissell, M.J. The significance of matrix metalloproteinases during early stages of tumor progression. *Ann. N. Y. Acad. Sci.* **1998**, *857*, 180–193. [CrossRef] [PubMed]
14. Mook, O.R.F.; Frederiks, W.M.; Van Noorden, C.J.F. The role of gelatinases in colorectal cancer progression and metastasis. *Biochim. Biophys. Acta* **2004**, *1705*, 69–89. [CrossRef] [PubMed]
15. Wagenaar-Miller, R.A.; Gorden, L.; Matrisian, L.M. Matrix metalloproteinases in colorectal cancer: Is it worth talking about? *Cancer Metast. Rev.* **2004**, *23*, 119–135. [CrossRef] [PubMed]
16. Cai, R.; Meng, G.; Li, Y.; Wang, W.; Diao, Y.; Zhao, S.; Feng, Q.; Tang, Y. The oncolytic efficacy and safety of avian reovirus and its dynamic distribution in infected mice. *Exp. Biol. Med.* **2019**, *244*, 983–991. [CrossRef] [PubMed]
17. Chiu, H.C.; Huang, W.R.; Liao, T.L.; Chi, P.I.; Nielsen, B.L.; Liu, J.H.; Liu, H.-J. Mechanistic insights into avian reovirus p17-modulated suppression of cell cycle CDK–cyclin complexes and enhancement of p53 and cyclin H interaction. *J. Biol. Chem.* **2018**, *293*, 12542–12562. [CrossRef] [PubMed]
18. Hsu, C.Y.; Chen, Y.H.; Huang, W.R.; Huang, J.W.; Chen, I.C.; Chang, Y.K.; Wang, C.Y.; Chang, C.D.; Liao, T.L.; Nielsen, B.L.; et al. Oncolytic avian reovirus sigma A-modulated fatty acid metabolism through the PSMB6/Akt/SREBP1/acetyl-CoA carboxylase pathway to increase energy production for virus replication. *Vet. Microbiol.* **2022**, *273*, 109545. [CrossRef] [PubMed]
19. Hsu, C.Y.; Huang, J.W.; Huang, W.R.; Chen, I.C.; Chen, M.S.; Liao, T.L.; Chang, Y.K.; Munir, M.; Liu, H.J. Oncolytic avian reovirus sigma A-modulated upregulation of the HIF-1a/C-myc/glut1 pathway to produce more energy in different cancer cell lines benefiting virus replication. *Viruses* **2023**, *15*, 523. [CrossRef] [PubMed]
20. Kozak, R.A.; Hattin, L.; Biondi, M.J.; Corredor, J.C.; Walsh, S.; Xue-Zhong, M.; Manuel, J.; McGilvray, I.D.; Morgenstern, J.; Lusty, E.; et al. Replication and oncolytic activity of an avian orthoreovirus in human hepatocellular carcinoma cells. *Viruses* **2017**, *9*, 90. [CrossRef] [PubMed]
21. Manocha, E.; Bugatti, A.; Belleri, M.; Zani, A.; Marsico, S.; Caccuri, F.; Presta, M.; Caruso, A. Avian reovirus p17 suppresses angiogenesis by promoting DPP4 secretion. *Cells* **2021**, *10*, 259. [CrossRef] [PubMed]
22. Shih, W.L.; Hsu, H.W.; Liao, M.H.; Lee, L.H.; Liu, H.J. Avian reovirus sigmaC protein induces apoptosis in cultured cells. *Virology* **2004**, *321*, 65–74. [CrossRef] [PubMed]
23. Chi, P.I.; Huang, W.R.; Lai, I.H.; Cheng, C.Y.; Liu, H.J. The p17 nonstructural protein of avian reovirus triggers autophagy enhancing virus replication via activation of phosphatase and tensin deleted on chromosome 10 (PTEN) and AMP activated protein kinase (AMPK), as well as dsRNA-dependent protein kinase (PKR)/eIF2a signaling pathways. *J. Biol. Chem.* **2013**, *288*, 3571–3584. [PubMed]
24. Chiu, H.C.; Huang, W.R.; Wang, Y.Y.; Li, J.Y.; Liao, T.L.; Nielsen, B.L.; Liu, H.J. Heterogeneous nuclear ribonucleoprotein A1 and lamin A/C modulate nucleocytoplasmic shuttling of avian reovirus p17. *J. Virol.* **2019**, *93*, e00851-19. [CrossRef] [PubMed]
25. Chiu, H.C.; Huang, W.R.; Liao, T.L.; Wu, H.Y.; Munir, M.; Shih, W.L.; Liu, H.J. Suppression of vimentin phos phorylation by the avian reovirus p17 through inhibition of CDK1 and Plk1 impacting the G2/M phase of the cell cycle. *PLoS ONE* **2016**, *11*, e0162356. [CrossRef] [PubMed]
26. Huang, W.R.; Chiu, H.C.; Liao, T.L.; Chuang, K.P.; Shih, W.L.; Liu, H.J. Avian reovirus protein p17 functions as a nucleoporin Tpr suppressor leading to activation of p53, p21 and PTEN and inactivation of PI3K/AKT/mTOR and ERK signaling pathways. *PLoS ONE* **2015**, *10*, e0133699. [CrossRef] [PubMed]
27. Huang, W.R.; Li, J.Y.; Wu, Y.Y.; Liao, T.L.; Nielsen, B.L.; Liu, H.J. p17-modulated Hsp90/Cdc37 complex governs avian reovirus replication by chaperoning p17, which promotes viral protein synthesis and accumulation of proteins σA and σC in viral factories. *J. Virol.* **2022**, *96*, e00074-22. [CrossRef] [PubMed]

28. Huang, W.R.; Li, J.Y.; Liao, T.L.; Yeh, C.M.; Wang, C.Y.; Wen, H.W.; Hu, N.J.; Wu, Y.Y.; Hsu, C.Y.; Chang, Y.K.; et al. Molecular chaperone TRiC governs avian reovirus replication by preventing outer-capsid protein σC and core protein s A and non-structural protein s NS from ubiquitin-proteasome degradation. *Vet. Microbiol.* **2022**, *264*, 109277. [CrossRef] [PubMed]
29. Díaz, B. Invadopodia Detection and Gelatin Degradation Assay. *Bio Protoc.* **2013**, *3*, e997. [CrossRef]
30. Schaller, M.D.; Hildebrand, J.D.; Shannon, J.D.; Fox, J.W.; Vines, R.R.; Parsons, J.T. Autophosphorylation of the focal adhesion kinase, pp125FAK, di rects SH2-dependent binding of pp60src. *Mol. Cell. Biol.* **1994**, *14*, 1680–1688. [PubMed]
31. Chen, H.C.; Guan, J.L. Association of focal adhesion kinase with its potential sub-strate phosphatidylinositol 3-kinase. *Proc. Natl. Acad. Sci. USA* **1994**, *91*, 10148–10152. [CrossRef] [PubMed]
32. Zhang, X.; Chattopadhyay, A.; Ji, Q.S.; Owen, J.D.; Ruest, P.J.; Carpenter, G.; Hanks, S.K. Focal adhesion kinase promotes phospholipase C-gamma1 activity. *Proc. Natl. Acad. Sci. USA* **1999**, *96*, 9021–9026. [CrossRef] [PubMed]
33. Chan, K.T.; Cortesio, C.L.; Huttenlocher, A. FAK alters invadopodia and focal adhesion composition and dynamics to regulate breast cancer invasion. *J. Cell Biol.* **2009**, *185*, 357–370. [CrossRef] [PubMed]
34. Saykali, B.A.; El-Sibai, M. Invadopodia, regulation, and assembly in cancer cell invasion. *Cell Commun. Adhes.* **2014**, *21*, 207–212. [CrossRef] [PubMed]
35. Tamura, M.; Gu, J.; Danen, E.H.J.; Takino, T.; Miyamotoi, S.; Yamada, K.M. PTEN interactions with focal adhesion kinase and suppression of the extracellular matrix-dependent phosphatidylinositol 3-kinase/Akt cell survival pathway. *J. Biol. Chem.* **1999**, *274*, 20693–20703. [CrossRef] [PubMed]
36. Tamura, M.; Gu, J.; Matsumoto, K.; Aota, S.; Parsons, R.; Yamada, K.M. Inhibition of cell migration, spreading, andfocal adhesions by tumor suppressor PTEN. *Science* **1998**, *280*, 1614–1617. [CrossRef]
37. Hoshino, D.; Jourquin, J.; Emmons, S.W.; Miller, T.; Goldgof, M.; Costello, K.; Tyson, D.R.; Brown, B.; Lu, Y.; Prasad, N.K.; et al. Network analysis of the focal adhesion to invadopodia transition identifies a PI3K-PKCa invasive signaling axis. *Sci. Signal.* **2012**, *5*, ra66. [CrossRef] [PubMed]
38. Yamaguchi, H.; Yoshida, S.; Muroi, E.; Yoshida, N.; Kawamura, M.; Kouchi, Z.; Nakamura, Y.; Sakai, R.; Fukami, K. Phosphoinositide 3-kinase signaling pathway mediated by p110a regulates invadopodia formation. *J. Cell Biol.* **2011**, *193*, 1275–1288. [CrossRef] [PubMed]
39. Fruman, A.; Meyers, R.E.; Cantley, L.C. Phosphoinositide kinases. *Annu. Rev. Bio Chem.* **1998**, *67*, 481–507. [CrossRef] [PubMed]
40. Cantley, L.C. The phosphoinositide 3-kinase pathway. *Science* **2002**, *296*, 1655–1657. [CrossRef] [PubMed]
41. Oikawa, T.; Itoh, T.; Takenawa, T. Sequential signals toward podosome formation in NIH-src cells. *J. Cell Biol.* **2008**, *182*, 157–169. [CrossRef] [PubMed]
42. Clark, E.S.; Weaver, A.M. New role for cortactin in invadopodia: Regulation of protease secretion. *Eur. J. Cell Biol.* **2008**, *87*, 581–590. [CrossRef] [PubMed]
43. Hsia, D.A.; Mitra, S.K.; Hauck, C.R.; Streblow, D.N.; Nelson, J.A.; Ilic, D.; Huang, S.; Li, E.; Nemerow, G.R.; Leng, J.; et al. Differential regulation of cell motility and invasion by FAK. *J. Cell Biol.* **2003**, *160*, 753–767. [CrossRef] [PubMed]
44. Sulzmaier, F.J.; Jean, C.; Schlaepfer, D.D. FAK in cancer: Mechanistic findings and clinical applications. *Nat. Rev. Cancer* **2014**, *14*, 598–610. [CrossRef]
45. Dunn, K.B.; Heffler, M.; Golubovskaya, V.M. Evolving therapies and FAK inhibitors for the treatment of cancer. *Anticancer Agents Med. Chem.* **2010**, *10*, 722–734. [CrossRef] [PubMed]
46. Buschman, M.D.; Bromann, P.A.; Cejudo-Martin, P.; Wen, F.; Pass, I.; Courtneidge, S.A. The novel adaptor protein Tks4 (SH3PXD2B) is required for functional podosome formation. *Mol. Biol. Cell* **2009**, *20*, 1302–1311. [CrossRef] [PubMed]
47. Kudlik, G.; Takacs, T.; Radnai, L.; Kurilla, A.; Szeder, B.; Koprivanacz, K.; Merő, B.L.; Buday, L.; Vas, V. Advances in Understanding TKS4 and TKS5: Molecular Scaffolds Regulating Cellular Processes from Podosome and Invadopodium Formation to Differentiation and Tissue Homeostasis. *Int. J. Mol. Sci.* **2020**, *21*, 8117. [CrossRef]
48. Seals, D.F.; Azucena, E.F.; Pass, I., Jr.; Tesfay, L.; Gordon, R.; Woodrow, M.; Courtneidge, S.A. The adaptor protein Tks5/Fish is required for podosome formation and function, and for the protease-driven invasion of cancer cells. *Cancer Cell* **2005**, *7*, 155–165. [CrossRef] [PubMed]
49. Zagryazhskaya-Masson, A.; Monteiro, P.; Mace, A.S.; Castagnino, A.; Ferrari, R.; Infante, E.; Chavrier, P. Intersection of TKS5 and FGD1/CDC42 signaling cascades directs the formation of invadopodia. *J. Cell. Biol.* **2020**, *219*, e201910132. [CrossRef] [PubMed]
50. Blouw, B.; Seals, D.F.; Pass, I.; Diaz, B.; Courtneidge, S.A. A role for the podosome/invadopodia scaffold protein Tks5 in tumor growth in vivo. *Eur. J. Cell Biol.* **2008**, *87*, 555–567. [CrossRef] [PubMed]
51. Iizuka, S.; Abdullah, C.; Buschman, M.D.; Diaz, B.; Courtneidge, S.A. The role of Tks adaptor proteins in invadopodia formation, growth and metastasis of melanoma. *Oncotarget* **2016**, *7*, 78473–78486. [CrossRef] [PubMed]
52. Leong, H.S.; Robertson, A.E.; Stoletov, K.; Leith, S.J.; Chin, C.A.; Chien, A.E.; Hague, M.N.; Ablack, A.; Carmine-Simmen, K.; McPherson, V.A.; et al. Invadopodia are required for cancer cell extravasation and are a therapeutic target for metastasis. *Cell Rep.* **2014**, *8*, 1558–1570. [CrossRef] [PubMed]
53. Yamaguchi, H.; Lorenz, M.; Kempiak, S.; Sarmiento, C.; Coniglio, S.; Symons, M.; Condeelis, J. Molecular mechanisms of invadopodium formation: The role of the N-WASP-Arp2/3 complex pathway and cofilin. *J. Cell Biol.* **2005**, *168*, 441–452. [CrossRef] [PubMed]
54. Yamaguchi, H.; Pixley, F.; Condeelis, J. Invadopodia and podosomes in tumor invasion. *Eur. J. Cell Biol.* **2006**, *85*, 213–218. [CrossRef] [PubMed]

55. Linder, S.; Wiesner, C.; Himmel, M. Degrading devices: Invadosomes in proteolytic cell invasion. *Annu. Rev. Cell Dev. Biol.* **2011**, *27*, 185–211. [CrossRef] [PubMed]
56. Oser, M.; Yamaguchi, H.; Mader, C.C.; Bravo-Cordero, J.J.; Arias, M.; Chen, X.; DesMarais, V.; van Rheenen, J.; Koleske, A.J.; Condeelis, J. Cortactin regulates cofilin and N-WASp activities to control the stages of invadopodium assembly and maturation. *J. Cell Biol.* **2009**, *186*, 571–587. [CrossRef] [PubMed]

viruses

MDPI

Article

Surveillance of Parrot Bornavirus in Taiwan Captive *Psittaciformes*

Brian Harvey Avanceña Villanueva [1], Jin-Yang Chen [2], Pei-Ju Lin [3,4], Hoang Minh [5], Van Phan Le [6], Yu-Chang Tyan [7,8,9,10,*], Jen-Pin Chuang [11,12,13,*] and Kuo-Pin Chuang [1,2,14,15,16,*]

1 International Degree Program in Animal Vaccine Technology, International College, National Pingtung University of Science and Technology, Pingtung 912, Taiwan; j11285355@mail.npust.edu.tw
2 Graduate Institute of Animal Vaccine Technology, College of Veterinary Medicine, National Pingtung University of Science and Technology, Pingtung 912, Taiwan
3 Livestock Disease Control Center of Chiayi County, Chiayi 612, Taiwan
4 Department of Veterinary Medicine, National Chiayi University, Chiayi 600, Taiwan
5 Department of Anatomy and Histology, Faculty of Veterinary Medicine, Vietnam National University of Agriculture, Hanoi 100000, Vietnam
6 Department of Microbiology and Infectious Diseases, Faculty of Veterinary Medicine, Vietnam National University of Agriculture, Hanoi 100000, Vietnam
7 Department of Medical Imaging and Radiological Sciences, Kaohsiung Medical University, Kaohsiung 807, Taiwan
8 Department of Medical Research, Kaohsiung Medical University Hospital, Kaohsiung 807, Taiwan
9 Center for Cancer Research, Kaohsiung Medical University, Kaohsiung 807, Taiwan
10 Center for Tropical Medicine and Infectious Disease Research, Kaohsiung Medical University, Kaohsiung 807, Taiwan
11 Chiayi Hospital, Ministry of Health and Welfare, Chiayi 600, Taiwan
12 Department of Surgery, Faculty of Medicine, College of Medicine, National Cheng Kung University, Tainan 701, Taiwan
13 Department of Surgery, National Cheng Kung University Hospital, Tainan 704, Taiwan
14 School of Medicine, Kaohsiung Medical University, Kaohsiung 807, Taiwan
15 School of Dentistry, Kaohsiung Medical University, Kaohsiung 807, Taiwan
16 Companion Animal Research Center, National Pingtung University of Science and Technology, Pingtung 912, Taiwan
* Correspondence: yctyan@kmu.edu.tw (Y.-C.T.); chuangjp@gmail.com (J.-P.C.); kpchuang@mail.npust.edu.tw (K.-P.C.)

check for updates

Citation: Villanueva, B.H.A.; Chen, J.-Y.; Lin, P.-J.; Minh, H.; Le, V.P.; Tyan, Y.-C.; Chuang, J.-P.; Chuang, K.-P. Surveillance of Parrot Bornavirus in Taiwan Captive *Psittaciformes*. *Viruses* **2024**, *16*, 805. https://doi.org/10.3390/v16050805

Academic Editor: Feng Li

Received: 23 April 2024
Revised: 10 May 2024
Accepted: 15 May 2024
Published: 18 May 2024

Correction Statement: This article has been republished with a minor change. The change does not affect the scientific content of the article and further details are available within the backmatter of the website version of this article.

Abstract: Parrot bornavirus (PaBV) is an infectious disease linked with proventricular dilatation disease (PDD) with severe digestive and neurological symptoms affecting psittacine birds. Despite its detection in 2008, PaBV prevalence in Taiwan remains unexplored. Taiwan is one of the leading psittacine bird breeders; hence, understanding the distribution of PaBV aids preventive measures in controlling spread, early disease recognition, epidemiology, and transmission dynamics. Here, we aimed to detect the prevalence rate of PaBV and assess its genetic variation in Taiwan. Among 124 psittacine birds tested, fifty-seven were PaBV-positive, a prevalence rate of 45.97%. Most of the PaBV infections were adult psittacine birds, with five birds surviving the infection, resulting in a low survival rate (8.77%). A year of parrot bornavirus surveillance presented a seasonal pattern, with peak PaBV infection rates occurring in the spring season (68%) and the least in the summer season (25%), indicating the occurrence of PaBV infections linked to seasonal factors. Histopathology reveals severe meningoencephalitis in the cerebellum and dilated cardiomyopathy of the heart in psittacine birds who suffered from PDD. Three brain samples underwent X/P gene sequencing, revealing PaBV-2 and PaBV-4 viral genotypes through phylogenetic analyses. This underscores the necessity for ongoing PaBV surveillance and further investigation into its pathophysiology and transmission routes.

Keywords: parrot bornavirus; proventricular dilatation diseases; prevalence rate; infectious disease

1. Introduction

Parrot bornaviruses (PaBV), namely parrot bornaviruses 1 to 8, are from the family of *Bornaviridae*, and the genus of *Orthobornavirus* has two viral species: *Orthobornavirus alphapsittaciforme* and *Orthobornavirus betapsittaciforme* [1]. *Orthobornavirus alphapsittaciforme* has six genotypes, which are PaBV-1 to -4, -7, and -8, while *Orthobornavirus betapsittaciforme* has two genotypes, PaBV-5 and -6 [1]. Although PaBV-1 to -8 are known in psittacine/parrot birds (order Psittaciformes), other avian bornaviruses host specific orders of birds. Canary bornaviruses 1 to 3 (CnBV-1 to CnBV-3) and munia bornavirus 1 (MuBV-1) belong to *Orthobornavirus serini* and estrildid finch bornavirus 1 (EsBV-1) belongs to *Orthobornavirus estrildidae* for passerine birds (order Passeriformes). In aquatic birds (orders Anseriformes and Charadriiformes), aquatic bornaviruses 1 and 2 (ABBV-1 and ABBV-2) are viral species of *Orthobornavirus avisaquaticae* [1]. Aside from avian host species, orthobornaviruses of mammalian and reptilian species were also reported. Orthobornaviruses of mammals such as Borna disease viruses 1 and 2 (BoDV-1 and -2) are viral species of *Orthobornavirus bornaense,* and variegated squirrel bornavirus 1 (VSBV-1) is a viral species of *Orthobornavirus sciuri*. Lastly, orthobornaviruses in snakes such as Caribbean watersnake bornavirus (CWBV) and Mexican black-tailed rattlesnake bornavirus (MRBV) are viral species of *Orthobornavirus caenophidiae* and Loveridge's garter snake virus 1 (LGSV-1) is a viral species of *Orthobornavirus elapsoideae* [1]. Recently, a new avian bornavirus was reported, barn owl bornavirus 1 (BoBV-1), with 83% viral sequence similarity with CnBV-2 and being detected in a barn owl (*Tyto* alba), suggesting a wider host range of *Orthobornavirus serini* [2]. Another report detected that avian bornaviruses in rgw Himalayan monal (*Lophophorus impedance*) and white-bellied caique (*Pionites leucogaster*) housed outside with eight other parrots (*Amazona* spp. and *Cacatua* spp.) have 100% matrix gene similarity with PaBV-4 [3]. Further surveillance, prevalence, and sequence reports on avian bornavirus are beneficial in further classifying and understanding their host range.

Parrot bornavirus is the causative agent of proventricular dilatation disease (PDD), and infection leads to a chronic neurological and digestive disorder in psittacine birds. PaBV presence has been reported in Brazil [4–6]; Germany [7–11]; France and Spain [9]; Portugal [12]; the Netherlands [8]; Sweden [13]; Austria, Switzerland, Hungary, and Australia [14]; the United States [15–18]; Canada [19,20]; South Africa [21]; the Czech Republic and Slovakia [22]; Qatar [23]; Israel [18]; Malaysia [24]; Thailand [25]; China [26]; South Korea [27]; and Japan [28,29]. The detection rates of PaBV vary significantly among these countries. Viral RNA detection through RT-qPCR has become the standard due to its low contamination risk and high sensitivity and specificity, while feces samples have been the most available for PaBV detection [1,30]. Currently, no studies have been available regarding the detection of PaBV infection cases in Taiwan.

In Taiwan, psittacine birds are the main pet birds and the majority of psittacine bird owners have more than one psittacine bird. Taiwan is also one of the leading exporters of parrots in global trade and has the largest number of naturalized or breeding psittacine birds [31,32]. With the great population of psittacine birds and the global lead in breeding, it is essential to understand the presence of infectious-disease-causing agents such as PaBV. This will provide insight into initial evidence of the potential risk that PaBV carries, especially in Taiwan's psittacine birds.

In Taiwan, there has been scarce available information regarding PaBV infection cases. Moreover, due to the high economic value of psittacine birds which are favored as companion pets in Taiwan, it is essential to further investigate the infectious virus, thus highlighting the importance of PaBV investigation. Hence, the presence and surveillance of PaBV across Taiwan are of significant importance in PaBV investigations and prevention. In this study, we screened one hundred twenty-four feces of captive psittacine birds collected for a year to report the prevalence rate of PaBV infection cases in Taiwan. Likewise, the sequencing of the PaBV X/P gene from a brain sample revealed the genotypes present in Taiwan. Furthermore, histopathology and radiograph images provide some insight into the nature of the proventriculus, cerebellum, and heart due to PaBV infection. This study underscores the critical need for ongoing surveillance and investigation into PaBV infection cases in Taiwan, particularly given the economic significance and popularity of psittacine birds as companion pets. By understanding the prevalence rates, genotypes, and pathological effects of PaBV, we can better inform prevention strategies and safeguard both psittacine birds of Taiwan.

2. Materials and Methods

2.1. Sample Collection

One hundred twenty-four psittacine feces samples used in this study were freshly collected by the veterinarian at Xing Yu Animal Hospital, Linyuan District, Kaohsiung City, Taiwan, or directly from the private psittacine owner's or breeder's house where the psittacine bird is housed and following the permission of the psittacine owners. For psittacine birds housed together, they were separated first and fresh feces were collected immediately after dropping. Clinal organs such as the brain, lung, pancreas, stomach, intestine, liver, eye, kidney, heart, muscle, and proventriculus from three psittacine birds that suffered from PaBV were donated for necropsy and RT-qPCR detection in different organ tissue. All the samples were placed in an ice bath right after collection and stored in a −80 °C Ultra-Low-Temperature Freezer (MDF-DU302VX-PA, TwinGuard, PHCBI, Gunma, Japan). The collection and sample handling guidelines were followed and approved by NPUST-IACUC. The sample collection started in June of 2022 and lasted until May 2023. Several psittacine birds with severe clinical symptoms of proventricular dilation disease (PDD) were screened through X-ray scans (E7239X, Rotanode^{TM}, Toshiba, Otawara, Japan) for their proventriculus size. Feces or clinical organ samples were prepared as 20% homogenates with 1x Phosphate-Buffered Solution (PBS), incubated for 30 min, and centrifuged (Centrisart A-14C, Sartorius, Göttingen, Germany) for 12,000× *g* for 15 min at 4 °C, and then the clarified supernatants were collected for RNA extraction and the excess was stored at −80 °C.

The 124 collected feces samples were as follows: 2 were from Taipei City (2/124; 1.61%), 2 were from Taoyuan City (2/124; 1.61%), 9 were from Taichung City (9/124; 7.26%), 1 was from Changhua County (1/124; 0.81%), 3 were from Yunlin County (3/124; 2.42%), 1 was from Nantou County (1/124; 0.81%), 7 were from Chiayi City (7/124; 5.65%), 3 was from Chiayi County (3/124; 2.42%), 16 were from Tainan City (16/124; 12.9%), 48 were from Kaohsiung City (48/124; 38.71%), and 32 were from Pingtung County (32/124; 25.81%). Altogether, the species of psittacine birds sampled were as follows: 2 *Agapornis* sp. (2/124; 1.61%), 1 *Agapornis pullarius* (1/124; 0.81%), 2 *Amazona aestiva* (2/124; 1.61%), 9 *Amazona ochrocephala* (9/124; 7.26%), 2 *Ara severus* (2/124; 1.61%), 3 *Ara auricollis* (3/124; 2.42%), 2 *Cacatua alba* (2/124; 1.61%), 3 *Cacatua ducorpsii* (3/124; 2.42%), 3 *Cacatua ophthalmica* (3/124; 2.42%), 1 *Cacatua moluccensis* (1/124; 0.81%), 10 *Diopsittaca nobilis* (10/124; 8.06%), 11 *Aratinga solstitialis* (11/124; 8.87%), 7 *Eclectus roratus* (7/124; 5.65%), 1 *Eolophus roseicapillus* (1/124; 0.81%), 1 *Ara ararauna* (1/124; 0.81%), 4 *Melopsittacus undulatus* (4/124; 3.23%), 7 *Myiopsitta monachus* (7/124; 5.65%), 16 *Nymphicus hollandicus* (16/124; 12.9%), 4 *Pionites leucogaster* (4/124; 3.23%), 2 *Pionus maximiliani* (2/124; 1.61%), 1 *Poicephalus gulielmi* (1/124; 0.81%), 5 *Psittacula krameri* (5/124; 4.03%), 26 *Psittacus erithacus* (26/124; 20.97%), and 1 *Pyrrhura molinae* (1/124; 0.81%).

2.2. Detection of Parrot Bornavirus

2.2.1. RNA Extraction

The RNA was extracted from the supernatant samples of 1XPBS homogenized feces of 124 psittacine birds following the manufacturer's instructions of R.T.U REzol^{TM} C&T (Protech, Taipei, Taiwan, KP200CT) with slight modification. An amount of 500 µL of the feces supernatant was mixed with 500 µL of REzol^{TM} C&T in 1.5 mL sterile microcentrifuge tubes (JetBiofil, Guangzhou, China, CFT100015), shaken vigorously for 15 s, and incubated for 5 min, and then 100 µL of chloroform was added, shaken for 15 s, incubated for 2 min, and centrifuged for 12,000× *g* for 15 min at 4 °C. A 500 µL colorless upper aqueous phase was collected and transferred in a new microcentrifuge tube, added with 500 μL of isopropanol (Honeywell Burdick & Jackson, Ulsan, Republic of Korea, AH323-4) with gentle mixing, incubated for 10 min, and centrifuged for 12, 000× *g* for 10 min at 4 °C, and isopropanol supernatant was discarded. The RNA precipitate pellets were washed with 1 mL of 75% ethanol (Echo, Miaoli, Taiwan) by vortex-mixing for 2 s and centrifuged for 5 min at 12,000× *g* for 4 °C, ethanol supernatant was discarded, and RNA pellets were air-dried for 15 min or more if required. Dried RNA pellets were dissolved in 50 μL of UltraPure DEPC (Protech, Taipei, Taiwan, PT-P560-500) and quantified using NanoDrop2000 Spectrophotometer (Thermo Fisher Scientific, Wilmington, DE, USA).

2.2.2. Reverse Transcription–Quantitative Polymerase Chain Reaction

The 124 freshly collected feces samples were extracted for RNA immediately and tested for PaBV through RT-qPCR. Clinical organ samples such as the brain, kidney, eyes, stomach, lung, intestine, liver, pancreas, and heart from three psittacine birds donated to our lab were also subjected to RT-qPCR. The RT-qPCR detection for parrot bornavirus (PaBV) was performed in a StepOne™ Real-Time PCR System Thermal Cycling Block (Applied Biosystems, Thermo Fisher Scientific, Marsiling, Singapore) using the qPCRBIO Probe 1-Step Go Hi-ROX kit (PCR Biosystems, London, UK, PB25.42) following the manufacturer's instructions with slight modification. Each reaction contained 5 μL of 2x qPCRBIO Probe 1-Step Go Mix, 0.4 μL of reverse and forward primers each with concentrations of 10 μM, 0.2 μL of the probe at 10 μM concentration, 1.5 μL of UltraPure DEPC water (Protech, Taipei, Taiwan, PT-P560-500), and 2.5 μL of RNA extracted from feces samples in a total reaction volume of 10 μL. The thermal cycle was as follows: 45 °C for 10 min for reverse transcription, 95 °C for 2 min for polymerase activation, and 40 cycles of 95 °C for 5 s and 60 °C for 30 s for denaturation and annealing/extension. The primers and the probe (Genomics BioSci & Tech, New Taipei City, Taiwan) used for RT-qPCR detection were as follows: for the forward primer, BornaPCA3 (5′-GATCCGCAGACAGYACGT-3′) was used; for the reverse primer; BornaPCA6 (5′-GAGATCATGGANGGRTTCTT-3′) was used; and for the probe, BornaP_Fam (5′-FAM-CGAATWCCCAGGGAGGCYCT-BHQ1-3′) was used, specific for PaBV-1, PaBV-2, PaBV-4, and PaBV-7 detection with a product size of 125 bp [30].

2.2.3. Gel Electrophoresis

The RT-qPCR products underwent gel electrophoresis to further confirm the detection of parrot bornavirus. An amount of 1.5 g of Biotechnology Grade Agarose I (VWR Chemicals, Solon, OH, USA, 97062-250) was dissolved in 100 mL of 0.5x Tris-borate-EDTA (TBE) solution, microwave-heated (RE-0711, Sampo, Taoyuan, Taiwan) for 2 min, shaken for 10 s, microwaved-heated for 2 min, shaken for 10 s, added with 5 μL of EtB"Out" Nucleic Acid Staining Solution 2.0 (Yeastern Biotech, Taipei City, Taiwan, FYD007-200P), shaken for 10 s to mix, and placed in a mold to solidify for 15 min. A Mupid®-2plus Submarine Electrophoresis System (Advance, Tokyo, Japan) was used for gel electrophoresis with a run time of 5 min for half voltage followed by 25 min for full voltage with 0.5x TBE running buffer, enough to submerge and cover the gel. The RT-qPCR products were added with 1 μL of 6x DNA Loading Dye (GeneMarkbiolab, Taichung, Taiwan, DL02), and 100 bp of DNA Ladder (Bio-Van, New Taipei City, Taiwan, M0100) was used. The gel band was viewed through a UV Transilluminator (MUV21-312, Major Science, Taoyuan City, Taiwan) compound with UV Imager (CI-01, Major Science, Taoyuan City, Taiwan), visualized with Major Science 1D Analysis software version 1.0 at 24x integration, and the gel band image was captured using a mono camera (MTV-12V6HE-R, Mintron, New Taipei City, Taiwan) with an 8.5–51 mm F1.2 lens (SSL85051M, Avenir Lens, Seiko, Tokyo, Japan).

2.3. Histopathological Examination

Donated clinical cerebellum and heart samples of deceased psittacine birds due to proventriculus dilatation disease were fixed with 10% phosphate buffer formalin solution and embedded in paraffin. A hematoxylin–eosin (H&E) stain was used for every 5 µm thick tissue sample. The samples were observed under a light microscope (Eclipse E200, Nikon, Shonan, Japan), and images were obtained using a Nikon DS-L2 camera (Nikon, Shonan, Japan).

2.4. Transmission Electron Microscope

1x PBS-homogenized brain samples were centrifuged for 10 min at 4000× *g* at 4 °C followed by 12,000× *g* at 4 °C for 30 min. The supernatant was passed through a 0.22 µm Millex®-GV filter (Merck Millipore, Carrigtwohill, Ireland, PR05099). Then, the virus was concentrated through polyethylene glycol 6000 (Alfa Aesar, Karlsruhe, Germany, 10212393) with 10% w/v, centrifuged at 3500× *g* for 5 min, and then 1.45 g of NaCl (Showa Chemical, Tokyo, Japan, KGE-343A) at 1 M was added for every 20 mL of virus supernatant. It was incubated overnight with shaking at 4 °C. Afterwards, it was centrifuged in 10,000× *g* for 30 min, the supernatant was discarded, and pellets were dissolved with 1x PBS. The virus solution was allowed to settle in a formvar/carbon 200-mesh copper grid (Ted Pella, Redding, CA, USA, 01800-F) for 30 s and coated with 2% aqueous uranyl acetate solution (Spi-Chem, Structure Probe, West Chester, PA, USA, 02624-AB) for 45 s. Excess stain was removed and the specimen was examined using an H-7500 transmission electron microscope (Hitachi, Tokyo, Japan).

2.5. PCR Amplification of the X/P Region and Sequencing

Following the manufacturer's instruction, RNA-extracted residue from three PaBV-positive donated brain samples was converted to cDNA using the qScript® cDNA Synthesis Kit (Quantabio, Hilden, Germany, 95047). PaBV X/P region primer (forward: 5′-CTCAATGGCACGGCCCTC-3′ and reverse: 5′-GGCCATCCAGGAACAATTACC-3′) was designed through NCBI Primer-BLAST using PaBV sequences with accession ID NC_039189.1, NC_028106.1, FJ620690.1, EU781967.1, NC_030688.1, JX065209.1, GU249596.2, and NC_030689.1. The P Fast-Pfu 2X PCR SuperMix (AllBio, Taichung, Taiwan, ABTGMBP03-100) produced X/P amplicons following the manufacturer's instructions. Each reaction has 1 µL of forward and reverse primer at 10 µM concentrations, 25 µL of P Fast-Pfu 2X PCR SuperMix, 18 µL of UltraPure DEPC water (Protech, Taipei, Taiwan, PT-P560-500), and 5 µL of cDNA in a total reaction of 50 µL. A Blue-Ray Biotech Turbo Cycler (Blue-Ray Biotech, Taipei City, Taiwan) was used for the PCR with thermal cycling conditions of 94 °C for 5 min as the initial denaturation, followed by 40 cycles of 94 °C for 30 s, 60 °C for 30 s, 72 °C for 1 min, and a final extension at 72 °C for 10 min. The PCR amplicon product size was 682 pb, amplicons were run in 1.5% agarose gel electrophoresis, and the band was sliced with a 200 mg weight and then sent to Genomics BioSci & Tech, New Taipei City, Taiwan, for sequencing. X/P amplicons were sequenced through the Sanger sequencing approach (Genomics BioSci & Tech, New Taipei City, Taiwan).

2.6. Phylogenetic Analysis

Alignments of X/P gene sequences were performed using the MUSCLE algorithm at 1000 bootstrap replicates of MEGA 11.0.13 software. Using available *Orthobornavirus* sequences, phylogenetic analyses were performed through the maximum likelihood algorithm and GTR + I model at 1000 bootstrap replicates.

3. Results

One hundred twenty-four (124) fecal samples were tested for PaBV, of which 2 were from Taipei City, 2 were from Taoyuan City, 9 were from Taichung City, 1 was from Changhua County, 3 were from Yunlin County, 1 was from Nantou County, 7 were from Chiayi City, 3 was from Chiayi County, 16 were from Tainan City, 48 were from Kaohsiung City, and 32 were from Pingtung County (Figure 1). Altogether, the feces-sampled psittacine birds were privately owned or breeding birds and were mostly contained in their appropriate cages. Not long after testing positive with PaBV RT-qPCR detection, the birds passed away (around 1 week–2 months). Most PaBV-positive birds were observed with digestive symptoms (loss of appetite, weight loss, emaciation, undigested seeds shedding in feces, diarrhea, proventriculus dilation, and delayed crop emptying) and neurological symptoms (incoordination, seizure, tremor, lameness, and retinitis).

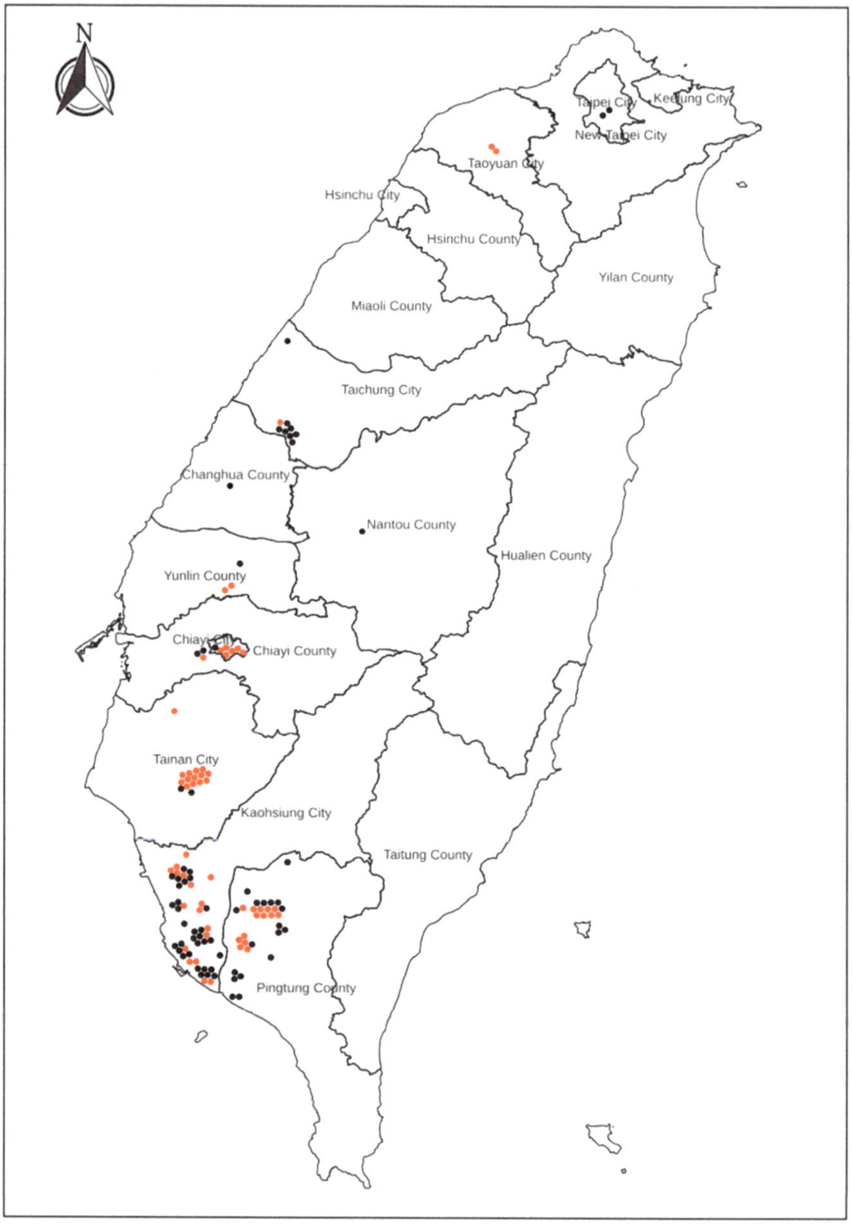

Figure 1. The map shows the geographical location of PaBV-positive (red dots) and PaBV-negative (black dots) psittacine birds in Taiwan; map was sourced from the National Land Surveying and Mapping Center (NLSC).

A total of 124 psittacine birds were subjected to PaBV detection, and 57 (57/124; 45.97%) were positive for PaBV. The C_T values ranged from 19.93 to 31.81. PaBV-positive cases were as follows: 2 from Taoyuan City (2/2; 100%), 1 from Taichung City (1/9; 11.11%), 2 from Yunlin County (2/3; 66.67%), 6 from Chiayi City (6/7; 85.71%), 1 from Chiayi County (1/1; 100%), 14 from Tainan City (14/16; 87.5%), 17 from Kaohsiung City (17/48; 35.42%), and 14 from Pingtung County (14/32; 43.75%) (Figure 1). Only five out of the fifty-seven PaBV-positive birds (5/57; 8.77%) survived PaBV infection, with observed proventricular dilatation, of which there were 2 from Tainan, 1 from Kaohsiung, and 2 from Pingtung, suggesting a high fatality rate (52/57; 91.23%) and mortality rate (52/124; 41.94%). Sample collection started from June of 2022 to May of 2023. The highest PaBV-positive rate was observed in April of 2023 (21/25; 84%) followed by October of 2022 and February of 2023 (2/3; 66.67% and 5/7; 71.4%), while zero positive cases were observed in January of 2023 (Figure 2). During the summer season (June to August), there were 25% (8/32) PaBV-positive cases, with 32% (8/25) during the fall season (September to November) and 41% (7/17) during the winter season (December to February), and an increasing trend was observed up to 68% (34/50) in the spring season (March to May). Most psittacine birds were companion birds, spending most of their time indoors or housed outdoors. These findings underscore the significant impact of PaBV infection on psittacine birds, highlighting the importance of continued monitoring and preventive measures to mitigate the high fatality and mortality rates associated with the disease.

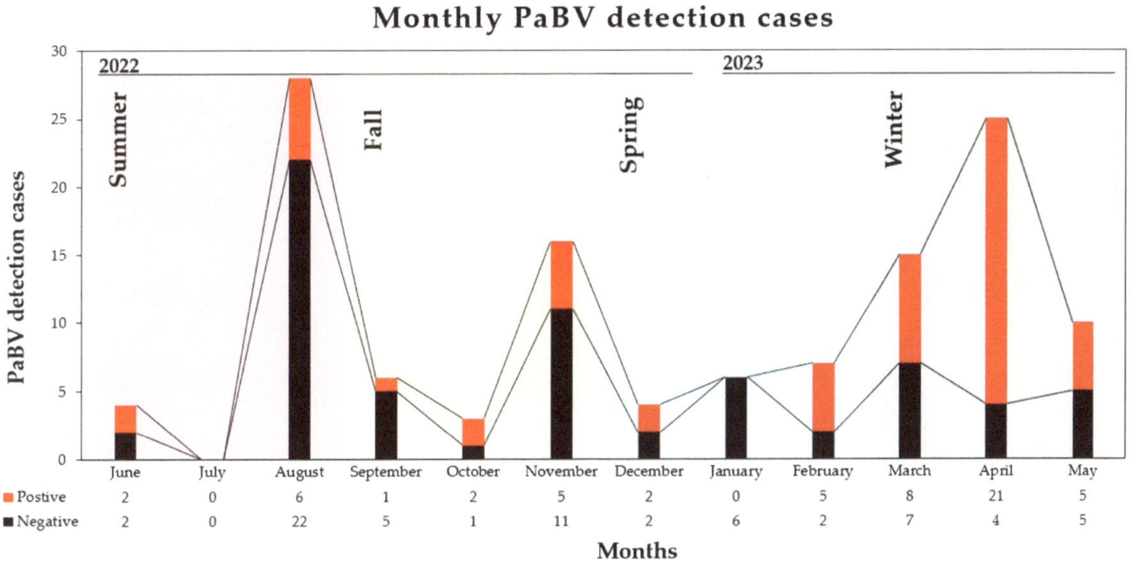

Figure 2. PaBV detection cases per month (June 2022 to May 2023); PaBV-positive case are in red while PaBV-negative cases are in black.

PaBV-infection cases were found to be highest with *Psittacus erithacus* psittacine bird species (11/57; 19%) followed by *Nymphicus hollandicus* (8/57; 14%) and *Aratinga solstitialis* (8/57; 14%) (Table 1). The rest of the PaBV-positive rates per psittacine species were as follows: 7% (4/57) for each species of *Myiopsitta monachus*, *Diopsittaca nobilis*, and *Amazona ochrocephala*; 4% (2/57) for each species of *Cacatua ophthalmica*, *Eclectus roratus*, *Ara severus*, *Pionites leucogaster*, *Amazona aestiva*, *Agapornis* sp., and *Psittacula krameri*; and 2% (1/57) for each species of *Poicephalus gulielmi*, *Pyrrhura molinae*, *Melopsittacus undulatus*, and *Cacatua moluccensis*.

Table 1. List of PaBV-positive rates in different psittacine species.

Psittacine Species of PaBV-Positive	Count	Rate
Psittacus erithacus	11	19%
Nymphicus hollandicus and *Aratinga solstitialis*	8	14%
Diopsittaca nobilis, *Myiopsitta monachus*, and *Amazona ochrocephala*	4	7%
Cacatua ophthalmica, *Eclectus roratus*, *Ara severus*, *Pionites leucogaster*, *Amazona aestiva*, *Agapornis* sp., and *Psittacula krameri*	2	4%
Poicephalus gulielmi, *Pyrrhura molinae*, *Melopsittacus undulatus*, and *Cacatua moluccensis*	1	2%

The ambiguity surrounding the age and sex of the psittacine birds often reflects on their adoption, mostly without prior information. Most of the PDD-suffering birds were adults, 1 year old and up. Based on thirty-one (31) identified sexes of the psittacine birds, 64.52% (20/31) were male and 35.48% (11/31) were female (Table 2). Mutual symptoms were weight loss, crop stasis, maldigestion, and proventriculus dilation followed by depression and regurgitation. Seizure was only observed in one identified male bird (case no. 2302013), while both ataxia and tremor were observed in 25% (5/20) of the males, and for females, and 18.18% (2/11) ataxia and 45.45% (5/11) tremor symptoms were observed.

Table 2. Summary of information for PaBV-positive cases. C_T values were obtained from feces samples.

Case Number	Bird Species	Location	Age	Sex	C_T	Symptoms
2206003	*Myiopsitta monachus*	Renwu, Kaohsiung	1 y	-	27.47	a b c d e
2208002+	*Amazona ochrocephala*	Changjhih, Pingtung	3.5 y	Female	27.83	a b d e
2208008+	*Amazona ochrocephala*	Changjhih, Pingtung	3.5 y	Male	24.54	a b d e
2208023	*Diopsittaca nobilis*	Changjhih, Pingtung	2 y	-	23.99	a b c d e
22080061+	*Cacatua ophthalmic*	Yongkang, Tainan	1 y	-	28.43	a b d e
22080071	*Cacatua ophthalmica*	Yongkang, Tainan	1 y	-	27.30	a b d e h
22080091	*Diopsittaca nobilis*	Changjhih, Pingtung	2 y	-	27.26	a b c d e h
2208013+	*Psittacus erithacus*	Renwu, Kaohsiung	4 y	Male	27.38	a b c d
2209009	*Pionites leucogaster*	Taibao, Chiayi	-	-	27.54	a b d e
2210003	*Nymphicus hollandicus*	Yongkang, Tainan	3 y	Male	26.81	a b c d e
2210004	*Eclectus roratus*	Linyuan, Kaohsiung	-	Male	27.89	a b d e
22110011	*Amazona ochrocephala*	Changjhih, Pingtung	3.5 y	Male	26.43	a b d e
22110012	*Ara severus*	Changjhih, Pingtung	1.5 y	Male	27.48	a b d e
22110013	*Ara severus*	Changjhih, Pingtung	1.5 y	Female	29.00	a b d e
22110014	*Amazona ochrocephala*	Changjhih, Pingtung	3.5 y	Female	27.40	a b d e
2301024	*Nymphicus hollandicus*	Gangshan, Kaohsiung	4 y	Female	26.36	a b c d e h
2212037	*Poicephalus gulielmi*	Alian, Kaohsiung	-	-	29.34	a b c d e
2212064	*Pyrrhura molinae*	Dapi, Yunlin	-	-	30.29	a b c d e
2302010	*Diopsittaca nobilis*	Pingtung, Pingtung	-	Female	23.47	a b c d e
2302013+	*Psittacus erithacus*	Yongkang, Tainan	5 y	Male	27.88	a b d e f g
2302017	*Psittacus erithacus*	Yongkang, Tainan	3 y	Female	27.66	a b c d e h
2302025	*Nymphicus hollandicus*	Gangshan, Kaohsiung	1 y	Female	28.25	a b c d e
2302026	*Nymphicus hollandicus*	Gangshan, Kaohsiung	1 y	Male	28.48	a b c d e h

Table 2. *Cont.*

Case Number	Bird Species	Location	Age	Sex	C_T	Symptoms
2303007	*Psittacus erithacus*	Yongkang, Tainan	3 y	Male	27.68	a b c d e
2303008	*Melopsittacus undulatus*	Chiayi, Chiayi	-	Female	28.31	a b c d e
2303013	*Agapornis* sp.	Gangshan, Kaohsiung	-	Male	29.30	a b d e g h
2303014	*Agapornis* sp.	Gangshan, Kaohsiung	-	Male	28.97	a b d e
2303017	*Eclectus roratus*	Linyuan, Kaohsiung	-	Male	24.34	a b c d e
2303019	*Psittacus erithacus*	Fengshan, Kaohsiung	3 y	Female	27.66	a b c d e h
2303023	*Nymphicus hollandicus*	Nanzi, Kaohsiung	-	Male	29.80	a b c d e
2303030	*Psittacula krameri*	Taoyuan, Taoyuan	-	Male	25.13	a b d e
2304002	*Nymphicus hollandicus*	Fengshan, Kaohsiung	-	-	22.80	a b c d e
2304003	*Psittacus erithacus*	Yongkang, Tainan	4 y	Male	31.32	a b d e
2304004011	*Myiopsitta monachus*	Xiaogang, Kaohsiung	-	-	24.91	a b c d e
2304004021	*Myiopsitta monachus*	Xiaogang, Kaohsiung	-	-	19.93	a b c d e
2304005	*Myiopsitta monachus*	Wantan, Pingtung	-	-	26.25	a b d e
2304006	*Aratinga solstitialis*	Wantan, Pingtung	-	-	23.51	a b d e
2304007	*Diopsittaca nobilis*	Taoyuan, Taoyuan	-	Male	28.68	a b c d e
2304008	*Psittacus erithacus*	Yanchao, Kaohsiung	-	Female	27.76	a b c d e g h
2304015	*Psittacula krameri*	Yongkang, Tainan	-	-	28.30	a b d e
2304018	*Pionites leucogaster*	Yongkang, Tainan	-	-	28.93	a b d e
2304019	*Aratinga solstitialis*	Yongkang, Tainan	-	-	29.78	a b d e
2304020	*Amazona aestiva*	Yongkang, Tainan	-	-	30.05	a b d e
2304021	*Aratinga solstitialis*	Yongkang, Tainan	-	-	30.15	a b d e
2304022	*Amazona aestiva*	Yongkang, Tainan	-	-	28.79	a b c d e
2304025	*Nymphicus hollandicus*	Wujih, Taichung	-	-	29.32	a b c d e
2304026	*Nymphicus hollandicus*	Qianzhen, Kaohsiung	-	-	29.49	a b c d e
2304028	*Aratinga solstitialis*	Chiayi, Chiayi	-	-	28.46	a b d e g h
2304029	*Aratinga solstitialis*	Chiayi, Chiayi	-	-	28.87	a b d e
2304030	*Aratinga solstitialis*	Chiayi, Chiayi	3 y	Male	28.94	a b d e
2304031	*Aratinga solstitialis*	Chiayi, Chiayi	-	-	31.15	a b d e
2304032	*Aratinga solstitialis*	Chiayi, Chiayi	-	-	30.16	a b d e
23050071	*Psittacus erithacus*	Wantan, Pingtung	-	Male	30.40	a b c d e g h
23050081	*Psittacus erithacus*	Wantan, Pingtung	-	Male	31.81	a b c d e g h
2305009	*Psittacus erithacus*	Wantan, Pingtung	-	Male	27.25	a b c d e g h
2305025	*Psittacus erithacus*	Dapi, Yunlin	-	Female	28.92	a b c d e g h
2305026	*Cacatua moluccensis*	Yanshui, Tainan	-	-	28.57	a b c d e g h

(-) The information is unknown. Symptoms: weight loss (a), crop stasis (b), regurgitation (c), maldigestion (d), depression (e), seizure (f), ataxia (g), and tremors (h). (+) The bird successfully recovered from the infection.

Additionally, psittacine birds with obvious and severe PDD clinical symptoms were subjected to X-ray scans to screen digestive organs, specifically proventriculus dilatation, observed in Figure 3A, while Figure 3B displays a proventriculus of a healthy psittacine bird. The proventriculus diameter could determine the short-term survival of psittacine birds with gastric implications. The normal range of the proventricular diameter-to-dorsoventral keel height ratio score was 0.200–0.476 [33,34], among the PDD-suffering birds a range from the proventricular diameter-to-dorsoventral keel height recorded exceeded the normal range, from 0.681–0.981 implying their poor survival.

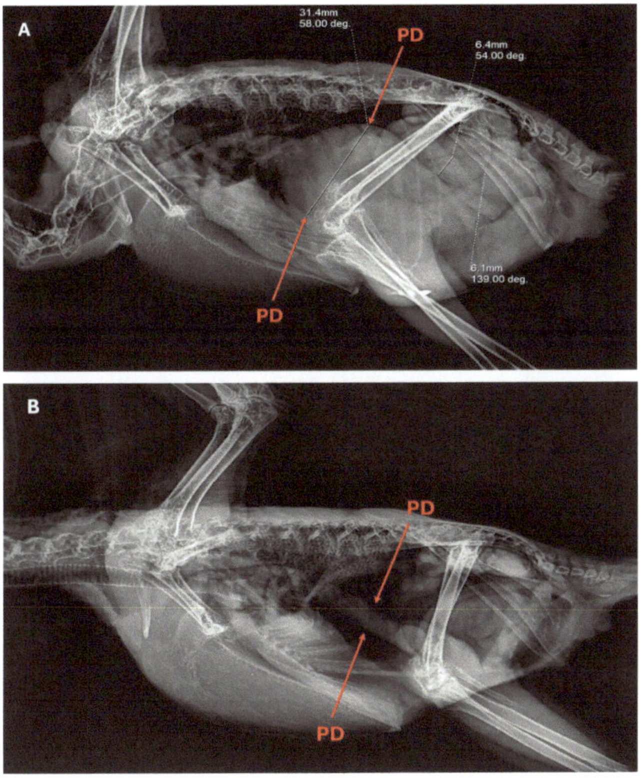

Figure 3. (**A**) X-ray scan of a proventriculus dilation (PD), 31.4 mm, and intestine, 6.4 mm and 6.1 mm; and (**B**) a normal proventriculus. Two radiographic images clearly illustrate the difference in the proventriculus diameter of a PDD-suffering psittacine bird compared to a healthy psittacine bird.

The elevated presence of lymphocytes in the cerebellum as shown in Figure 4A uncovers that PaBV-positive birds had a severe and diffused meningoencephalitis in contrast with a PaBV-negative cerebellum of a psittacine bird in Figure 4B. In Figure 4C, the psittacine bird suffered from PDD/AGN and PaBV-positive birds demonstrate dilated cardiomyopathy in the heart and extensive degeneration to necrosis of the myocardium. A transmission electron image of the PaBV is observed in Figure 5A, where the size ranges from 82.9 nm to 113 nm. Parrot bornaviruses are membrane viruses that allow them to enlarge or contract in size. The shedding of undigested seeds and diarrhea symptoms in feces were observed among PDD-suffering psittacine birds as a clinical symptom of gastric implications or digestive disorder (Figure 5B). At the same time, physiological symptoms such as tilting of the head, twitching of the eyes, and loss of balance were observed (Figure 5C,F). The twitching of the eyes and the rousing of the feathers indicate the discomfort of the bird (Figure 5C). Typical loss of balance is due to ataxia or loss of muscle, limiting the bird from grabbing and climbing. A 125 bp RT-qPCR product for PaBV detection was further confirmed in gel electrophoresis for gel band viewing. Figure 5D displays the gel band image for the lung, intestine, brain, eye, proventriculus, stomach, heart, kidney, liver, pancreas, muscle, and feces samples. Likewise, a clinical symptom of proventriculus dilation causing thinning of the gastrointestinal wall with undigested seeds was observed in Figure 5E of a PaBV-positive bird after suffering from PDD. The proventriculus measured about 6 cm in length over one-third to the overall length of the bird (about 18 cm) and had a 0.915 proventricular diameter-to-dorsoventral keel height ratio, exceeding the normal range for the proventricular diameter-to-dorsoventral keel height score. The diverse clinical manifestations observed in PaBV-positive psittacine birds, ranging from severe meningoencephalitis to gastrointestinal complications, underscore the multifaceted nature of the disease and the need for comprehensive veterinary care and management strategies.

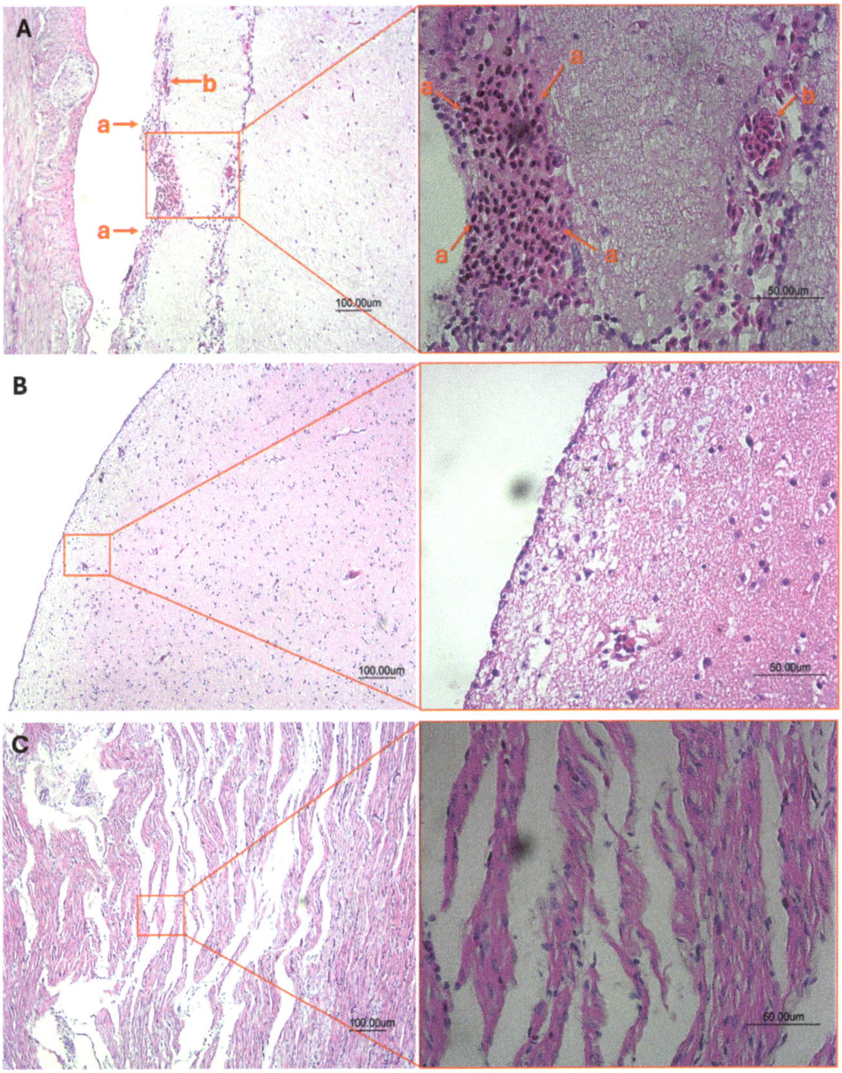

Figure 4. (**A**) Histopathological image at 10× and 40× magnification of the cerebellum with severe and diffuse lymphocytes indicating severe meningoencephalitis of PaBV-infected psittacine bird suffering from PDD/AGN (a: lymphocytes and b: red blood cells), and (**B**) histopathological image of the cerebellum of psittacine birds negative to PaBV infection or any signs of digestive or neurological disorders. (**C**) Histopathological image at 10× and 40× magnification of the heart from a PaBV-positive psittacine bird suffering from PDD/AGN with extensive degeneration to necrosis of the myocardium and dilated cardiomyopathy can be observed.

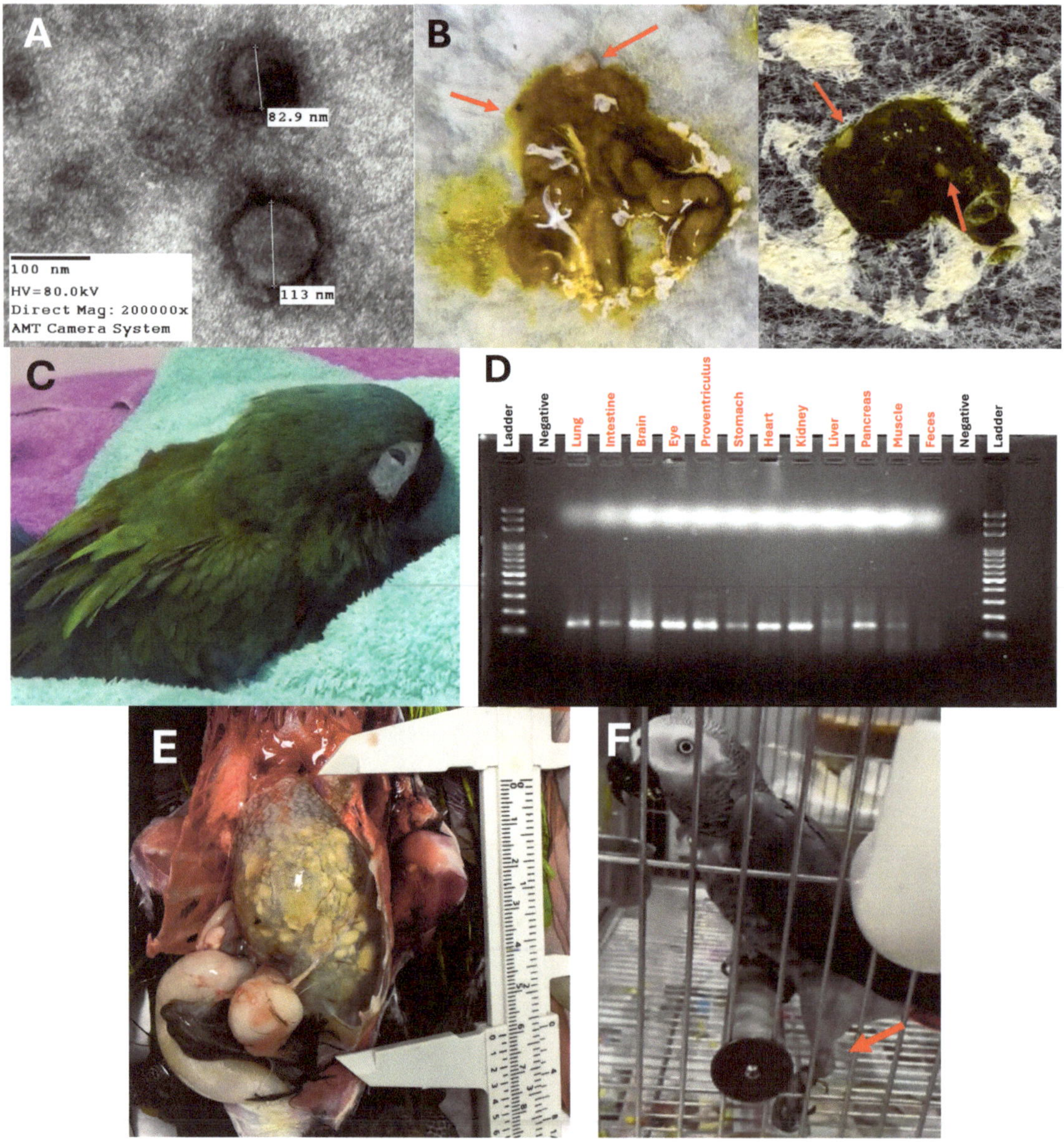

Figure 5. (**A**) Transmission electron microscopy image of the PaBV at 200,000× magnification, with a diameter of 82.9 nm and 113 nm. (**B**) Feces droppings with shedding of undigested seeds (red arrow). (**C**) Red-shouldered macaw (*Diopsittaca nobilis*) suffering from proventriculus dilation and showing neurological signs; discomfort can be seen in the twitching of the eyes. (**D**) Gel band image of the RT-qPCR product, 125 bp, for PaBV detection in lung, intestine, brain, eye, proventriculus, stomach, heart, kidney, liver, pancreas, muscle, and feces samples from case number 2301024. (**E**) Dilated proventriculus with a thin wall containing undigested seeds, about 6 cm in length, of a red-shouldered macaw (*Diopsittaca nobilis*) enduring proventriculus dilatation disease. (**F**) Photo of an African grey parrot (*Psittacus erithacus*) unable to balance right before it fell due to loss of control of the left leg (red arrow).

For further analysis, the three brain samples (Bird cases 2208023, 2301024, and 2302010) were amplified for their X/P gene with 682 bp in length. Prior to X/P gene amplifications, the brain samples were tested for PaBV through RT-qPCR with C_T values of 18.59, 12.49, and 5.15 (Table 3 and Figure 5D). The organs were collected several days after the decease of the psittacine birds affecting viral RNA load and C_T values in different organs. The brain has consistently low C_T values reflecting high viral load and a much more suitable source for PCR amplification of the X/P gene. Therefore, it was selected for X/P gene amplification.

Table 3. Summary of the C_T values in different organs for PaBV detection.

Case No.	Genotype	Brain	Lung	Pancreas	Stomach	Intestine	Liver	Eye	Kidney	Heart	Muscle	Proven.
2208023	PaBV-4	18.59	23.3	23.38	23.98	24.29	27.98	-	-	-	-	-
2301024	PaBV-2	12.94	24.35	25.3	26.43	25.76	29.17	18.52	21.6	24.15	29.24	20.22
2302010	PaBV-4	5.15	6.09	7.88	4.27	7.57	7.75	4.94	4.4	25.97	-	-

(-) The information is unknown as the organ is not tested or the organ is unavailable.

NCBI BLASTn search provided the homology analysis, which revealed that two of the Taiwan strains (NPUSTIAVT-PaBV/Brain-2208023 and NPUSTIAVT-PaBV/Brain-2302010) were PaBV-4, with both originating from Changzhi, Pingtung, and isolated from *Diopsittaca nobilis* (red-shouldered macaw), and one (NPUSTIAVT-PaBV/Brain-2301024) PaBV-2 was isolated from *Nymphicus hollandicus* (cockatiel) in Kangshan, Kaohsiung. The sequences were submitted and deposited in GenBank with accession numbers PP529446-PP529448.

The Taiwan strain PaBV-2 X/P gene (PP529446.1: NPUSTIAVT-PaBV/Brain-2301024) has 99.41% sequence similarity with the Germany strain PaBV-2 X/P gene (KU748803.1: L55595) from a *Psittacus erithacus* (African grey parrot). The two Taiwan strain PaBV-4 X/P genes, NPUSTIAVT-PaBV/Brain-2208023 (PP529447.1) and NPUSTIAVT-PaBV/Brain-2302010 (PP529448.1), have 95.89% sequence similarity with each other, with 85.51% and 84.77% sequence similarity with the Taiwan strain PaBV-2 X/P gene. The Taiwan strain PaBV-4 X/P gene, NPUSTIAVT-PaBV/Brain-2208023 (PP529447.1), has 99.71% sequence similarity with the Japan strain (LC486412.1: AR18A) isolated from the brain of an *Ara ararauna* (blue-and-yellow macaw), Germany strains (MK291400.1: L62637) from a *Psittacula cyanocephala* (plum-headed parakeet), (MK291396.1: DR-15) *Cacatua galerita* (sulfur-crested cockatoo), (KU748815.1: TiHo-154) *Ara glaucogularis* (blue-throated macaw), (KU748814.1: TiHo-40) *Ara chloroptera* (red-and-green macaw), Spain strain (MK291399.1: G-18720) from a *Psittacula alexandri* (red-breasted parakeet), and South Korea strains (MZ310179.1: CBNU_PaBV_04 and MZ310182.1: CBNU_PaBV_07) from an *Amazona ochrocephala* (yellow-crowned amazon). Lastly, the Taiwan strain PaBV-4 X/P gene, NPUSTIAVT-PaBV/Brain-2302010 (PP529448.1), has a 99.85% sequence similarity with Germany strain (KU748811.1: L63115) from an *Ara macao* (scarlet macaw).

A phylogenetic tree was applied, using our sequenced X/P gene and all the available X/P gene sequences (682 nucleotides) of *Orthobornavirus alphapsittaciformes*, *Orthobornavirus betapsittaciformes*, and other genotypes of *Orthobornavirus*, with one representative per species isolates in each country. The analysis conclusively shows that our X/P gene sequence, Taiwan strain NPUSTIAVT-PaBV/Brain-2301024, belongs to the PaBV-2 genotype, and Taiwan strains NPUSTIAVT-PaBV/Brain-2302010 and NPUSTIAVT-PaBV/Brain-2208023 belong to the PaBV-4 genotype (Figure 6).

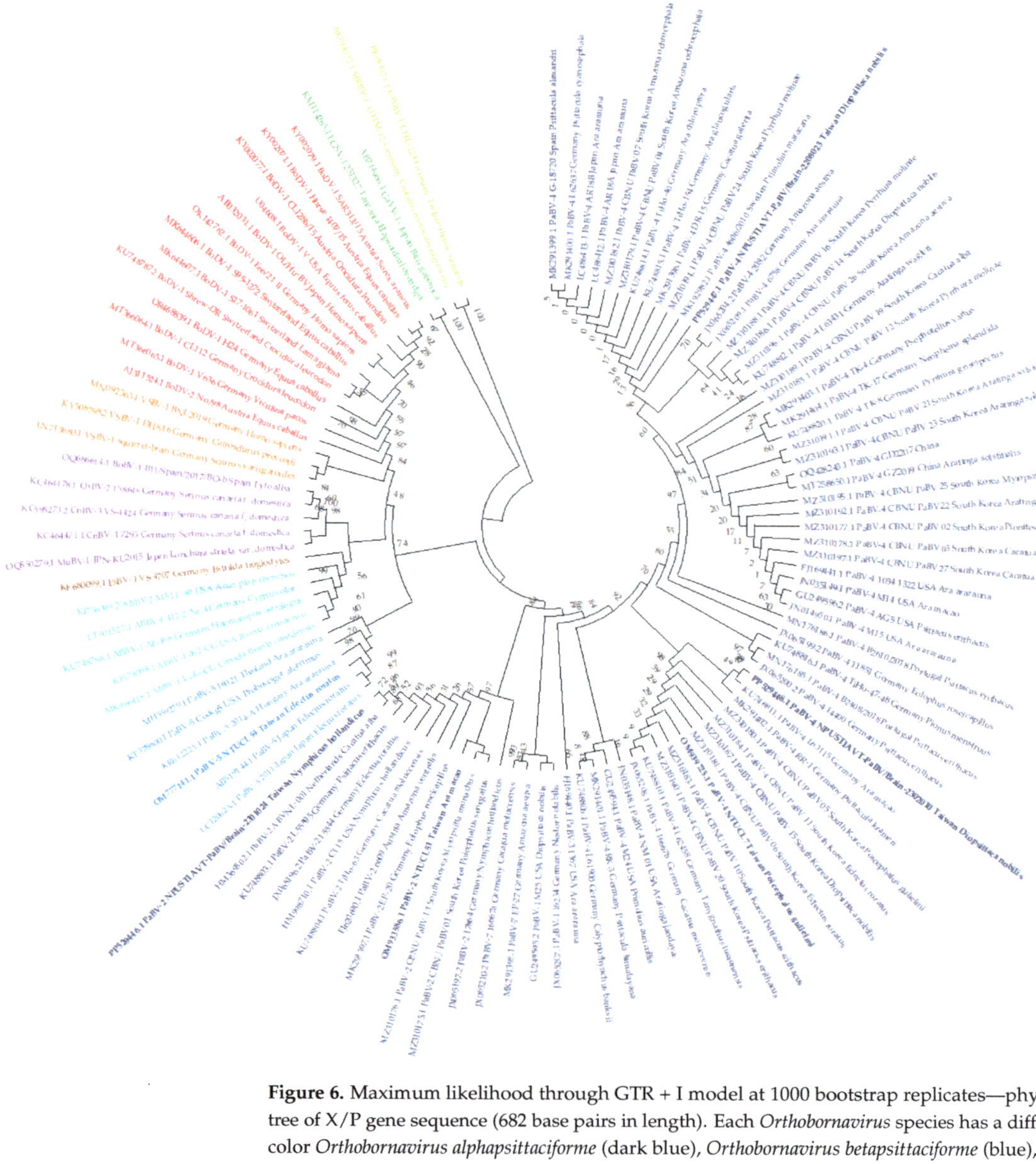

Figure 6. Maximum likelihood through GTR + I model at 1000 bootstrap replicates—phylogenetic tree of X/P gene sequence (682 base pairs in length). Each *Orthobornavirus* species has a different font color *Orthobornavirus alphapsittaciforme* (dark blue), *Orthobornavirus betapsittaciforme* (blue), *Orthobornavirus serini* (purple), *Orthobornavirus estrildidae* (brown), *Orthobornavirus avisaquaticae* (light blue), *Orthobornavirus bornaense* (red), *Orthobornavirus sciuri* (orange), *Orthobornavirus caenophidiae* (light green), and *Orthobornavirus elapsoideae* (dark green). The Taiwan strain X/P genes are highlighted in bold.

4. Discussion

Since the first report of avian bornaviruses in 2008, there has been an increase in the number of countries reporting the presence of PaBV, a novel infectious viral agent causing proventricular dilatation disease affecting psittacine birds [1,11,14,16–19,21,35–41]. In Taiwan, the presence of PaBV has been known through the submitted sequences of the matrix protein (M) gene (MK736729.1-MK736782.1), nucleoprotein (N) gene (MK770085.1-

MK770118.1), and PaBV-2 (OM933586.1), PaBV-4 (OM939725.1), and PaBV-5 (OM777141.1) complete genome in GenBank [42]. To further elucidate the PaBV presence in Taiwan, we screened feces samples from 124 psittacine birds collected for a year (June 2022 to May 2023), and demonstrated that 57 were PaBV-positive, with a prevalence of 45.97% and a low survival rate of 8.77%. Feces samples were collected freshly and tested for RT-qPCR immediately to secure the presence of PaBV in the feces and reduce false negative results. The majority of the tested feces were collected in a local animal hospital where the psittacine owners brought them for either regular health evaluation or veterinary care concerns due to diarrhea or loss of appetite. This may influence the prevalence rate determined in this study, which may require further surveillance of parrot bornavirus in Taiwan.

In the detection of PaBV through RT-qPCR assay, $C_T < 21$ is strongly positive [30]; however, viral RNA present in the feces samples were observed to have a higher C_T, carried out with the impurities in feces samples [11]. In the RT-qPCR detection, C_Ts higher than 21 were also observed as a possible outcome [20,30]. Gel electrophoresis of the RT-qPCR product may be suitable in securing and further confirming detection results to reduce false-negative or -positive results. Tissue samples such as the proventriculus, kidney, colon, cerebrum, and cerebellum have the most viral RNA, much more suitable for RT-qPCR detection [20]. However, viral RNA extraction and PCR detection should be performed promptly to minimize false results due to the unstable nature of the virus as single-strand negative-sense RNA. Delays can lead to degradation of the RNA, potentially yielding inaccurate results. Due to the sampling limitations, it is crucial to conduct further surveillance studies of PaBV in Taiwan. This would help in understanding the transmission dynamics and potential impact of PaBV on parrot populations, especially in Taiwan. Enhanced surveillance can provide valuable insights for disease management and prevention strategies, safeguarding both companion and wildlife psittacine birds.

Young psittacine birds are the most vulnerable to PaBV infection or PDD [43,44]; however, they may have no clinical signs but are the probable source of seroconversion and PaBV-RNA shedding [45]. In most cases, psittacine birds are housed together with other birds. Viral transmission sources to housed birds may come from newly introduced young bird/s in the enclosure, a potential carrier of PaBV. Then, PaBV shedding in the enclosure infects adult birds and possibly introduces the PaBV to the brood or clutch [44,46]. Adult psittacine birds appeared to have more clinical symptoms [43] and sex appeared to have no significant influence on PaBV infection. The age and sex of psittacine birds are often unknown to owners since most were adopted without any preexisting information. Moreover, among the tested PaBV-positive psittacine birds in Taiwan, it was more common in *Psittacus erithacus* or the African grey parrots (19%). Similar PaBV host species cases were reported in the United States, Japan, South Korea, China, Portugal, Thailand, Germany, Canada, Austria, Hungary, Switzerland, and Israel [10,12,14,25–28].

PDD affects the overall digestive health of the psittacine bird such as body weight, crop emptying, and seed digestion, alongside neurological problems such as severe meningoencephalitis [27,43,47]. Proventriculus dilation displayed thinning of the gastrointestinal wall and a build-up of undigested seeds that may cause pain and discomfort to psittacine birds, leading to a loss of appetite and further causing malnutrition, weight loss, depression, loss of balance, and tremors. Through radiograph scans, the proventricular diameter-to-dorsoventral keel height is determined, from 0.681 to 0.981, indicating the poor survival of the psittacine birds. The highly enlarged proventriculus and thinning wall are clinical signs of neurogenic atrophy. Histopathology of the cerebellum in deceased psittacine birds due to PaBV infection elucidates severe diffuse meningoencephalitis due to accumulated lymphocytes. The PaBV infection could cause PDD due to gastrointestinal crisis; however, neurological damage was more likely to appear in PaBV infection. Recently, it has become more appropriate to address this neurological crisis as avian ganglioneuritis (AGN) [48,49]. Probable mechanisms of PaBV leading to PDD/AGN were attributed to CD8+ T-cells, causing injury to neurons and ganglia recruiting CD4 T-cells, facilitating the antibody-mediated phagocytosis of axons [48]. This leads to persistent damage in the nervous system, suggesting an autoimmune response to gangliosides [48]. Histopathology of the heart showed a dilated cardiomyopathy or myocardium. This highlights the etiological implications of PaBV in neurological disorders other than PDD [38].

The spring season (68%) has the highest cases of PaBV infection while the summer season (28%) has the least, which might suggest that PaBV has a cycle transmission with regard to the season. Low PaBV infection during the summer season could be due to dry air, while the fall season could potentially allow the spread of PaBV in the environment, most probably due to dry feces particles in the air or fecal–oronasal route [11], viral trace contamination of waters, and residues of PaBV that are already present in the surroundings [1]. An increase in moisture or humidity during the winter season could contribute to viral persistence, spread, and incubation leading to contamination in feeds or drinking water, resulting in high cases of PaBV in the spring season and permitting a continuous incubation life cycle of PaBV [1]. The presence of PaBV in the environment and horizontal transmission to companion psittacine birds is still a challenge to understand [8]. Potential viral reservoirs such as wild free-ranging psittacine birds or other potential host carriers have not been fully illustrated, similar to PaBV host species which are most prevalent, and surveillance reports were carried out in captive, breeding, or companion psittacine birds [1,2,4–29,39,42,44,50,51]. In Taiwan, all psittacine birds were introduced, mostly kept as captive, companion, or breeding birds. Certainly, preventive measures targeting both horizontal and vertical transmission are vital for successfully managing PaBV infection cases [8,17,44,46,52,53], particularly in Taiwan.

Furthermore, our X/P gene sequences confirmed the presence of PaBV-2 and PaBV-4 genotypes in Taiwan strains. The two identified PaBV-4 X/P genes have 95.89% similarity from each other. Among our sequenced X/P genes, Germany strains were found to be consistently similar to our sequences. Taiwan strain NTUCL7 PaBV-4 has 95.89% sequence similarity with NPUSTIAVT-PaBV/Brain-2208023 and 99.7% sequence similarity with NPUSTIAVT-PaBV/Brain-2302010, while Taiwan strain NTUCL51 PaBV-2 has 97.80% sequence similarity with NPUSTIAVT-PaBV/Brain-2301024. Recently, phylogeographic analysis revealed that the South American ancestor could be the origin of PaBV-1, -2, and -8 genotypes [42]. This highlights the importance of further surveillance of *Orthobornavirus* for captive *Psittaciformes*, similar to Taiwan.

Moreover, avian bornavirus, specifically parrot bornavirus, causes severe neurological and digestive disorders or death in infected birds [14,16,36,54], a threat to psittacine birds of Taiwan. Additionally, it could disrupt local ecosystems affecting unique and vulnerable bird species and have economic implications for industries reliant on bird populations, such as agriculture, bird breeding farms, and tourism.

The findings of this study highlight the importance of the ongoing monitoring of Parrot bornavirus in Taiwan's psittacine populations to monitor new strains or potential recombinants, as demonstrated in a recent report [2].

Author Contributions: Conceptualization, K.-P.C. and B.H.A.V.; methodology, B.H.A.V.; validation, B.H.A.V., J.-Y.C., K.-P.C., P.-J.L., Y.-C.T., J.-P.C., H.M., and V.P.L.; formal analysis, B.H.A.V.; investigation, B.H.A.V., K.-P.C., and J.-Y.C.; resources, K.-P.C., B.H.A.V., and J.-Y.C.; data curation, B.H.A.V. and J.-Y.C.; writing—original draft preparation, B.H.A.V. and K.-P.C.; writing—review and editing, B.H.A.V., J.-Y.C., K.-P.C., J.-P.C., Y.-C.T., P.-J.L., H.M., and V.P.L. visualization, B.H.A.V.; supervision, K.-P.C.; funding acquisition, K.-P.C. All authors have read and agreed to the published version of the manuscript.

Funding: This research was funded by the Joint Research Program of the National Pingtung University of Science and Technology and Kaohsiung Medical University serial numbers NPUST-KMU-113-P004 and KMU-TC112B01, from Kaohsiung Medical University.

Institutional Review Board Statement: The animal handling, guidelines, and study protocols followed the National Pingtung University of Science and Technology—Institutional Animal Care and Use Committee (NPUST-IACUC) guidelines, with approval numbers NPUST-111-082 and NPUST-112-183.

Informed Consent Statement: Not applicable.

Data Availability Statement: All data generated and analyzed in this study are included in this article. PaBV X/P gene nucleotide sequences were deposited in GenBank with accession numbers PP529446-PP529448.

Acknowledgments: The authors thank Benji Brayan Ilagan Silva and Ching-Yi Tsai for their assistance and guidance. We are grateful for the Precision Instruments Center of the National Pingtung University of Science and Technology in which the Transmission Electron Microscope was performed. We thank Xing Yu Animal Hospital, Kaohsiung, Taiwan, where sample collection and X-ray scans were performed. We thank the Kaohsiung Medical University and the National Pingtung University of Science and Technology for their financial support on this project, KMU-TC112B01 and NPUST-KMU-113-P004.

Conflicts of Interest: The authors declare no conflicts of interest. The funders had no role in the design of the study; in the collection, analyses, or interpretation of data; in the writing of the manuscript; or in the decision to publish the results.

References

1. Rubbenstroth, D. Avian Bornavirus Research—A Comprehensive Review. *Viruses* **2022**, *14*, 1513. [CrossRef] [PubMed]
2. Aguilera-Sepúlveda, P.; Llorente, F.; Rosenstierne, M.W.; Bravo-Barriga, D.; Frontera, E.; Fomsgaard, A.; Fernández-Pinero, J.; Jiménez-Clavero, M. Detection of a New Avian Bornavirus in Barn Owl (*Tyto alba*) by Pan-Viral Microarray. *Veter. Microbiol.* **2024**, *289*, 109959. [CrossRef] [PubMed]
3. Bourque, L.; Laniesse, D.; Beaufrère, H.; Pastor, A.; Ojkic, D.; Smith, D.A. Identification of Avian Bornavirus in a Himalayan Monal (*Lophophorus impejanus*) with Neurological Disease. *Avian Pathol.* **2015**, *44*, 323–327. [CrossRef] [PubMed]
4. Encinas-Nagel, N.; Enderlein, D.; Piepenbring, A.; Herden, C.; Heffels-Redmann, U.; Felippe, P.A.; Arns, C.; Hafez, H.M.; Lierz, M. Avian Bornavirus in Free-Ranging Psittacine Birds, Brazil. *Emerg. Infect. Dis.* **2014**, *20*, 2103–2106. [CrossRef] [PubMed]
5. Philadelpho, N.A.; Rubbenstroth, D.; Guimarães, M.B.; Ferreira, A.J.P. Survey of Bornaviruses in Pet Psittacines in Brazil Reveals a Novel Parrot Bornavirus. *Veter. Microbiol.* **2014**, *174*, 584–590. [CrossRef] [PubMed]
6. Silva, A.S.G.; Raso, T.F.; Costa, E.A.; Gómez, S.Y.M.; Martins, N.R.d.S. Parrot Bornavirus in Naturally Infected Brazilian Captive Parrots: Challenges in Viral Spread Control. *PLoS ONE* **2020**, *15*, e0232342. [CrossRef] [PubMed]
7. Rubbenstroth, D.; Rinder, M.; Kaspers, B.; Staeheli, P. Efficient Isolation of Avian Bornaviruses (ABV) from Naturally Infected Psittacine Birds and Identification of a New ABV Genotype from a Salmon-Crested Cockatoo (*Cacatua moluccensis*). *Veter. Microbiol.* **2012**, *161*, 36–42. [CrossRef] [PubMed]
8. Rubbenstroth, D.; Schmidt, V.; Rinder, M.; Legler, M.; Twietmeyer, S.; Schwemmer, P.; Corman, V.M. Phylogenetic Analysis Supports Horizontal Transmission as a Driving Force of the Spread of Avian Bornaviruses. *PLoS ONE* **2016**, *11*, e0160936. [CrossRef] [PubMed]
9. Kessler, S.; Heenemann, K.; Krause, T.; Twietmeyer, S.; Fuchs, J.; Lierz, M.; Corman, V.M.; Vahlenkamp, T.M.; Rubbenstroth, D. Monitoring of Free-Ranging and Captive *Psittacula* Populations in Western Europe for Avian Bornaviruses, Circoviruses and Polyomaviruses. *Avian Pathol.* **2020**, *49*, 119–130. [CrossRef]
10. Lierz, M.; Hafez, H.M.; Honkavuori, K.S.; Gruber, A.D.; Olias, P.; Abdelwhab, E.M.; Kohls, A.; Lipkin, W.I.; Briese, T.; Hauck, R. Anatomical Distribution of Avian Bornavirus in Parrots, Its Occurrence in Clinically Healthy Birds and ABV-Antibody Detection. *Avian Pathol.* **2009**, *38*, 491–496. [CrossRef]
11. Rinder, M.; Ackermann, A.; Kempf, H.; Kaspers, B.; Korbel, R.; Staeheli, P. Broad Tissue and Cell Tropism of Avian Bornavirus in Parrots with Proventricular Dilatation Disease. *J. Virol.* **2009**, *83*, 5401–5407. [CrossRef] [PubMed]
12. Pinto, M.C.; Craveiro, H.; Wensman, J.J.; Carvalheira, J.; Berg, M.; Thompson, G. Bornaviruses in Naturally Infected *Psittacus erithacus* in Portugal: Insights of Molecular Epidemiology and Ecology. *Infect. Ecol. Epidemiol.* **2019**, *9*, 1685632. [CrossRef]
13. Pinto, M.C.; Rondahl, V.; Berg, M.; Ågren, E.; Carvalheira, J.; Thompson, G.; Wensman, J.J. Detection and Phylogenetic Analysis of Parrot Bornavirus 4 Identified from a Swedish Blue-Winged Macaw (*Primolius maracana*) with Unusual Nonsuppurative Myositis. *Infect. Ecol. Epidemiol.* **2019**, *9*, 1547097. [CrossRef] [PubMed]
14. Weissenböck, H.; Bakonyi, T.; Sekulin, K.; Ehrensperger, F.; Doneley, R.J.; Dürrwald, R.; Hoop, R.; Erdélyi, K.; Gál, J.; Kolodziejek, J.; et al. Avian Bornaviruses in Psittacine Birds from Europe and Australia with Proventricular Dilatation Disease. *Emerg. Infect. Dis.* **2009**, *15*, 1453–1459. [CrossRef] [PubMed]
15. Murray, O.; Turner, D.; Streeter, K.; Guo, J.; Shivaprasad, H.; Payne, S.; Tizard, I. Apparent Resolution of Parrot Bornavirus Infection in Cockatiels (*Nymphicus hollandicus*). *Veter. Med. Res. Rep.* **2017**, *8*, 31–36. [CrossRef] [PubMed]
16. Gray, P.; Hoppes, S.; Suchodolski, P.; Mirhosseini, N.; Payne, S.; Villanueva, I.; Shivaprasad, H.; Honkavuori, K.S.; Briese, T.; Reddy, S.M.; et al. Use of Avian Bornavirus Isolates to Induce Proventricular Dilatation Disease in Conures. *Emerg. Infect. Dis.* **2010**, *16*, 473–479. [CrossRef]

17. Kistler, A.L.; Smith, J.M.; Greninger, A.L.; DeRisi, J.L.; Ganem, D. Analysis of Naturally Occurring Avian Bornavirus Infection and Transmission during an Outbreak of Proventricular Dilatation Disease among Captive Psittacine Birds. *J. Virol.* **2010**, *84*, 2176–2179. [CrossRef] [PubMed]
18. Kistler, A.L.; Gancz, A.; Clubb, S.; Skewes-Cox, P.; Fischer, K.; Sorber, K.; Chiu, C.Y.; Lublin, A.; Mechani, S.; Farnoushi, Y.; et al. Recovery of Divergent Avian Bornaviruses from Cases of Proventricular Dilatation Disease: Identification of a Candidate Etiologic Agent. *Virol. J.* **2008**, *5*, 88. [CrossRef]
19. Raghav, R.; Taylor, M.; DeLay, J.; Ojkic, D.; Pearl, D.L.; Kistler, A.L.; DeRisi, J.L.; Ganem, D.; Smith, D.A. Avian Bornavirus is Present in Many Tissues of Psittacine Birds with Histopathologic Evidence of Proventricular Dilatation Disease. *J. Veter. Diagn. Investig.* **2010**, *22*, 495–508. [CrossRef]
20. Delnatte, P.; Mak, M.; Ojkic, D.; Raghav, R.; DeLay, J.; Smith, D.A. Detection of Avian Bornavirus in Multiple Tissues of Infected Psittacine Birds Using Real-Time Reverse Transcription Polymerase Chain Reaction. *J. Veter. Diagn. Investig.* **2014**, *26*, 266–271. [CrossRef]
21. Last, R.D.; Weissenböck, H.; Nedorost, N.; Shivaprasad, H. Avian Bornavirus Genotype 4 Recovered from Naturally Infected Psittacine Birds with Proventricular Dilatation Disease in South Africa. *J. South Afr. Veter. Assoc.* **2012**, *83*, 4. [CrossRef] [PubMed]
22. Vondráčková, M.; Tukač, V.; Grymová, V.; Hájková, P.; Knotek, Z.; Dorrestein, G.M. Detection of Anti-Avian Bornavirus Antibodies in Parrots in the Czech Republic and Slovakia. *Acta Veter. Brno* **2014**, *83*, 195–199. [CrossRef]
23. Hammer, S.; Watson, R. The Challenge of Managing Spix Macaws (*Cyanopsitta spixii*) at Qatar—An Eleven-Year Retrospection. *Zool. Garten N.F* **2012**, *81*, 81–95. [CrossRef]
24. Lutpi, S.M.; Abu, J.; Arshad, S.S.; Rahaman, N.Y. Molecular Detection, Risk Factors and Public Awareness of Avian Bornavirus among Captive and Non-Captive Birds in Peninsular Malaysia. *J. Veter. Res.* **2022**, *66*, 523–535. [CrossRef] [PubMed]
25. Sa-Ardta, P.; Rinder, M.; Sanyathitiseree, P.; Weerakhun, S.; Lertwatcharasarakul, P.; Lorsunyaluck, B.; Schmitz, A.; Korbel, R. First Detection and Characterization of Psittaciform Bornaviruses in Naturally Infected and Diseased Birds in Thailand. *Veter. Microbiol.* **2019**, *230*, 62–71. [CrossRef] [PubMed]
26. Zhang, L.-N.; Huang, Y.-H.; Liu, H.; Li, L.-X.; Bai, X.; Yang, G.-D. Molecular Detection of Bornavirus in Parrots Imported to China in 2022. *BMC Veter. Res.* **2023**, *19*, 259. [CrossRef]
27. Hong, S.S.; Kim, S.; Seo, M.-K.; Han, M.-N.; Kim, J.; Lee, S.-M.; NA, K.-J. Genetic Trends in Parrot Bornavirus: A Clinical Analysis. *J. Veter. Med Sci.* **2024**, *86*, 239–246. [CrossRef]
28. Sassa, Y.; Bui, V.N.; Saitoh, K.; Watanabe, Y.; Koyama, S.; Endoh, D.; Horie, M.; Tomonaga, K.; Furuya, T.; Nagai, M.; et al. Parrot Bornavirus-2 and -4 RNA Detected in Wild Bird Samples in Japan are Phylogenetically Adjacent to Those Found in Pet Birds in Japan. *Virus Genes* **2015**, *51*, 234–243. [CrossRef]
29. Horie, M.; Ueda, K.; Ueda, A.; Honda, T.; Tomonaga, K. Detection of Avian bornavirus 5 RNA in Eclectus Roratus with Feather Picking Disorder. *Microbiol. Immunol.* **2012**, *56*, 346–349. [CrossRef]
30. Sigrist, B.; Geers, J.; Albini, S.; Rubbenstroth, D.; Wolfrum, N. A New Multiplex Real-Time RT-PCR for Simultaneous Detection and Differentiation of Avian Bornaviruses. *Viruses* **2021**, *13*, 1358. [CrossRef]
31. Chan, D.T.C.; Poon, E.S.K.; Wong, A.T.C.; Sin, S.Y.W. Global Trade in Parrots—Influential Factors of Trade and Implications for Conservation. *Glob. Ecol. Conserv.* **2021**, *30*, e01784. [CrossRef]
32. Preston, C.E.C.; Pruett-Jones, S. The Number and Distribution of Introduced and Naturalized Parrots. *Diversity* **2021**, *13*, 412. [CrossRef]
33. Dennison, S.E.; Paul-Murphy, J.R.; Adams, W.M. Radiographic Determination of Proventricular Diameter in Psittacine Birds. *J. Am. Vet. Med. Assoc.* **2008**, *232*, 709–714. [CrossRef] [PubMed]
34. Dennison, S.E.; Adams, W.M.; Johnson, P.J.; Yandell, B.S.; Paul-Murphy, J.R. Prognostic Accuracy of the Proventriculus: Keel Ratio for Short-Term Survival in Psittacines with Proventricular Disease. *Veter. Radiol. Ultrasound* **2009**, *50*, 483–486. [CrossRef] [PubMed]
35. Gancz, A.Y.; Kistler, A.L.; Greninger, A.L.; Farnoushi, Y.; Mechani, S.; Perl, S.; Berkowitz, A.; Perez, N.; Clubb, S.; DeRisi, J.L.; et al. Experimental Induction of Proventricular Dilatation Disease in Cockatiels (*Nymphicus hollandicus*) Inoculated with Brain Homogenates Containing Avian Bornavirus 4. *Virol. J.* **2009**, *6*, 100–111. [CrossRef] [PubMed]
36. Hoppes, S.M.; Tizard, I.; Shivaprasad, H.L. Avian Bornavirus and Proventricular Dilatation Disease: Diagnostics, Pathology, Prevalence, and Control. Veterinary Clinics of North America. *Exot. Anim. Pract.* **2013**, *16*, 339–355, Update on *Exot. Anim. Pract.* **2020**, *23*, 337–351.
37. Weissenböck, H.; Fragner, K.; Nedorost, N.; Mostegl, M.; Sekulin, K.; Maderner, A.; Bakonyi, T.; Nowotny, N. Localization of Avian Bornavirus RNA by In Situ Hybridization in Tissues of Psittacine Birds with Proventricular Dilatation Disease. *Veter. Microbiol.* **2010**, *145*, 9–16. [CrossRef] [PubMed]
38. Ouyang, N.; Storts, R.; Tian, Y.; Wigle, W.; Villanueva, I.; Mirhosseini, N.; Payne, S.; Gray, P.; Tizard, I. Histopathology and the Detection of Avian Bornavirus in the Nervous System Of Birds Diagnosed with Proventricular Dilatation Disease. *Avian Pathol.* **2009**, *38*, 393–401. [CrossRef]
39. Heffels-Redmann, U.; Enderlein, D.; Herzog, S.; Herden, C.; Piepenbring, A.; Neumann, D.; Müller, H.; Capelli, S.; Müller, H.; Oberhäuser, K.; et al. Occurrence of Avian Bornavirus Infection in Captive Psittacines in Various European Countries and Its Association with Proventricular Dilatation Disease. *Avian Pathol.* **2011**, *40*, 419–426. [CrossRef]

40. Wünschmann, A.; Honkavuori, K.; Briese, T.; Lipkin, W.I.; Shivers, J.; Armien, A.G. Antigen Tissue Distribution of Avian Bornavirus (ABV) in Psittacine Birds with Natural Spontaneous Proventricular Dilatation Disease and ABV Genotype 1 Infection. *J. Veter. Diagn. Investig.* **2011**, *23*, 716–726. [CrossRef]
41. Payne, S.; Shivaprasad, H.L.; Mirhosseini, N.; Gray, P.; Hoppes, S.; Weissenböck, H.; Tizard, I. Unusual and Severe Lesions of Proventricular Dilatation Disease in Cockatiels (*Nymphicus hollandicus*) Acting as Healthy Carriers of Avian Bornavirus (ABV) and Subsequently Infected with a Virulent Strain of ABV. *Avian Pathol.* **2011**, *40*, 15–22. [CrossRef] [PubMed]
42. Chacón, R.D.; Sánchez-Llatas, C.J.; Forero, A.J.D.; Guimarães, M.B.; Pajuelo, S.L.; Astolfi-Ferreira, C.S.; Ferreira, A.J.P. Evolutionary Analysis of a Parrot Bornavirus 2 Detected in a Sulphur-Crested Cockatoo (*Cacatua galerita*) Suggests a South American Ancestor. *Animals* **2024**, *14*, 47. [CrossRef]
43. Petzold, J.; Gartner, A.M.; Malberg, S.; Link, J.B.; Bücking, B.; Lierz, M.; Herden, C. Tissue Distribution of Parrot Bornavirus 4 (PaBV-4) in Experimentally Infected Young and Adult Cockatiels (*Nymphicus hollandicus*). *Viruses* **2022**, *14*, 2181. [CrossRef] [PubMed]
44. Link, J.; Herzog, S.; Gartner, A.M.; Bücking, B.; König, M.; Lierz, M. Factors Influencing Vertical Transmission of Psittacine Bornavirus in Cockatiels (*Nymphicus hollandicus*). *Viruses* **2022**, *14*, 2721. [CrossRef]
45. Gartner, A.M.; Link, J.; Bücking, B.; Enderlein, D.; Herzog, S.; Petzold, J.; Malberg, S.; Herden, C.; Lierz, M. Age-Dependent Development and Clinical Characteristics of an Experimental Parrot Bornavirus-4 (PaBV-4) Infection in Cockatiels (*Nymphicus hollandicus*). *Avian Pathol.* **2021**, *50*, 138–150. [CrossRef] [PubMed]
46. Delnatte, P.; Nagy, É.; Ojkic, D.; Crawshaw, G.; Smith, D.A. Investigation into the Possibility of Vertical Transmission of Avian Bornavirus in Free-Ranging Canada Geese (*Branta canadensis*). *Avian Pathol.* **2014**, *43*, 301–304. [CrossRef]
47. Jorge, K.; Loeber, S.; Hawkins, S.; Elsmo, E.; Mans, C. Computed Tomography Enterography of Jejunal Infarction in a Timneh African Grey Parrot (*Psittacus timneh*). *J. Exot. Pet Med.* **2022**, *41*, 62–66. [CrossRef]
48. Boatright-Horowitz, S.L. Avian Bornaviral Ganglioneuritis: Current Debates and Unanswered Questions. *Veter. Med. Int.* **2020**, *2020*, 6563723. [CrossRef] [PubMed]
49. Rossi, G.; Dahlhausen, R.D.; Galosi, L.; Orosz, S.E. Avian Ganglioneuritis in Clinical Practice. *Veter. Clin. N. Am. Exot. Anim. Pr.* **2018**, *21*, 33–67. [CrossRef]
50. de Kloet, A.H.; Kerski, A.; de Kloet, S.R. Diagnosis of Avian Bornavirus Infection in Psittaciformes by Serum Antibody Detection and Reverse Transcription Polymerase Chain Reaction Assay Using Feather Calami. *J. Veter. Diagn. Investig.* **2011**, *23*, 421–429. [CrossRef]
51. Chen, D.-S.; Wu, Y.-Q.; Zhang, W.; Jiang, S.-J.; Chen, S.-Z. Horizontal Gene Transfer Events Reshape the Global Landscape of Arm Race between Viruses and Homo Sapiens. *Sci. Rep.* **2016**, *6*, 26934. [CrossRef]
52. Rubbenstroth, D.; Brosinski, K.; Rinder, M.; Olbert, M.; Kaspers, B.; Korbel, R.; Staeheli, P. No Contact Transmission of Avian Bornavirus in Experimentally Infected Cockatiels (*Nymphicus hollandicus*) and Domestic Canaries (*Serinus canaria forma domestica*). *Veter. Microbiol.* **2014**, *172*, 146–156. [CrossRef]
53. Nielsen, A.M.W.; Ojkic, D.; Dutton, C.J.; Smith, D.A. Aquatic Bird Bornavirus 1 Infection in a Captive Emu (*Dromaius novaehollandiae*): Presumed Natural Transmission from Free-Ranging Wild Waterfowl. *Avian Pathol.* **2018**, *47*, 58–62. [CrossRef]
54. de Araujo, J.L.; Rech, R.R.; Heatley, J.J.; Guo, J.; Giaretta, P.R.; Tizard, I.; Rodrigues-Hoffmann, A. From Nerves to Brain to Gastrointestinal Tract: A Time-Based Study of Parrot Bornavirus 2 (PaBV-2) Pathogenesis in Cockatiels (*Nymphicus hollandicus*). *PLoS ONE* **2017**, *12*, e0187797. [CrossRef]

viruses

MDPI

Article

Host Immune Response Modulation in Avian Coronavirus Infection: Tracheal Transcriptome Profiling In Vitro and In Vivo

Kelsey O'Dowd [1], Ishara M. Isham [1], Safieh Vatandour [2], Martine Boulianne [3,4], Charles M. Dozois [3,5], Carl A. Gagnon [3,6], Neda Barjesteh [3,†] and Mohamed Faizal Abdul-Careem [1,*]

1. Health Research Innovation Centre, Faculty of Veterinary Medicine, University of Calgary, Calgary, AB T2N 4N1, Canada; kelsey.odowd@ucalgary.ca (K.O.); fathimaishara.muhamm@ucalgary.ca (I.M.I.)
2. Department of Animal and Poultry Science, Islamic Azad University, Qaemshahr Branch, Qaem Shahr 4765161964, Iran; svatandour@gmail.com
3. Swine and Poultry Infectious Diseases Research Centre–Fonds de Recherche du Québec (CRIPA-FRQ), Faculty of Veterinary Medicine, Université de Montréal, Saint-Hyacinthe, QC J2S 2M2, Canada; martine.boulianne@umontreal.ca (M.B.); charles.dozois@inrs.ca (C.M.D.); carl.a.gagnon@umontreal.ca (C.A.G.); neda.barjesteh@zoetis.com (N.B.)
4. Department of Clinical Sciences, Faculty of Veterinary Medicine, Université de Montréal, Saint-Hyacinthe, QC J2S 2M2, Canada
5. Institut National de Recherche Scientifique-Centre Armand-Frappier Santé Biotechnologie, Laval, QC H7V 1B7, Canada
6. Molecular Diagnostic and Virology Laboratories, Centre de Diagnostic Vétérinaire de l'Université de Montréal (CDVUM), Faculty of Veterinary Medicine, Université de Montréal, Saint-Hyacinthe, QC J2S 2M2, Canada

* Correspondence: faizal.abdulcareem@ucalgary.ca; Tel.: +1-(403)-220-4462

† Current address: Global Companion Animal Therapeutics, Zoetis, Kalamazoo, Michigan, MI 49007, USA.

Citation: O'Dowd, K.; Isham, I.M.; Vatandour, S.; Boulianne, M.; Dozois, C.M.; Gagnon, C.A.; Barjesteh, N.; Abdul-Careem, M.F. Host Immune Response Modulation in Avian Coronavirus Infection: Tracheal Transcriptome Profiling In Vitro and In Vivo. *Viruses* **2024**, *16*, 605. https://doi.org/10.3390/v16040605

Academic Editor: Chi-Young Wang

Received: 21 March 2024
Revised: 5 April 2024
Accepted: 10 April 2024
Published: 14 April 2024

Abstract: Infectious bronchitis virus (IBV) is a highly contagious *Gammacoronavirus* causing moderate to severe respiratory infection in chickens. Understanding the initial antiviral response in the respiratory mucosa is crucial for controlling viral spread. We aimed to characterize the impact of IBV Delmarva (DMV)/1639 and IBV Massachusetts (Mass) 41 at the primary site of infection, namely, in chicken tracheal epithelial cells (cTECs) in vitro and the trachea in vivo. We hypothesized that some elements of the induced antiviral responses are distinct in both infection models. We inoculated cTECs and infected young specific pathogen-free (SPF) chickens with IBV DMV/1639 or IBV Mass41, along with mock-inoculated controls, and studied the transcriptome using RNA-sequencing (RNA-seq) at 3 and 18 h post-infection (hpi) for cTECs and at 4 and 11 days post-infection (dpi) in the trachea. We showed that IBV DMV/1639 and IBV Mass41 replicate in cTECs in vitro and the trachea in vivo, inducing host mRNA expression profiles that are strain- and time-dependent. We demonstrated the different gene expression patterns between in vitro and in vivo tracheal IBV infection. Ultimately, characterizing host–pathogen interactions with various IBV strains reveals potential mechanisms for inducing and modulating the immune response during IBV infection in the chicken trachea.

Keywords: transcriptome; tracheal epithelial cell; trachea; infectious bronchitis virus; chicken; immune response

1. Introduction

Infectious bronchitis virus (IBV) is a highly contagious virus that causes mild to severe respiratory infections in chickens. The severity of the disease is dependent on several factors, such as environment, IBV strain, vaccination program, and coinfections [1]. The resulting disease is known as infectious bronchitis (IB) and is characterized by tracheitis and loss of ciliary activity in the upper respiratory tract of chickens [2]. Chickens of all ages are susceptible to IBV infection; however, the disease is more severe in young chicks [3]. IB is an acute disease transmitted via the respiratory tract by inhalation or by direct contact with contaminated poultry, litter, or equipment. The incubation period is short, 18 to 36 h, and clinical signs develop around 24 to 48 h post exposure [3,4]. Clinical manifestations of the respiratory tract include sneezing, gasping, coughing, tracheal rales, nasal discharge, and dyspnea [5]. In older chickens and in laying hens, respiratory signs can be mild or even absent [1]. Although initial infection typically occurs in the epithelial layer of the upper respiratory tract, IBV can disseminate and infect the gastrointestinal, renal, reproductive, and immune systems [5–10], potentially via the lymph or blood [6,11,12]. Depending on the IBV strain, this can lead to other clinical and pathological manifestations, such as nephritis [13], a decline in egg production and quality of the egg and egg shell in layer/breeder flocks [14–16], and a depletion of immune cells [7].

IBV is a positive-sense, single-stranded RNA virus and, typical of many RNA viruses, it is associated with rapid mutation rates and recombination in the genome, leading to the emergence of genetically diverse strains at a global level [17,18]. Vaccination with live attenuated/killed vaccines is one of the most important methods for the control of IB, along with rigorous biosecurity measures, but the aforementioned genetic diversity of these viruses is a significant obstacle for efficient and effective protection of flocks from potential outbreaks, as there is poor cross protection between heterologous strains [19]. A novel IBV variant, IBV Delmarva (DMV)/1639, emerged in 2011 [20]. Since 2015, IBV DMV/1639 strains have become more prevalent in Eastern Canada, namely in Quebec and Ontario [21–23]. Recent work has been conducted to characterize the underlying immunopathogenesis of this Canadian IBV DMV/1639 strain [21,24,25]. This DMV strain, among other IBV strains, such as the Massachusetts (Mass)-type IBVs, have been associated with the failure of a previously infected flock to reach peak lay due to a variable number of birds with severe developmental oviduct lesions, also known as false layers [14,23,24,26–28]. In addition, flock depopulation and secondary bacterial infections of the respiratory system following IBV infection cause significant economic losses to the poultry industry [1]. This highlights the importance in understanding the detailed mechanism of pathogenesis and host defense during IBV infection at the primary site of infection, namely, the airway epithelial cells.

The chicken immune system is a complex system designed to fight off invading pathogens, including viruses such as IBV. When the virus crosses the primary mucosal barriers, the innate immune responses provide the first line of defense and the airway epithelial cells become the primary target for the pathogen. In birds and mammals alike, airway epithelial cells have many important immune functions, which include the secretion of antimicrobial substances, cytokines and growth factors, cell-to-cell communication with immune cells, and modulation of early adaptive immunity during viral infections [29,30]. The induction of the innate response is dependent on many factors, including the detection of viral pathogen-associated molecular patterns (PAMPs) through pattern recognition receptors (PRRs), including Toll-like receptors (TLRs) [31]. The primary antiviral innate immune responses are characterized by this recognition and activation, resulting in the transcriptional activation of type I interferons (IFNs) and IFN-stimulated genes (ISGs), such as IFN-induced proteins with tetratricopeptide repeats (IFIT), myxovirus-resistance protein (MX), protein kinase R (PKR), and 2′-5′ oligoadenylate synthase-like (OASL) proteins [32,33]. These proteins are important for protecting the host and conferring resistance to RNA viral infections [34,35]. On the other hand, IBV has been shown to inhibit type 1 IFN response in primary chicken renal and tracheal epithelial cells and a chicken fibroblast cell line [36].

Since the early 2000s, researchers have aimed to map the host gene expression patterns involved in IBV infection [37–39]. More recent transcriptomic studies have looked at chicken spleen tissues [40–42], tracheal tissues [43–45], lung tissues [41], human lung epithelial-like cells [46], chicken kidney tissues and cells [47–51], dendritic cells [52,53], macrophages [54], and fibroblasts [55] upon infection with various strains of IBV. Currently, there are no RNA-seq studies specifically looking at IBV infection in chicken tracheal epithelial cells (cTECs), nor using the IBV DMV/1639 strain, which has been the dominant IBV genotype circulating in Canada [21,22] and the United States of America (USA) in recent years [20,56]. Despite extensive research on the pathogenicity of these different strains of the virus [7,24,28,57–60], there is a lack of knowledge regarding the regulation of molecular mechanisms involved in the initial induction of the host antiviral responses at the level of the trachea and tracheal epithelial cells upon infection with different strains of IBV, which may help to explain the differing pathogenesis in the tracheal tissues of infected birds. To this end, we aimed to characterize the impact of IBV DMV/1639 and IBV Mass41 at the primary site of infection, namely, in cTECs in vitro and the trachea in vivo, and to evaluate the impact of infection on the host gene expression. We hypothesized that the host antiviral reactions elicited by IBV DMV/1639 and IBV Mass41 exhibit unique characteristics in terms of differential expression of immune-related genes in the infection models presented in this study.

2. Materials and Methods

2.1. Virus Propagation and Titration

The Canadian IBV DMV/1639 clinical isolate IBV/Ck/Can/17-036989 (GenBank accession no. MN512435), isolated from the kidneys of infected layers (Ontario, Canada) [21], and the Canadian IBV Mass41 clinical isolate IBV/Ck/Can/21-2455844 (GenBank accession no. PP373115), obtained from a pool of tissues from infected broilers (Quebec, Canada) (Dr. Carl A. Gagnon, CDVUM), were propagated by inoculation in 10-day-old specific-pathogen-free (SPF) embryonated chicken (layer chickens, white Leghorn) eggs obtained from the Canadian Food Inspection Agency (CFIA), Ottawa, ON, Canada [61,62]. Allantoic fluid was harvested at 3 days post-infection (dpi) and viral titers were determined by 50% embryo infectious dose (EID_{50}), as described previously [21,61]. The viral titer was calculated using the Reed and Muench method and expressed as EID_{50}/mL [63]. The viral titers were determined to be $10^{6.0}$ EID_{50}/mL for IBV DMV/1639 and $10^{6.5}$ EID_{50}/mL for IBV Mass41.

2.2. cTEC Preparation

Primary cTEC isolation was performed as previously described with some modifications [64–66]. Briefly, tracheas were aseptically dissected from 19-day-old SPF chicken embryos (CFIA, Ottawa, ON, Canada) and digested with filter-sterilized protease from Streptomyces griseus (Pronase, Sigma-Aldrich Oakville, ON, Canada) (2 mg/mL) in complete Medium 199 (Sigma-Aldrich Oakville, ON, Canada) supplemented with 2 mM GlutaMax supplement, 25 mM 4-(2-hydroxyethyl)-1-piperazineethanesulfonic acid (HEPES) buffer, 100 U/mL penicillin/100 μg/mL streptomycin, 50 μg/mL gentamicin, and 0.25 μg/mL amphotericin B (Gibco, Burlington, ON, Canada). The cells were treated with a filter-sterilized 0.5 mg/mL DNase solution (Deoxyribonuclease I from bovine pancreas, Sigma-Aldrich, Oakville, ON, Canada) in complete Medium 199, followed by a brief incubation period in complete Dulbecco's Modified Eagle Medium/Nutrient Mixture F-12 (DMEM/F-12), containing 10% FBS, 2 mM GlutaMax supplement, 100 U/mL penicillin/100 μg/mL streptomycin, 50 μg/mL gentamicin, 0.25 μg/mL amphotericin B, 1 mM β-mercaptoethanol (BME), and 1% non-essential amino acids (MEM NEAA) (Gibco, Burlington, ON, Canada), as a negative selection step for fibroblast growth. Finally, the cells were resuspended in complete DMEM/F-12 medium supplemented with 10% chicken embryo extract. The chicken embryo extract was prepared in-house from 11-day-old SPF chicken embryos as previously described in the protocol developed by Pajtler and colleagues [67]. The cTECs were seeded at a viable cell density (determined by trypan blue exclusion test) of 3×10^5 cells per well into wells of 5% MatriGel-coated (Corning Inc., Corning, NY, USA) 24-well culture plates. After 4 days of incubation at 37 °C 5% CO_2, the cells were subjected to further experiments as described in Section 2.3 below.

2.3. Infection of cTECs with IBV

Tracheal epithelial cells were cultured in complete DMEM/F-12 (serum-free) infection medium containing 2 mM GlutaMax supplement, 100 U/mL penicillin/100 μg/mL streptomycin, 50 μg/mL gentamicin, 25 mM HEPES buffer, and 2.5% bovine serum albumin (BSA 7.5% solution) (Gibco, Burlington, ON, Canada) and incubated at 37 °C 5% CO_2 for all steps. Prior to infection, cells were washed twice with medium and then infected with 200 μL with a low (2×10^4 EID_{50}/mL), intermediate (1×10^5 EID_{50}/mL), or high (5×10^5 EID_{50}/mL) dose, diluted in phosphate-buffered saline (PBS), of either IBV DMV/1639 or IBV Mass41. The control groups received DMEM/F-12 infection medium only. Subsequently, cells were washed twice two hours post-infection (hpi) following the adsorption period and incubated in fresh DMEM/F-12 infection medium. These doses were selected in part based on a previous study [65]. At 0, 18, 24, and 48 h, supernatants were collected in TRIzol™ LS reagent (Invitrogen, Burlington, ON, Canada), to determine viral genome load. Based on the results of this preliminary study, in a separate experiment, the cells were infected with the different IBV isolates at a high (5×10^5 EID_{50}/mL) dose and the cells were collected in QIAzol™ reagent (QIAGEN, Toronto, ON, Canada) at an early time point, 3 h, and at a later time point near the peak of viral genome load detected, 18 h, for RNA sequencing.

2.4. Chickens

One-day-old SPF chickens (layer chickens, white Leghorn) (n = 60) were purchased from the CFIA, Ottawa, ON, and housed and closely monitored in the animal facilities by staff at the National Experimental Biology Laboratory (NEBL) of the Institut national de la recherche scientifique (INRS) Armand-Frappier Santé Biotechnologie Research Centre, where the experiments were conducted in temperature-controlled poultry isolators in negative pressure rooms. The chickens were divided into 5 groups (n = 12 chickens/group). The groups were named as follows: IBV DMV/1639 low dose, IBV DMV/1639 high dose, IBV Mass41 low dose, IBV Mass41 high dose, and uninfected control. The experimental protocols were approved by the Institutional Animal Care and Use Committee (IACUC) of the Université de Montréal (ethics protocol no. 21-Rech-2120) and the INRS (ethics protocol no. 2106-03). The tracheal tissue samples used for the real-time quantitative polymerase chain reaction (qPCR) mRNA gene expression validation experiments were from chickens that were housed at the Veterinary Science Research Station (VSRS), Spyhill, Campus, University of Calgary, and subjected to the same experimental conditions as those in the NEBL INRS Armand-Frappier Santé Biotechnologie Research Centre animal facility. The experimental protocols for these experiments were approved by the Veterinary Science Animal Care Committee (VSACC) and the Health Science Animal Care Committee (HSACC) of the University of Calgary (ethics protocol no. AC22-0012).

2.5. Infections of Chickens with IBV

The IBV stocks were diluted in PBS to the appropriate doses for inoculation. Six-day-old SPF chickens were inoculated with a low dose (10^4 EID_{50}/bird) or a high dose (10^5 EID_{50}/bird) of either IBV DMV/1639 or IBV Mass41 through the intranasal and intraocular routes (100 μL). The negative control group received PBS. Samples from the upper half of the trachea were collected at 4 (n = 6 chickens/group) and 11 dpi (n = 6 chickens/group) and stored in RNAlater® (Invitrogen, Burlington, ON, Canada).

2.6. Quantification of IBV Viral Genome Load and Host mRNA Gene Expression

From cTEC cell culture supernatants, total RNA was extracted from the samples using the TRIzol™ LS reagent (Invitrogen, Burlington, ON, Canada), according to the manufacturer's protocol. For the tracheas collected from IBV DMV/1639-infected chickens at 4 dpi and 11 dpi, the samples were lysed in TRIzol™ reagent (Invitrogen, Burlington, ON, Canada) and homogenized using 0.5 mm glass beads and a tissue homogenizer (MP FastPrep-24 Classic Instrument, MP Biomedicals, Solon, OH, USA). Total RNA was extracted according to the manufacturer's protocol. Isolated RNA was resuspended in

20 μL RNase-free water. Assessment of RNA concentration and quality was performed using the NanoDrop ND-1000 spectrophotometer (Thermo Scientific, Wilmington, DE, USA). Using the High-Capacity Reverse Transcription Kit with random primers (Applied Biosystems, Waltham, MA, USA) according to manufacturer's instructions, complementary deoxyribonuclease (cDNA) synthesis was performed for 500 ng (cTEC supernatants) or 2000 ng (tracheas) of RNA per sample. qPCR targeting the IBV nucleoprotein gene (N) was performed for quantification of IBV viral genome load in cTEC supernatants and trachea and for host mRNA gene expression in the tracheal tissues, using gene-specific primers (Table S1, [68–75]) at a final concentration of 5 nM (Sigma-Aldrich, Saint-Louis, MO, USA) and PowerUp SYBR Green Master Mix (Applied Biosystems, Burlington, ON, Canada) in a 20 μL reaction according to the manufacturer's instructions. Furthermore, a 10-fold dilution series of the IBV-N gene plasmid was used to generate the standard curve, as previously described [68]. The IBV-N gene plasmid DNA was generated from a stock prepared in-house. IBV-N plasmid transformation was performed using the Subcloning Efficiency™ DHα Competent cells (Thermo Scientific, Burlington, ON, Canada) and purification was performed using the GeneJET Plasmid miniprep kit (Thermo Scientific, Burlington, ON, Canada), according to manufacturers' instructions. The qPCR cycling program for quantification of all genes consisted of a pre-incubation at 95 °C for 20 s, and amplification/extension at 95 °C for 3 s and 60 °C for 30 s, repeated for 40 cycles. Melting curve analysis was assessed at 95 °C for 10 s (segment 1), 65 °C for 5 s (segment 2), and 9 °C for 5 s (segment 3). Fluorescence acquisition was performed at 60 °C for 30 s and the results for IBV genome load are presented as $\log_{10}$ IBV genome copies per 1 μL of reaction/cDNA [68]. Fold-changes for host mRNA gene expression were calculated using the $2^{-\Delta\Delta Ct}$ method [76] and quantified relative to the β-actin housekeeping gene.

2.7. RNA Isolation, cDNA Library Preparations and High-Throughput Sequencing

For the RNA-sequencing (RNA-seq) experiments, total RNA was isolated from cTECs, and lysed and homogenized tracheal tissues using QIAzol™ reagent (QIAGEN, Toronto, ON, Canada) and the miRNeasy Mini Kit (QIAGEN, Toronto, ON, Canada) according to the miRNeasy Mini Kit Quick-Start protocol. The purified RNA was eluted in 30 μL RNase-free water. Prior to sequencing, RNA quality control was performed by automatic electrophoresis-based analysis (TapeStation RNA Screen Tape, Agilent, Santa Clara, CA, USA).

For the cTEC samples, RNA library preparations and sequencing were performed at Plateforme de séquençage de nouvelle génération of the Université Research Center of the CHU de Québec-Université Laval. Twenty-four libraries were prepared for RNA-seq, with 4 replicates per treatment group: IBV DMV/1639 3 h, IBV DMV/1639 18 h, IBV Mass41 3 h, IBV Mass 18 h, control (CTRL) 3 h, CTRL 18 h. Each replicate consisted of a pool of cells from 2 individual embryos. Infected samples are from cTECs infected with a high dose (5×10^5 EID_{50}/mL) of IBV.

For the tracheal samples, RNA library preparations and sequencing were performed at the McGill Applied Genomics Innovation Core (MAGIC) of the McGill Genome Centre, McGill University. Eighteen libraries were prepared for RNA-seq, with 3 replicates per treatment group: IBV DMV/1639 4 dpi, IBV DMV/1639 11 dpi, IBV Mass41 4 dpi, IBV Mass41 11 dpi, control (CTRL) 4 dpi, CTRL 11 dpi. Each replicate consisted of a pool of tracheal tissue from 2 individual chickens. Infected samples were from tracheal tissues that originated from chickens infected with a high dose (10^5 EID_{50}/bird) of IBV. The RNA libraries were sequenced on a NovaSeq 6000 S4 (Illumina, San Diego, CA, USA) platform to generate 100 base pair (bp) paired-end reads.

2.8. RNA-Seq Differential Expression, Gene Ontology (GO), and Pathway Analysis

Analysis for RNA-seq data was performed using the open-source framework GenPipes [77]. Analyses were conducted using RStudio [78,79], unless stated otherwise. The R packages knitr [80], ggrepel [81], tibble [82], tidyverse [83], magrittr [84], hablar [85], and kableExtra [86] were used for analysis and formatting. RNA-SeQC [87] was used to assess the quality of the generated reads. Trimmomatic [88] was used to process raw sequencing reads and trim adaptor sequences and low-quality score-containing bases (Phred score < 30) from reads. The resulting reads were aligned to the Ensembl chicken (Gallus gallus) reference genome (ASM223467v1, GRCg6a, INSDC Assembly GCA_000002315.5) from http://aug2020.archive.ensembl.org/Gallus_gallus/Info/Index (accessed on 7 June 2022). This was conducted using Spliced Transcripts Alignment to a Reference (STAR) [89] and read counts were obtained using HTSeq [90]. The R package DESeq2 [91] was then used to identify differences in expression levels between the groups using negative binomial generalized linear model (GLM) fitting and Wald statistics: nbinomWaldTest. Data were batched normalized and log transformed. The R package "ashr" [92] was used to shrink $\log_2$ fold-changes ($\log_2$FC) for gene expression data. For the purpose of this study, differential gene expression was based on an infected group compared to the uninfected control group at the same time point and genes were considered differentially expressed (DE) if the adjusted p-value was <0.05 and $\log_2$FC was $\geq |1|$ or fold-change (FC) $\geq |2|$. Principle Component Analysis (PCA) plots, heatmaps using the R packages ComplexHeatmap [93] and tidyHeatmap [94], and volcano plots using the R package EnhancedVolcano [95] were created in R [78,79]. Venn diagram analysis and visualization were created using the online tools https://bioinformatics.psb.ugent.be/webtools/Venn/ and Venny (accessed on 9 January 2024) [96].

All genes that were DE were considered (separated by down- and up-regulated genes) for further analyses. GO functional enrichment analyses, or over-representation analyses (ORA), and visualizations for Biological Process (BP), Molecular Function (MF), and Cellular Component (CC) were performed using the R packages gprofiler2 (g:Profiler) [97,98], enrichplot [99], DOSE [100], and ggplot2 [101]. Enrichment p-values were based on a hypergeometric test, the g:GOSt method, using the default g:SCS method applied for multiple testing correction. This corresponds to an experiment-wide threshold of $\alpha = 0.05$, wherein at least 95% of matches above the threshold are statistically significant. The background used was the set of known genes and terms with GO evidence codes Inferred from Electronic Annotation (IEA) were excluded. The R package GOfuncR [102] was used to investigate relationships between enriched GO term parent and child nodes. Kyoto Encyclopedia of Genes and Genomes (KEGG) [103] pathway analysis and visualization for key enriched pathways was performed using the R packages gprofiler2 (g:Profiler) [97,98], pathview [104], and org.Gg.eg.db [105].

2.9. Statistical Analysis

Statistical analysis for IBV genome loads for each strain was assessed using two-way analysis of variance (ANOVA), followed by Tukey's post hoc test. The differences were considered significant if the p-value was <0.05. Statistical analysis was performed using GraphPad Prism 10 software (GraphPad, La Jolla, CA, USA). Statistical methods for sequence data analysis are contained within the software used.

3. Results

3.1. IBV Genome Load in cTEC Supernatants and the Trachea

The effects of the different doses and time points on IBV genome loads in the cTEC supernatants were assessed by qPCR for both IBV strains and are shown in Figure 1. No IBV genome was detected for the uninfected controls. Upon cTEC infection with different doses of IBV DMV/1639 (Figure 1a) or IBV Mass41 (Figure 1b), it was found that there was a significant increase in IBV genome load between the time point 0 h and the time points 18 h, 24 h, and 48 h for the three doses evaluated (p-value < 0.05). No significant differences were observed between the time points 18 h, 24 h, and 48 h within each respective dose (p-value > 0.05). In addition, a significantly higher IBV genome load was observed with the IBV DMV/1639 high dose group compared to the low dose group at 24 h (p-value < 0.05).

The IBV genome loads in the trachea samples collected during the in vivo experiment are shown in Figure 2. The samples from all infected groups were IBV-positive. No IBV was detected in uninfected controls at 4 dpi and 11 dpi. The IBV genome load in the trachea was significantly higher (p-value < 0.05) in high dose IBV DMV/1639-infected chickens at 4 dpi compared to 11 dpi (Figure 2a). In the IBV Mass41-infected group, there was a significant decrease (p-value < 0.05) in viral genome load from 4 dpi to 11 dpi in the tracheas of chickens challenged with a low dose of virus (Figure 2b).

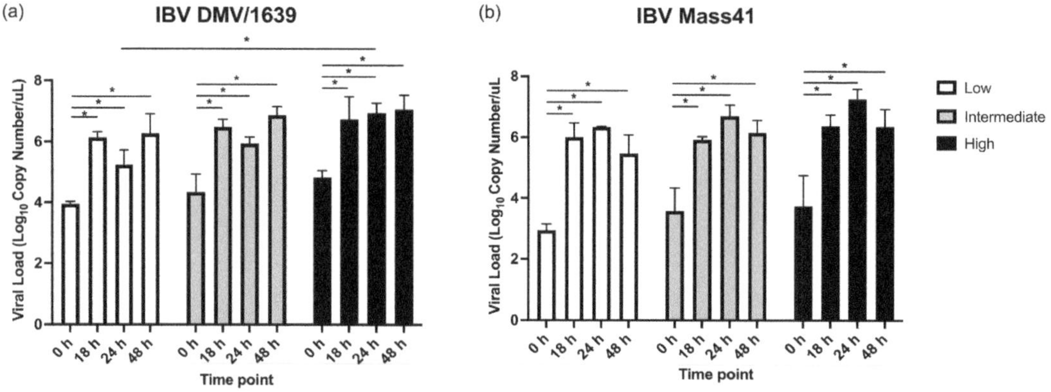

Figure 1. IBV genome load in the supernatants of cTECs infected with IBV DMV/1639 or IBV Mass41 strains. The cTECs were inoculated with a low (2×10^4 EID_{50}/mL), intermediate (1×10^5 EID_{50}/mL), or high (5×10^5 EID_{50}/mL) dose of either IBV DMV/1639 (**a**) or IBV Mass41 (**b**). At 0, 18, 24, and 48 h, supernatants were collected, RNA extracted, and cDNA synthesized to determine viral genome loads using a qPCR assay. Statistical analysis for IBV viral genome loads for each strain was assessed using two-way ANOVA followed by Tukey's post hoc test. Significant differences (p-value < 0.05) are denoted by *. The error bars represent standard deviation (SD).

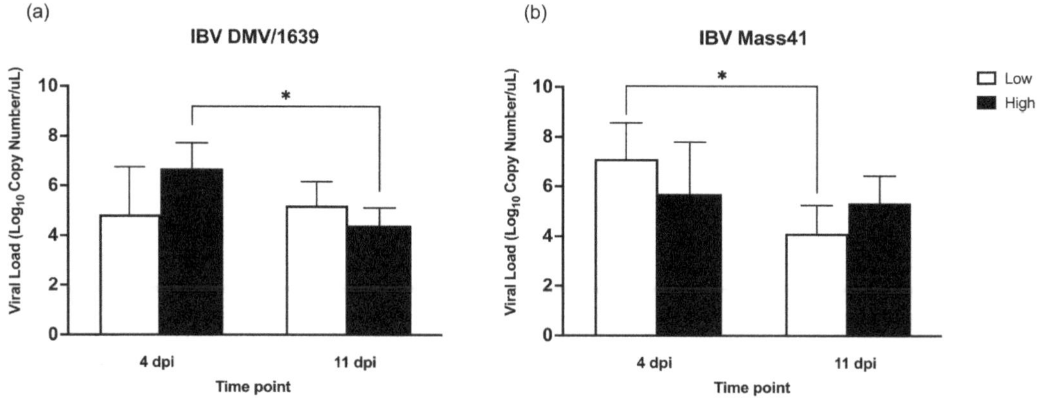

Figure 2. IBV viral genome in tracheal tissues from chickens infected with IBV DMV/1639 or IBV Mass41. Six-day-old chickens were infected with a low (10^4 EID_{50}/bird) or a high (10^5 EID_{50}/bird) dose of either IBV DMV/1639 (**a**) or IBV Mass41 (**b**). At 4 dpi and 11 dpi, tracheal tissue samples were collected, RNA extracted, and cDNA synthesized to determine viral genome load using a qPCR assay. Statistical analysis for differences in IBV genome loads for each strain was conducted using two-way ANOVA followed by Tukey's post hoc test, and significant differences (p-value < 0.05) are denoted by *. The error bars represent SD.

3.2. mRNA Expression and Functional Profiles from cTECs Infected with Different IBV Strains

The mRNA expression profiles of cTECs infected with the high dose (5×10^5 EID_{50}/mL) of IBV DMV/1639 or IBV Mass41 at 3 h and 18 h were evaluated to determine strain-specific and temporal-related changes in gene expression. All RNA-seq differential expression results are compiled in Table S2, which includes the following comparisons: CTRL 18 h vs. CTRL 3 h, IBV DMV/1639 3 h vs. CTRL 3 h, IBV DMV/1639 18 h vs. CTRL 18 h, IBV DMV/1639 18 h vs. IBV DMV/1639 3 h, IBV Mass41 3 h vs. CTRL 3 h, IBV Mass41 18 h vs. CTRL 18 h, IBV Mass41 18 h vs. IBV Mass41 3 h. For this study, comparisons of the treatment groups and the control groups at the same respective time point were considered (IBV DMV/1639 3 h vs. CTRL 3 h, IBV DMV/1639 18 h vs. CTRL 18 h, IBV Mass41 3 h vs. CTRL 3 h, IBV Mass41 18 h vs. CTRL 18 h). The results filtered for significantly DE mRNAs (defined by an adjusted p-value < 0.05 and a $\log_2FC \geq |1|$) are summarized in Table S3.

The variance in log counts across all samples by group is shown in Figure 3a. In addition, the heatmaps provided in the Supplementary Files (Figure S1) demonstrate the relationships between cTECs infected with IBV DMV/1639 at 3 h (Figure S1a) and 18 h (Figure S1b) or IBV Mass41 at 3 h (Figure S1c) and 18 h (Figure S1d), relative to their respective control groups. The clustering is based on the similarity of normalized log counts, rather than differential expression, and there are differences in counts between the virus-treated groups and uninfected control groups. Overall, there are a higher number of DE mRNAs at 18 h as compared to the 3 h groups for both virus strains (Figure 3b). Among all treatment groups, including IBV DMV/1639- and IBV Mass41-infected cTECs at 3 h and 18 h, a total of 1653 DE mRNAs were identified among all treatment groups (Table S3). Figure 3c–f shows the number of down- and up-regulated mRNAs per group which passed the adjusted p-value < 0.05 and $\log_2FC \geq |1|$ thresholds. Briefly, a total of 248 and 1322 DE mRNAs, 30 and 821 down-regulated mRNAs, and 218 and 501 up-regulated mRNAs were identified for IBV DMV/1639 3 h and IBV DMV/1639 18 h, respectively. Furthermore, 114 and 1093 DE mRNAs, 32 and 628 down-regulated mRNAs, and 82 and 465 up-regulated mRNAs were identified for IBV Mass41 3 h and IBV Mass41 18 h, respectively. At the 3 h time point, fewer genes were down-regulated than up-regulated, while at the 18 h time point, more genes were down-regulated than up-regulated.

Some DE mRNAs were present in several treatment groups, as shown in Figure 4a, for down-regulated mRNAs, and in Figure 4b for up-regulated mRNAs. Details of the Venn diagram results are summarized in Table S4. There were 3 down-regulated mRNAs, namely solute carrier family 6 member 4 (SLC6A4), Kruppel-like factor (KLF) 1 (KLF1), and ENSGALG00000008599, and 35 up-regulated mRNAs common to all treatment groups (for both IBV strains at both time points). The commonly up-regulated mRNAs among all groups included immune response-related genes zinc finger NFX1-type-containing 1 (ZNFX1), poly(adenosine diphosphate-ribose) polymerase family member 9 (PARP9), deltex E3 ubiquitin ligase 3L (DTX3L), tripartite motif-containing 25 (TRIM25), IFIT5, MX1, OASL, IFN regulatory factor (IRF)7, TLR3, DExH-box helicase 58 (DHX58), also known as Laboratory of Genetics and Physiology 2 (LPG2), IFN induced with helicase C domain 1 (IFIH1), also known as melanoma differentiation-associated protein 5 (MDA5), radical S-adenosyl methionine domain-containing 2 (RSAD2), also known as viperin, and eukaryotic translation initiation factor 2 α kinase 2 (EIF2AK2), also known as PKR. Furthermore, IFN-induced transmembrane protein 3-like (IFITM3) is down-regulated in the IBV DMV/1639 and IBV Mass41 3 h groups but up-regulated in the IBV DMV/1639 and IBV Mass41 18 h groups. In addition, signal transducer and activator of transcription (STAT) 1 (STAT1), STAT2, tumor necrosis factor (TNF) receptor-associated factor (TRAF)-type zinc finger domain-containing 1 (TRAFD1), IFITM5, adenosine deaminase that acts on RNA (ADAR), Moloney leukemia virus 10 (MOV10), and DExD/H box helicase 60 (DDX60) were up-regulated in the IBV DMV/1639 3 h, IBV DMV/1639 18 h, and IBV Mass41 18 h groups, while suppressor of cytokine signaling (SOCS) 1 (SOCS1) was up-regulated in the IBV DMV/1639 3 h, IBV Mass41 3 h, and IBV Mass41 18 h groups. Moreover, myeloid differentiation primary response (MYD)88 was up-regulated in the IBV DMV/1639 3 h and IBV Mass41 18 h groups.

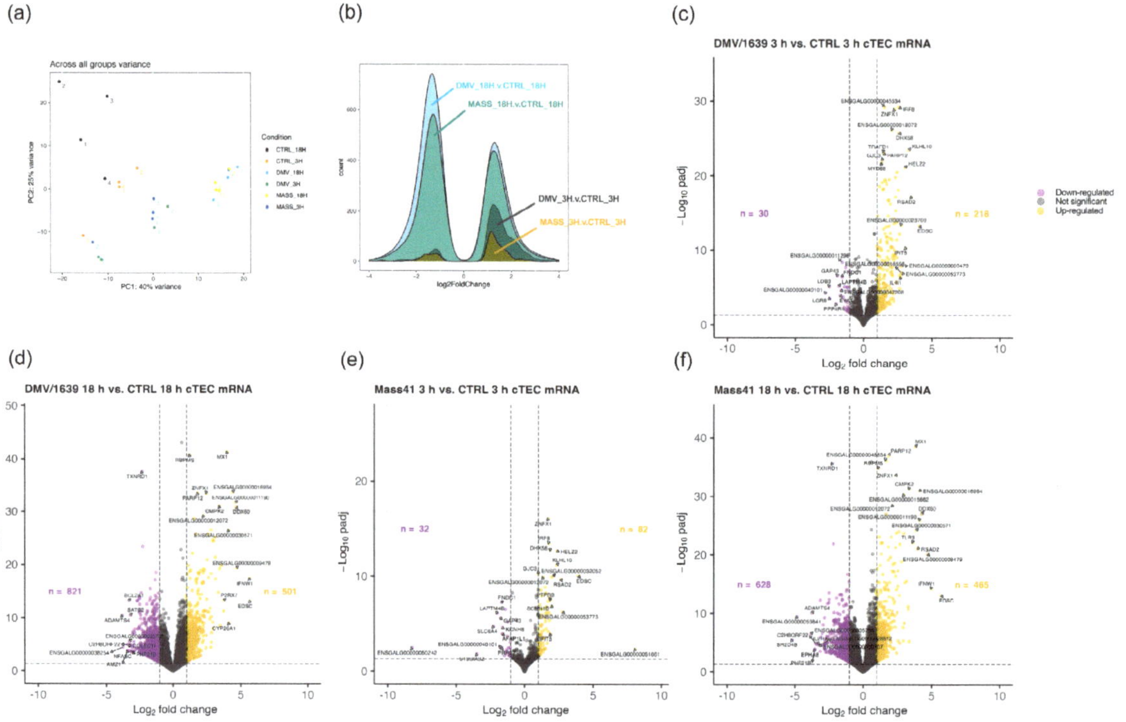

Figure 3. Differential expression of mRNAs from cTECs infected with IBV DMV/1639 or IBV Mass41. The PCA plot (**a**) evaluates the variance across all samples based on the log counts of all mRNAs. The histogram (**b**) represents the $\log_2$FC distribution of fluorescence signal intensity ratios for DE mRNAs of cTECs infected with IBV DMV/1639 or IBV Mass41 at 3 h and 18 h. The volcano plots show DE mRNAs of cTECs infected with IBV DMV/1639 at 3 h (**c**) and 18 h (**d**) or IBV Mass41 at 3 h (**e**) and 18 h (**f**), relative to their respective control groups. The horizontal dotted line represents the adjusted p-value < 0.05 threshold. The vertical dotted lines represent the $\log_2\text{FC} \geq |1|$ ($\text{FC} \geq |2|$) threshold. The x-axis limits are set from −10 to 10 $\log_2$FC. Down-regulated mRNAs are represented by purple data points and up-regulated mRNAs are represented by yellow data points. The list of all up- and down-regulated mRNAs for each treatment group are shown in Table S3.

Few common DE mRNAs were identified between time points for the same IBV strains. Protein phosphatase 4 regulatory subunit 4 (PPP4R4) was down-regulated, and two mRNAs, complement component 1r (C1R) and ENSGALG00000046098, were up-regulated in the IBV DMV/1639 3 h and 18 h groups. Furthermore, TNF superfamily member (TNFSF) 15 (TNFSF15) was down-regulated in the IBV DMV/1639 18 h group but up-regulated in the IBV DMV/1639 3 h group. Potassium voltage-gated channel subfamily D member 2 (KCND2) was up-regulated in the IBV Mass41 3 h and 18 h groups. The IBV DMV/1639 3 h and IBV Mass41 3 h groups shared 8 down-regulated mRNAs and 33 up-regulated mRNAs, including IRF1 and IRF8. Of all the intersecting groups, the IBV DMV/1639 18 h and IBV Mass41 18 h groups had the highest number of common DE mRNAs, with 527 down-regulated mRNAs and 326 up-regulated mRNAs.

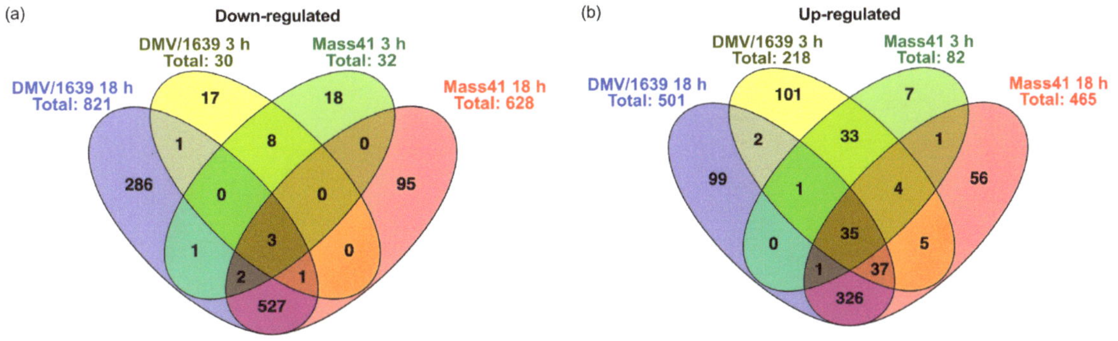

Figure 4. Common and unique DE mRNAs of cTECs infected with IBV DMV/1639 or IBV Mass41. The Venn diagram illustrates common and unique down-regulated (**a**) and up-regulated (**b**) DE mRNAs among cTECs infected with IBV DMV/1639 or IBV Mass41 at 3 h and 18 h. Lists of common and unique DE mRNAs are found in Table S4.

At 18 h, the common down-regulated mRNAs included interleukins (IL)-1β (IL1B), IL-21 receptor (IL21R), IL-8-like 1 (IL8L1), IL-2 receptor subunit α (IL2RA), IL-31 receptor subunit α (IL3RA), IL-10 receptor subunit α (IL10RA), ISG20, TNF receptor superfamily (TNFRSF) 18 (TNFRSF18), TNFRSF1B, TNFRSF8, TRAF3, tripartite motif-containing 9 (TRIM9), SOCS3, activator protein (AP)-1 transcription factor subunits Jun proto-oncogene (JUN) and Fos proto-oncogene (FOS), and nuclear factor of κ light polypeptide gene enhancer in B-cells (NFKB) inhibitor, α (NFKBIA), also known as IκBα. The common up-regulated mRNAs at 18 h included IFN ω 1 (IFNW1), IFN α-inducible protein 6 (IFI6), IFN α-inducible protein 27-like 2 (IFI27L2), IL-18 receptor 1 (IL18R1), thioredoxin reductase 1 (TXNRD1), and sterile α motif and histidine–aspartate domain-containing protein 1 (SAMHD1).

In total, 17, 286, 18, and 95 mRNAs were uniquely down-regulated and 101, 99, 7, and 56 mRNAs were uniquely up-regulated in the IBV DMV/1639 3 h, IBV DMV/1639 18 h, IBV Mass41 3 h, and IBV Mass41 18 h groups, respectively. Up-regulated mRNAs in the IBV DMV/1639 3 h group included TNFRSF4, TLR21, IRF9, IL-6 (IL6), colony-stimulating factor 3 (CSF3), chemokine ligand (CCL) 4 (CCL4), nucleotide-binding oligomerization domain (NOD)-like receptor family caspase activation and recruitment domain (CARD)-containing (NLRC) 5 (NLRC5), inducible nitric oxide synthase (iNOS or NOS2), and aconitate decarboxylase 1 (ACOD1). FOSB was down-regulated in the IBV DMV/1639 18 h group. Up-regulated mRNAs in the IBV DMV/1639 18 h group included cathepsin S (CTSS) and cluster of differentiation (CD) 38 (CD38). For the IBV Mass41 3 h group, IL-19 (IL19) was down-regulated. Finally, IL-8 (IL8) and transforming growth factor beta receptor III (TGFBR3) were down-regulated and IL-7 (IL7) and C5 were up-regulated in the IBV Mass41 18 h group.

Figure 5 illustrates the enriched GO terms (BP) for DE RNAs. The full details for the GO enrichment analysis are summarized in Table S5. At the earlier time point, 3 h, GO terms associated with the down-regulated RNAs (Figure 5a,c) tended to be more associated with cell signaling and metabolism, while those associated with the up-regulated RNAs (Figure 5e,g) tended to be associated with defense responses. For example, some of the top GO terms included response to stimulus, regulation of the immune response, and response to virus. At the 18 h time point, the GO terms for down-regulated RNAs (Figure 5b,d) were generally associated with cell signaling and metabolism, or development and cell proliferation. For up-regulated RNAs (Figure 5f,h), GO terms were also associated with defense responses. Pathways are considered enriched when multiple genes from that pathway are up- or down-regulated upon IBV infection.

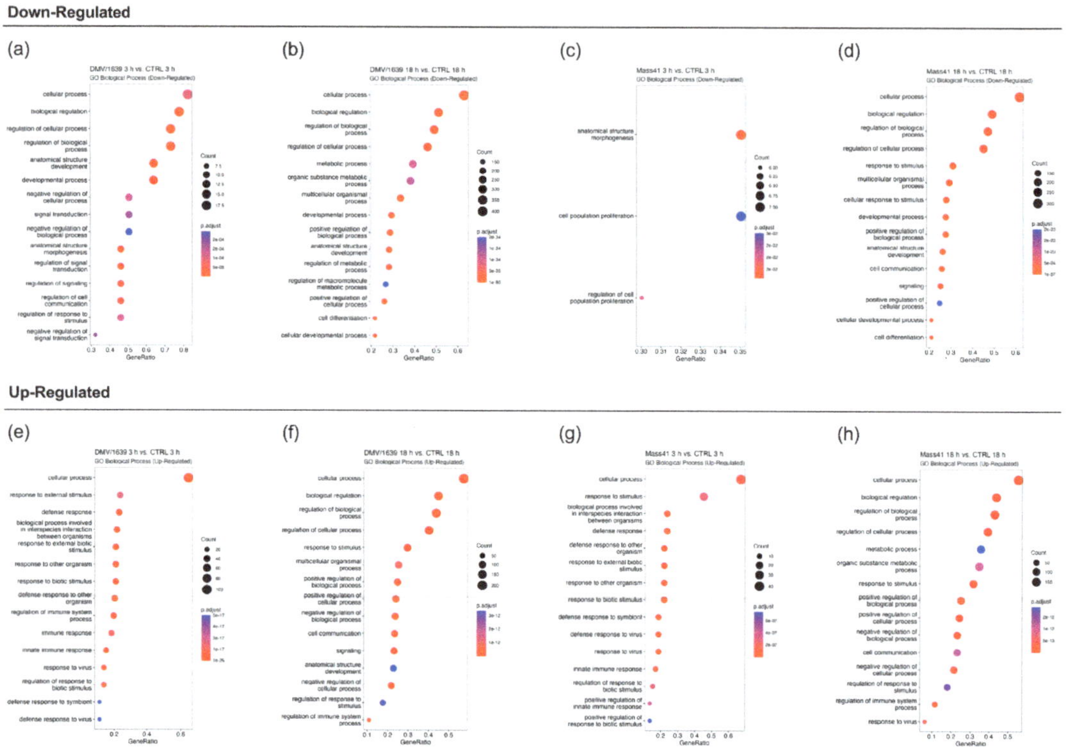

Figure 5. GO functional enrichment analysis for DE mRNAs from cTECs infected with IBV DMV/1639 or IBV Mass41. The dot plots represent the enriched GO Biological Process terms for down-regulated mRNAs from the IBV DMV/1639 at 3 h (**a**), IBV DMV/1639 at 18 h (**b**), IBV Mass41 at 3 h (**c**), and IBV Mass41 at 18 h (**d**) groups, and for up-regulated mRNAs from the IBV DMV/1639 at 3 h (**e**), IBV DMV/1639 at 18 h (**f**), IBV Mass41 at 3 h (**g**), and IBV Mass41 at 18 h (**h**) groups. Count is the number of genes enriched in a GO term and GeneRatio is the percentage of total DE mRNAs in the given GO term. The color intensities represent the adjusted *p*-values. The list of all GO terms for DE mRNAs is found in Table S5.

All treatment groups, except the IBV Mass41 3 h group, were significantly enriched in immune signaling pathways such as TLR signaling, cytokine–cytokine receptor interaction, RIG-I-like receptor signaling, and cytosolic DNA-sensing. At 3 h, the differences between the enriched pathways of the different strains were marked. The subset of DE genes for the IBV DMV/1639 group was enriched for many pathways, including the ones mentioned above and the NOD-like receptor signaling, calcium signaling, C-type lectin receptor signaling, mitogen-activated protein kinase (MAPK) signaling, and focal adhesion, while the IBV Mass41 group was enriched only for the RIG-I-like receptor signaling pathway. At 18 h, necroptosis was enriched for the IBV DMV/1639 group, while regulation of actin cytoskeleton and TGFβ signaling pathways were enriched for the IBV Mass41 group. The enriched pathways showing the specifically enriched genes for IBV DMV/1639 18 h and IBV Mass41 18 h for the TLR signaling pathway are shown in Figure 6. While many of the DE genes in this pathway are common to both treatment groups, we can observe that, for example, IFN α and β receptor subunit 1 (IFNAR1) and MAPK10, also known as c-Jun N-terminal kinase 3 (JNK3), are down-regulated only in the IBV DMV/1639 18 h group and that inhibitor of nuclear factor κ-B kinase subunit ε (IKBKE) and MYD88 are up-regulated only in the IBV Mass41 18 h group. Full details for KEGG enrichment analysis are summarized in Table S5.

(a)

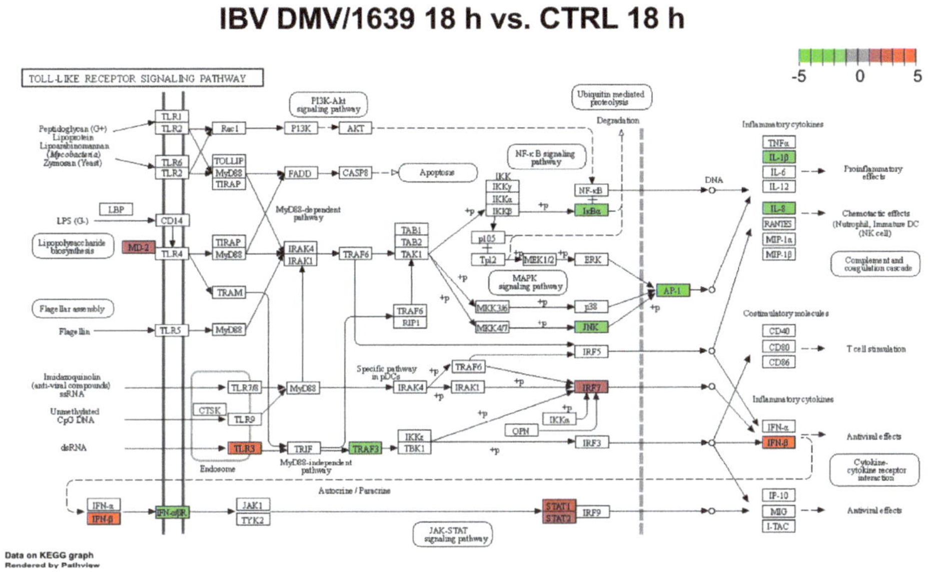

(b)

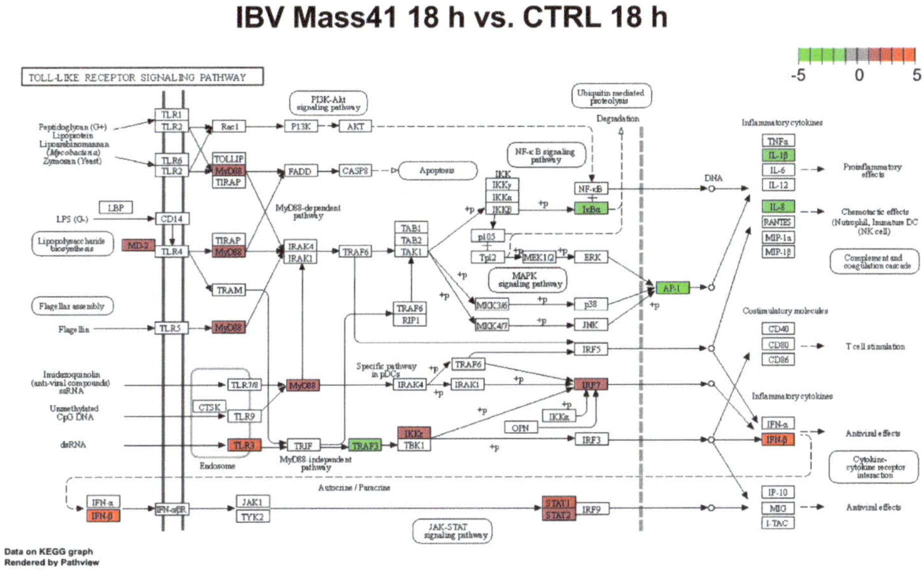

Figure 6. KEGG pathway analysis for DE mRNAs from cTECs infected with IBV DMV/1639 or IBV Mass41. The KEGG pathway figures illustrate the genes within the enriched TLR signaling pathway for IBV DMV/1639 at 18 h (**a**) and for IBV Mass41 at 18 h (**b**). The color intensities represent the log_2FC. Full details for the pathway analysis are found in Table S5.

3.3. mRNA Expression and Functional Profiles in the Tracheal Tissues of IBV DMV/1639- and IBV Mass41-Infected Chickens

The mRNA expression profiles in tracheal tissues from chickens infected with a high dose (10^5 EID_{50}/bird) of IBV DMV/1639 or IBV Mass41 collected at 4 dpi and 11 dpi were evaluated to determine the effect of the IBV virus strain and collection time point on gene expression. The heatmaps (Figure S2) provided in the Supplementary Files demonstrate the relationships between samples from chickens infected with IBV DMV/1639 at 4 (Figure S2a) and 11 dpi (Figure S2b) or IBV Mass41 at 4 (Figure S2c) and 11 dpi (Figure S2d), relative to their respective control groups (based on differences in mRNA normalized log counts).

For the trachea, the RNA-seq differential expression results are compiled in Table S6. Included in this table are the following comparisons: CTRL 11 dpi vs. CTRL 4 dpi, IBV DMV/1639 4 dpi vs. CTRL 4 dpi, IBV DMV/1639 11 dpi vs. CTRL 11 dpi, IBV DMV/1639 11 dpi vs. IBV DMV/1639 4 dpi, IBV Mass41 4 dpi vs. CTRL 4 dpi, IBV Mass41 11 dpi vs. CTRL 11 dpi, IBV Mass41 11 dpi vs. IBV Mass41 4 dpi. Only the comparisons of the treatment groups and the control groups at the same respective time point were considered (IBV DMV/1639 4 dpi vs. CTRL 4 dpi, IBV DMV/1639 11 dpi vs. CTRL 11 dpi, IBV Mass41 4 dpi vs. CTRL 4 dpi, IBV Mass41 11 dpi vs. CTRL 11 dpi). The results filtered for significantly DE mRNAs (defined by an adjusted *p*-value < 0.05 and a $\log_2FC \geq |1|$) are summarized in Table S7.

The variance in log counts across all tracheal samples, shown in Figure 7a, demonstrates the differences in normalized log counts between the virus-treated groups and uninfected control groups. Among all treatment groups, including IBV DMV/1639- and IBV Mass41-infected samples at 4 dpi and 11 dpi, a total of 751 DE mRNAs were identified (Table S7). Overall, there are a lower number of down-regulated mRNAs as compared to up-regulated mRNAs at both the 4 dpi and 11 dpi time points for both virus strains (Figure 7b). The numbers of DE mRNAs which passed the adjusted *p*-value < 0.05 and $\log_2FC \geq |1|$ thresholds were 479 and 335 DE mRNAs, 25 and 88 down-regulated mRNAs, and 454 and 247 up-regulated mRNAs for the IBV DMV/1639 4 dpi and IBV DMV/1639 11 dpi groups, respectively (Figure 7c,d). Furthermore, 536 and 110 DE mRNAs, 60 and 53 down-regulated mRNAs, and 476 and 57 up-regulated mRNAs were identified for the IBV Mass41 4 dpi and 11 dpi groups, respectively (Figure 7e,f).

Seven down-regulated (Figure 8a) and forty-four up-regulated (Figure 8b) mRNAs were identified in all the treatment groups, for both IBV strains at both time points. Details of the Venn diagram trachea results are summarized in Table S8. The commonly down-regulated mRNAs included contactin-associated protein 1 (CNTNAP1) and fibromodulin (FMOD). On the other hand, the commonly up-regulated mRNAs among all groups included IFI6, MX1, CD8 subunit α (CD8A), CD8 subunit β family member 2 (CD8BP), CD3 δ subunit of T cell receptor complex (CD3D), CD7, IL21R, IL-12 receptor subunit β 2 (IL12RB2), CCL19, CX3C motif chemokine receptor 1 (CX3CR1), C-C chemokine receptor (CCR) 8 (CCR8), chemokine (C motif) ligand (XCL1), STAT1, cytidine/uridine monophosphate kinase 2 (CMPK2), NLRC3, granzyme K (GZMK, ENSGALG00000013546), granzyme A (GZMA), granulysin (GNLY), epithelial stromal interaction 1 (EPSTI1, ENSGALG00000016964), 9L sterile a motif domain-containing 9 like (SAMD9L, ENSGALG00000009479), ζ chain of T cell receptor-associated protein kinase 70 (ZAP70), lymphocyte antigen 6 family member E (LY6E), T cell receptor (TCR) β chain (TCRB, ENSGALG00000014754), cytotoxic and Regulatory T cell molecule (CRTAM), and TCR γ alternate reading frame protein (TARP).

Furthermore, there were 125 mRNAs up-regulated in the IBV DMV/1639 4 dpi and 11 dpi and IBV Mass41 4 dpi groups but not in the IBV Mass41 11 dpi group, which included IRF4, IRF8, STAT4, Burton's tyrosine kinase (BTK), IFI27L2, Eomesodermin (EOMES), LY96, also known as myeloid differentiation factor 2 (MD-2), IL-2 receptor subunit β (IL2RB), IL-2 receptor subunit γ (IL2RG), IL-4 inducible 1 gene (IL4I1), IL7, IL-7 receptor (IL7R), TNFRSF18, TNFR13B, TNFRSF8, CCL21, CCR2, CCR5, CCR7, C-X-C chemokine receptor (CXCR) 4, CXCR5, C-X-C chemokine ligand (CXCL) 13 (CXCL13), CXCL13-like (CXCL13L)

2 (CXCL13L2), and CD proteins (CD247, CD28, CD38, CD3 ε/CD3E, CD4, CD48, CD72, CD74, CD79 β/CD79B, and CD83). In addition, OASL and DDX60 were the only up-regulated mRNAs shared among the IBV DMV/1639 4 dpi and 11 dpi and IBV Mass41 11 dpi groups, and IFIT5 was the only up-regulated mRNA shared among the IBV DMV/1639 4 dpi and IBV Mass41 4 dpi and 11 dpi groups.

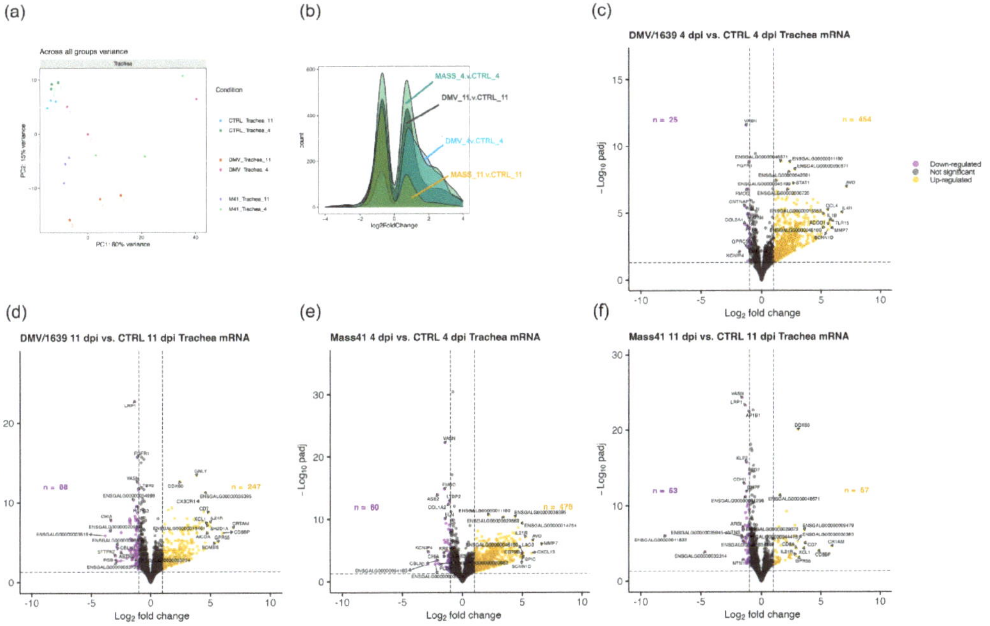

Figure 7. Differential expression of mRNAs in tracheal tissues from chickens infected with IBV DMV/1639 or IBV Mass41. The PCA plot (**a**) evaluates the variance across all samples based on the log counts of all mRNAs. The histogram (**b**) represents the $\log_2$FC distribution of fluorescence signal intensity ratios for DE mRNAs in tracheal tissues from chickens infected with IBV DMV/1639 or IBV Mass41 at 4 dpi and 11 dpi. The volcano plots show DE mRNAs in tracheal tissues from chickens infected with IBV DMV/1639 at 4 (**c**) and 11 dpi (**d**) or IBV Mass41 at 4 (**e**) and 11 dpi (**f**) relative to their respective control groups. The horizontal dotted line represents the adjusted p-value < 0.05 threshold. The vertical dotted lines represent the $\log_2\text{FC} \geq |1|$ ($\text{FC} \geq |2|$) threshold. The x-axis limits are set from −10 to 10 $\log_2$FC. Down-regulated mRNAs are represented by purple data points and up-regulated mRNAs are represented by yellow data points. The list of all up- and down-regulated mRNAs for each treatment group are shown in Table S7.

Few similarities in gene expression were observed between the different time points for each IBV strain. For the IBV DMV/1639-infected tissues, there were two commonly down-regulated mRNAs, namely, fibroblast growth factor receptor 1 (FGFR1) and collagen (COL) type XVI α 1 chain (COL16A1, ENSGALG00000026836), and three commonly up-regulated mRNAs, including placenta-associated 8-like 1 (PLAC8L1) and hepatitis A virus cellular receptor 1 (HAVCR1), also known as T cell immunoglobulin. As for the IBV Mass41-infected groups, COL type I α 2 chain (COL1A2) was the only down-regulated mRNA, and no mRNAs were commonly up-regulated at both the 4 dpi and 11 dpi time points.

At 4 dpi, 4 mRNAs were down-regulated, and 201 mRNAs were up-regulated (the largest intersecting group) in both the IBV DMV/1639 and IBV Mass41-infected groups. Up-regulated mRNAs from this group included IRF1, IRF9, TLR1A, TLR2B, TLR3, TLR4, TLR15, IFIH1 (MDA5), IFN-γ (IFNG), IL-1β, IL-22, IL-6, IL-8, IL10RA, IL18R1, IL-18 receptor accessory protein (IL18RAP), IL-1 receptor 2 (IL1R2), IL-20 receptor subunit α (IL20RA),

IL-22 receptor subunit α 1 and 2 (IL22RA, IL22RA2), IL8L1, TNFRSF25, TNFRSF4, TNFRSF6B, PARP9, RSAD2 (viperin), MOV10, DTX3L, SAMHD1, NLRC5, TNF α-induced protein 3 (TNFAIP3), TNFAIP3-interacting protein 2 (TNIP2), a disintegrin and metalloproteinase (ADAM) domain 8 (ADAM8), Spi-1 proto-oncogene/hematopoietic transcription factor PU.1 (SPI1), Tyrosine-protein kinase Lyn (LYN), negative regulator of reactive oxygen species (NRROS), ACOD1, CCL4, CD proteins (CD180, CD200R1, CD40 molecule-like family member G/CD40LG, and CD72 antigen/CD72AG), complement components (C1QA, C1QB, C1QC, C1R, and C1S), SOCS1, SOCS3, NFKB inhibitor ε (NFKBIE), and helicase with zinc finger domain 2 (HELZ2). At 11 dpi, there were 15 down-regulated mRNAs, including nuclear receptor subfamily 4 group A member 1 (NR4A1), low-density lipoprotein receptor-related protein 1 (LRP1), and epithelial cadherin (CDH1), and 6 up-regulated mRNAs, including activation-induced cytidine deaminase (AICDA) and synaptotagmin Like 3 (SYTL3), common to the IBV DMV/1639- and IBV Mass41-infected groups.

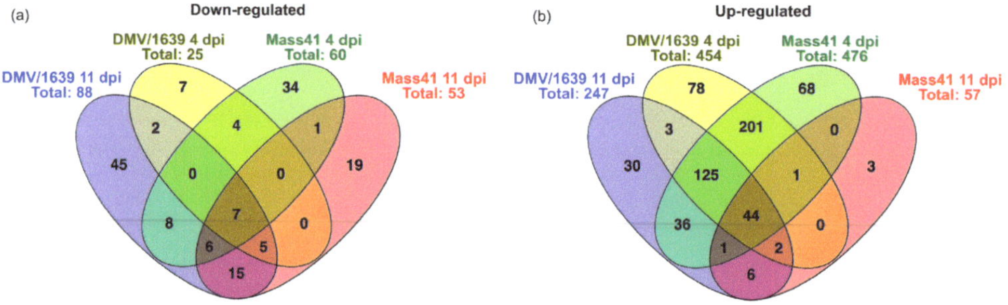

Figure 8. Common and unique DE mRNAs in tracheal tissues from chickens infected with IBV DMV/1639 or IBV Mass41. The Venn diagram shows the common and unique down-regulated (**a**) and up-regulated (**b**) DE mRNAs among tracheal tissues from chickens infected with IBV DMV/1639 or IBV Mass41 at 4 dpi and 11 dpi. Lists of common and unique DE mRNAs are found in Table S8.

In total, 7, 45, 34, and 19 mRNAs were uniquely down-regulated and 78, 30, 68, and 3 mRNAs were uniquely up-regulated in the IBV DMV/1639 4 dpi, IBV DMV/1639 11 dpi, IBV Mass41 4 dpi, and IBV Mass41 11 dpi groups, respectively. The 78 up-regulated mRNAs in the IBV DMV/1639 4 dpi group included IRF7, TLR1B, STAT2, CD80, CD300LG, CXCR1, IFI35, TRIM25, TNFSF10, TRAFD1, ZNFX1, MAP3K8, IKBKE, DHX58 (LPG2), and EIF2AK2 (PKR). The 30 up-regulated mRNAs in the IBV DMV/1639 11 dpi group included CXCL13L3 and zinc finger CCCH-type-containing 12D (ZC3H12D). The 68 up-regulated mRNAs in the IBV Mass41 4 dpi group included TLR2A, TLR7, signal-transducing adaptor family member 1 (STAP1), CD1C, CD86, cytotoxic T-lymphocyte associated protein 4 (CTLA4), phospholipase Cg 2 (PLCG2), IL-12 subunit β (IL12B), CCL20, CCR4, and TNFSF11. Finally, the 22 down-regulated mRNAs in the IBV Mass41 11 dpi group included KLF2 and NR4A2.

Gene ontology (GO) terms associated with the DE mRNAs revealed functional insights into the gene subsets identified for the different treatment groups (Figure 9). Details of the GO functional analyses for DE mRNAs from tracheal samples are compiled in Table S9. Overall, the down-regulated mRNAs from all infected groups relative to the respective control groups were enriched in BP GO terms mainly related to developmental processes and anatomical structures (Figure 9a–d). On the other hand, the top BP GO terms associated with the up-regulated mRNAs from all groups were related to immune system processes (Figure 9e–j). More specifically, at 4 dpi, the top BP GO terms for both the IBV DMV/1639 (Figure 9e) and IBV Mass41 (Figure 9g) groups included regulation of immune system process, defense response, cell activation, and leucocyte activation. At 11 dpi, in terms of the up-regulated mRNAs from the IBV DMV/1639 group (Figure 9f), the top BP GO terms included lymphocyte activation, leucocyte activation, and T cell response. For the up-regulated mRNAs from the IBV Mass41 (Figure 9h) group, the top BP GO terms included defense response, innate immune response, and cytokine-mediated signaling. Furthermore, the top enriched BP GO terms for up-regulated mRNAs found in all treatment groups (Figure 9i) in the 4 dpi groups only (Figure 9j) were associated with immune system processes and defense response.

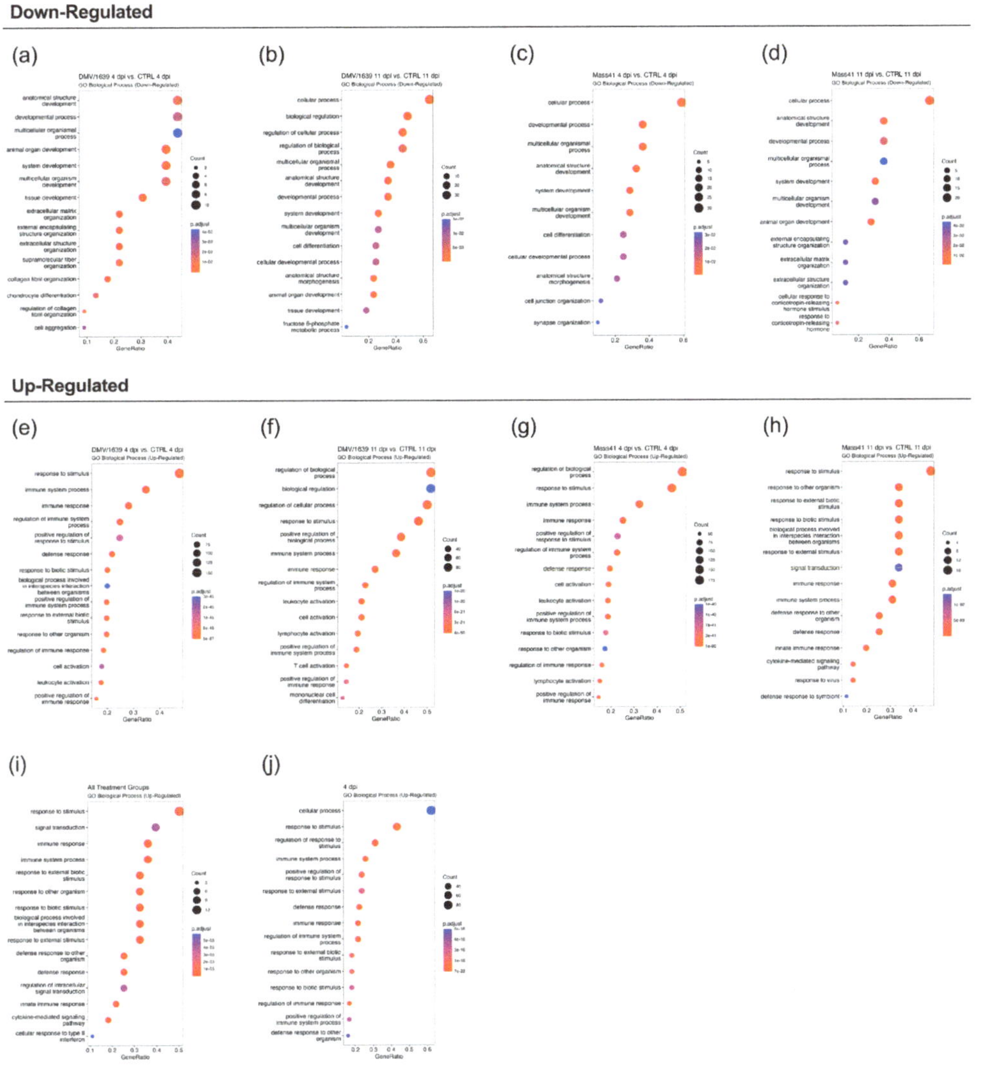

Figure 9. GO functional enrichment analysis for mRNAs in tracheal tissues from chickens infected with IBV DMV/1639 or IBV Mass41. The dot plots represent the enriched GO Biological Process terms for down-regulated mRNAs from the IBV DMV/1639 at 4 dpi (**a**), IBV DMV/1639 at 11 dpi (**b**), IBV Mass41 at 4 dpi (**c**), and IBV Mass41 at 11 dpi (**d**) groups, and for up-regulated mRNAs from the IBV DMV/1639 at 4 dpi (**e**), IBV DMV/1639 at 11 dpi (**f**), IBV Mass41 at 4 dpi (**g**), and IBV Mass41 at 11 dpi (**h**) groups. Enriched GO Biological Process terms for gene subsets common to all treatment groups (**i**) and the 4 dpi groups (**j**) are also shown. Count is the number of genes enriched in a GO term and GeneRatio is the percentage of total DE mRNAs in the given GO term. The color intensities represent the adjusted *p*-values. Full details for mRNA GO enrichment analysis are found in Table S9.

Upon further KEGG pathway analysis, all treatment groups were found to be enriched for the cytokine–cytokine receptor interaction and cell adhesion molecule pathways (Table S9). The enriched pathways for both 4 dpi groups included TLR signaling, necroptosis, NOD-like receptor signaling, retinoic acid-inducible gene I (RIG-I)-like receptor signaling, apoptosis, and cytosolic DNA sensing. The p53 signaling pathway was enriched for the IBV DMV/1639 4 dpi group only, while the regulation of actin cytoskeleton and focal adhesion pathways was enriched for the IBV Mass41 4 dpi group only. The IBV DMV/1639 11 dpi group was also enriched for cell adhesion molecules, endocytosis, and C-type lectin receptor signaling pathways, while the IBV Mass41 11 dpi group for cell adhesion molecules and extracellular matrix (ECM)–receptor interaction pathways. Enrichment and expression of the specific components in the TLR signaling (Figure 10a,b) and cytokine–cytokine receptor interaction (Figure 10c,d) pathways are shown for the IBV DMV/1639 4 dpi and IBV Mass41 4 dpi treatment groups. The pathway enrichment analysis revealed that several DE genes are common to both 4 dpi groups, but some important differences are observed. For example, IKBKE, IRF7, and STAT2 are up-regulated in the IBV DMV/1639 4 dpi group but not in the IBV Mass41 4 dpi group.

IBV DMV/1639 4 dpi vs. CTRL 4 dpi

(a)

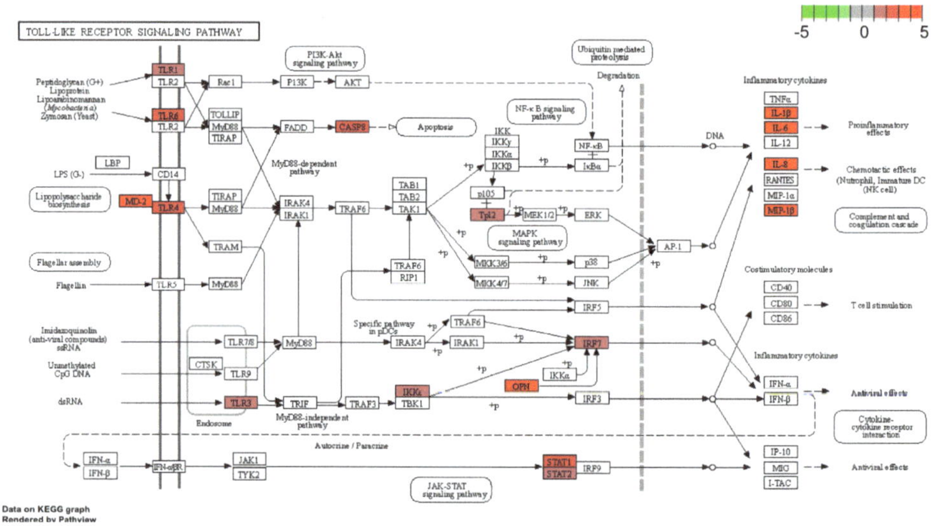

Figure 10. *Cont.*

IBV Mass41 4 dpi vs. CTRL 4 dpi

(b)

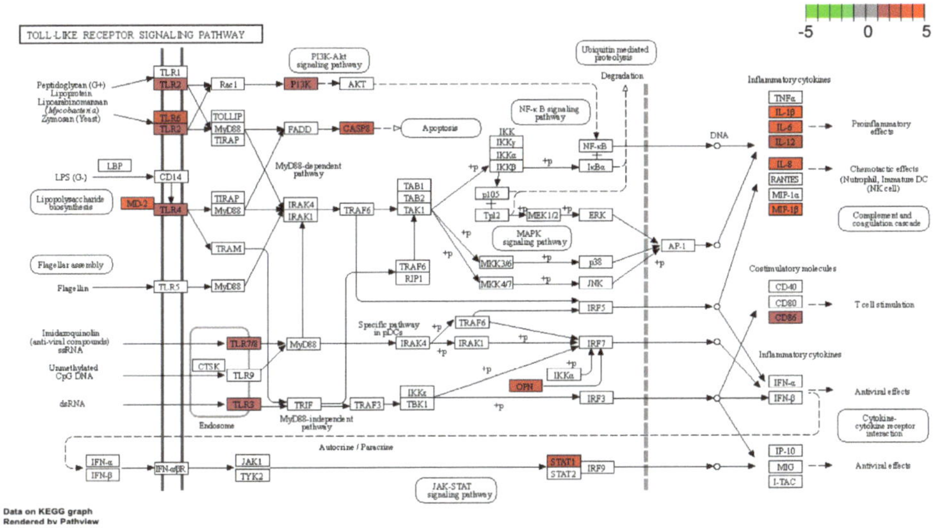

IBV DMV/1639 4 dpi vs. CTRL 4 dpi

(c)

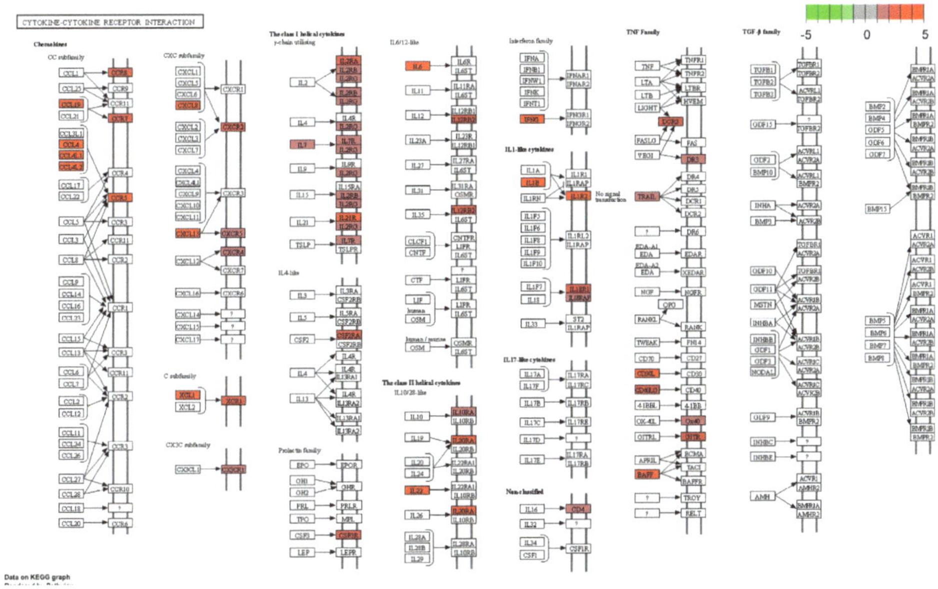

Figure 10. *Cont.*

IBV Mass41 4 dpi vs. CTRL 4 dpi

(d)

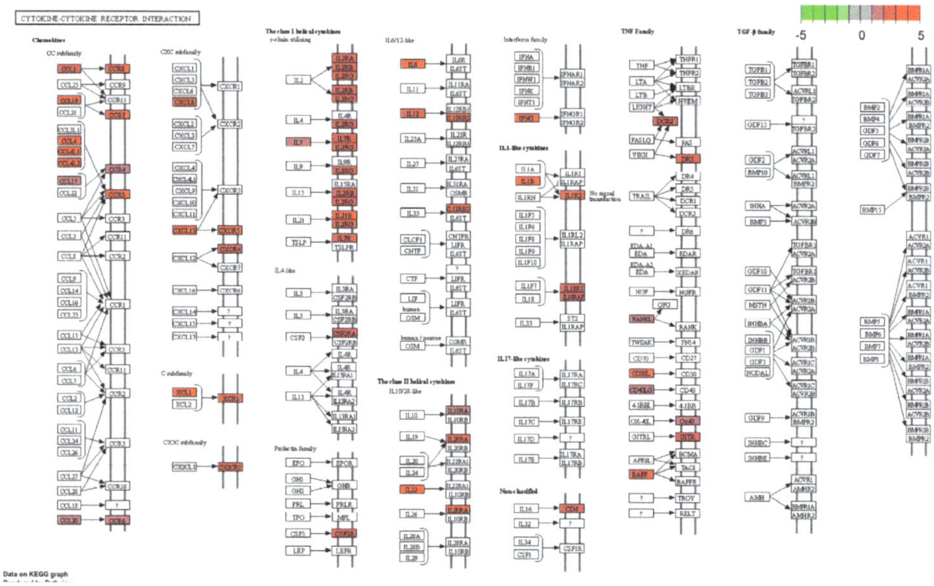

Figure 10. KEGG pathway analysis for DE mRNAs in tracheal tissues from chickens infected with IBV DMV/1639 or IBV Mass41. DE genes in the enriched KEGG pathways are shown for IBV DMV/1639 4 dpi TLR signaling (**a**), IBV Mass41 4 dpi TLR signaling (**b**), IBV DMV/1639 4 dpi cytokine-cytokine receptor interaction (**c**), and IBV Mass41 4 dpi cytokine-cytokine receptor interaction (**d**). KEGG pathway analysis figures were generated using the R package pathview. The color intensities represent the expression levels of the DE mRNAs identified in the RNA-seq analysis. Full details for mRNA KEGG enrichment analysis are found in Table S9.

3.4. Comparisons of DE mRNAs in In Vitro and In Vivo Infection Models

Overall, upon comparing the expression patterns in in vitro and in vivo RNA-seq datasets, a total of 162 DE mRNAs were found to be common to both infection models in at least one treatment group (Table S10). In total, 21 of these DE mRNAs were down-regulated and 141 were up-regulated. The down-regulated mRNAs included kelch-like family member 30 (KLHL30), KLF2, NR4A1, and NR4A2. Up-regulated mRNAs included SAMHD1, NLRC5, TRAFD1, IL18R1, IL-6, IRF7, IRF1, ACOD1, TRIM25, CCL4, DDX60, DHX58 (LPG2), TLR3, STAT1, STAT2, PARP9, IFIH1 (MDA5), CD38, LY96 (MD-2), SOCS1, RSAD2 (viperin), EIF2AK2 (PKR), OASL, MX1, CMPK2, IFIT5, and sodium channel epithelial 1 subunit δ (SCNN1D).

More specifically, Figure 11 illustrates the gene overlaps at the early time points post-infection, 3 h (in vitro), or 4 dpi (in vivo), for down-regulated (Figure 11a) and up-regulated (Figure 11b) mRNAs and at the late time points post-infection, 18 h or 11 dpi, for down-regulated (Figure 11c) and up-regulated (Figure 11d) mRNAs, for both IBV infection models. At the earlier time points post-infection, we did not observe any overlap with down-regulated mRNAs; however, 27 up-regulated mRNAs were common to all early treatment groups, including TLR3, IFIT5, IFIH1 (MDA5), MX1, RSAD2 (viperin), CMPK2, SOCS1, and SCNN1D. Two mRNAs were down-regulated in all treatment groups at the later time points post-infection, namely, CNTNAP1 and NR4A1, while twenty mRNAs were up-regulated in all later time point treatment groups, including IFI6, LY6E, MX1, OASL, STAT1, and CMPK2.

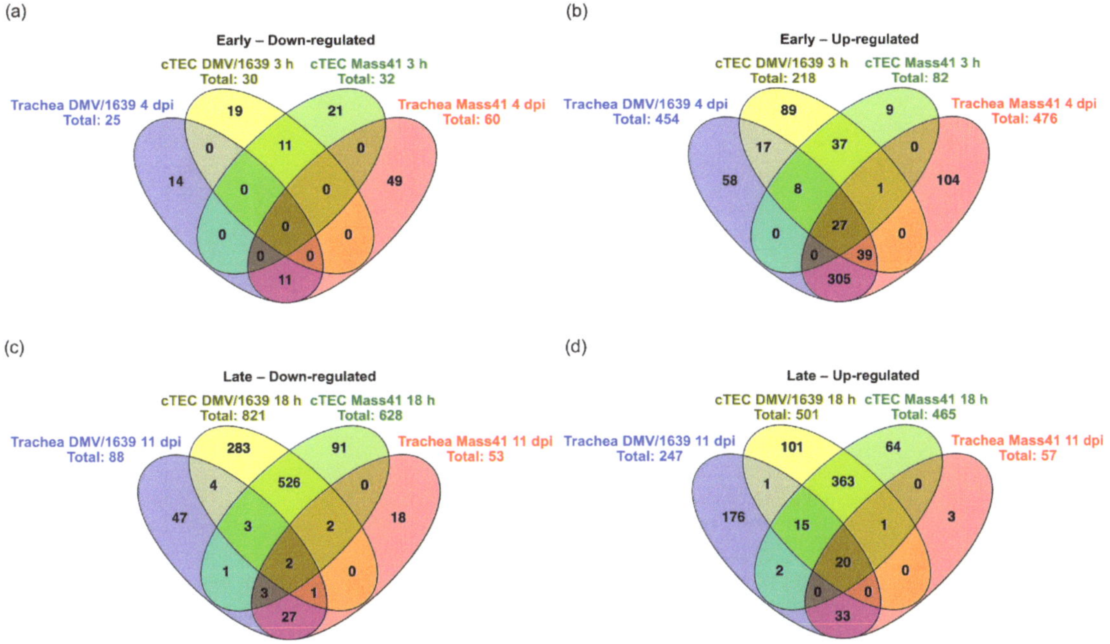

Figure 11. Common and unique DE mRNAs from cTECs and the trachea in the context of IBV DMV/1639 or IBV Mass41 infection at early and late time points post-infection. The Venn diagram illustrates common and unique down-regulated (**a**) and up-regulated (**b**) mRNAs at the early time points post-infection and down-regulated (**c**) and up-regulated (**d**) at the late time points post-infection. Lists of common and unique DE mRNAs are found in Table S10.

Although we observed these important overlaps in gene expression among the two infection models, 938 down-regulated mRNAs and 567 up-regulated mRNAs were identified in the IBV-infected cTECs only. Down-regulated mRNAs included SLC6A4, PPP4R4, TRAF3, JUN, and NFKBIA. Up-regulated mRNAs included IFITM5, ADAR, and MOV10. In contrast, we observed 132 down-regulated mRNAs and 457 up-regulated mRNAs in the IBV-infected tracheal tissues only. COL1A2, COL2A1, COL16A1, elastin (ELN), and LRP1 were among the down-regulated mRNAs and TLR4, TLR7, CCR2, CCL17, CCL20, IL-22, NLRC3, IFN-γ, GZMA, and GNLY were among the up-regulated mRNAs. Finally, we observed some cases of differential dysregulation for certain mRNAs in vitro versus in vivo. For example, CDH1 was up-regulated in the cTEC IBV DMV/1639 and IBV Mass41 18 h groups, but down-regulated in the trachea IBV DMV/1639 and IBV Mass41 11 dpi groups. IL-1β and SOCS3, on the other hand, were down-regulated in the cTEC IBV DMV/1639 and IBV Mass41 18 h groups and up-regulated in the tracheas of IBV DMV/1639- and IBV Mass41-infected 4 dpi groups.

3.5. Host mRNA Gene Expression Validation

To validate the RNA-seq results, qPCR was performed to detect expression of a subset of DE mRNAs using tracheal samples from IBV DMV/1639-infected chickens. Three down-regulated and four up-regulated mRNAs were selected, and the relative expression of these genes was measured (Table 1). The qPCR results demonstrate that the patterns of host mRNA expression are similar to the patterns determined by RNA-seq, with little variation in the magnitude of the expressions.

Table 1. Comparison of host mRNA expression fold-changes (FC) of selected genes between RNA-seq and qPCR in tracheas from IBV DMV/1639-infected chickens relative to the uninfected control group at 4 dpi and 11 dpi.

		IBV DMV/1639 4 dpi		**IBV DMV/1639 11 dpi**	
	Gene	**RNA-Seq FC**	**qPCR FC**	**RNA-Seq FC**	**qPCR FC**
Down-regulated	KLHL30	−1.012	−3.230	−1.147	−1.826
	FMOD	−2.283	−2.987	−2.181	−1.401
	NR4A1	−1.005	−3.131	−2.516	−2.829
Up-regulated	SOCS1	6.538	3.030	1.057	1.633
	TLR3	2.192	1.697	1.704	1.061
	STAT1	6.167	1.636	2.635	1.168
	STAT2	2.749	4.224	1.141	2.269

4. Discussion

Understanding the different factors which can affect the underlying mechanisms of IBV pathogenesis, particularly at the primary site of infection, airway epithelial cells, is key in developing new strategies for IBV control. In the present study, we aimed to characterize the induction of the antiviral response following IBV infection in vitro and in vivo. We expected that IBV infection would impact the overall induction and initiation of the host immune responses and wanted to investigate the specific factors and mediators involved. First, we demonstrated that IBV DMV/1639 and IBV Mass41 replicate in cTECs in vitro and in the trachea in vivo and induce strain- and time-dependent expression of host mRNAs. Second, these observations also provided insight into the regulation of expressed transcripts involved in immune system signaling pathways upon IBV infection of cTECs and the trachea. Finally, we demonstrated the differences in gene expression patterns between in vitro and in vivo tracheal IBV infection models.

Tracheal organ culture has long been used to investigate IBV infection [106–112]. While this ex vivo model offers many benefits, understanding the mechanisms specifically at the level of tracheal epithelial cells is useful for studying immediate host responses under highly controlled conditions. Our findings shed light on the replication dynamics of IBV in cTECs, providing valuable insights into host–pathogen interactions under specific conditions. Both IBV DMV/1639 and IBV Mass41 strains demonstrated a comparable replication capability in this in vitro model. Few studies have evaluated IBV infection in cTEC models, despite the significance of airway epithelial cells as the primary target for IBV during initial infection. Shen and colleagues established a primary cTEC culture system as a means to study viral cytopathogenesis and showed that these cells were susceptible to IBV Taiwan (TW)-type infection [65]. In addition, Kint and colleagues infected cTECs with IBV Mass41-type to demonstrate the delayed induction of the type I IFN response [36]. The latter two studies did not provide data of IBV replication kinetics that can be used for comparison of our IBV replication kinetic data. Although the cTECs were closely monitored for growth and viability over the course of the experiments, a cell viability assay to confirm our visual observations would be an important addition for future work.

Generally, the in vivo inoculation doses of IBV used in this study, low (10^4 EID_{50}/bird) and high (10^5 EID_{50}/bird), did not have an impact on the viral genome load detected in the trachea. This 10-fold difference in IBV inoculation dose may not be enough to see a difference in resulting viral genome load in the trachea. Several similar studies infecting young or adult chickens with IBV use an inoculation dose of 10^6 EID_{50}/bird [24,113,114] and we may have seen greater differences between the groups if this upper limit had been used for the high dose. Typically, the highest concentration of IBV is found in the trachea at 3–5 dpi; however, IBV has been detected as early as 3 dpi in various tissues [115]. As a result, we chose the 4 dpi time point and a later time point of 11 dpi for sample collection. Given that the upper respiratory tract of the chicken is known to mount strong innate antiviral responses against invading respiratory pathogens [6,64,116], the significant decrease (p-value < 0.05) in viral genome load from 4 dpi to 11 dpi in the trachea for the high-dose IBV DMV/1639 and low-dose IBV Mass41 groups may indicate the dissemination of the virus to establish infection and persist at distal sites.

Previously, RNA-seq analyses have been conducted studying the interaction between IBV strains such as Beaudette, Mass41 strains [49], and K047-12 [51] in chicken kidney cells and focused on only one time point following IBV inoculation. Our data are different since we focused on cTECs involved at the IBV entry site (respiratory mucosa) and included an additional IBV strain which has recently become endemic in North America, IBV DMV/1639 [21,22]. Furthermore, we included an early time point and a later time point for both of our in vitro and in vivo studies, which allowed us to observe changes in host transcripts over the course of IBV infection in different models. The mRNA expression profiles of IBV DMV/1639- or IBV Mass41-infected cTECs or tracheas provide evidence that there are distinct interactions between the IBV strains and the host. Collection time points further separate expression profiles, indicating a switch in gene expression from a naïve to activated antiviral state.

Dinan and colleagues observed 579 up-regulated and 132 down-regulated genes in response to IBV Beaudette and Mass41 strains in kidney cells 24 h following infection [49], whereas Lee and colleagues observed 787 up-regulated and 297 down-regulated genes in response to IBV K047-12 infection in kidney cells 48 h following infection [51]. In comparison, we observed 30 (3 h) and 821 (18 h) down-regulated genes, and 218 (3 h) and 501 (18 h) up-regulated genes, for IBV DMV/1639 infection of cTECs and 32 (3 h) and 628 (18 h) down-regulated genes, and 82 (3 h) and 465 (18 h) up-regulated genes, for IBV Mass41 infection of cTECs. Another 2013 microarray study by Cong and colleagues determined that IL6, STAT1, MYD88, and IRF1, all of which were present in our IBV-infected cTEC data, were key genes in chicken kidneys during IBV infection [47]. Our data show more genes are turned on or off as the infection progresses from 3 h to 18 h in cTECs following IBV DMV/1639 or IBV Mass41 infection. This is expected, as viral infection disturbs the host homeostasis, triggering the activation of several downstream signaling pathways and factors involved in host defense against the invading pathogen [117,118].

Downstream of TLR and ligand engagement, two pathways can be activated: MYD88-dependent and MYD88-independent pathways [119]. In the current study, we observed that the MYD88 gene is enriched following IBV DMV/1639 infection at 3 h and IBV Mass41 infection at 18 h. Previously, it has been shown that IBV infection in kidneys and trachea up-regulates MYD88 expression [47,68]. Up-regulation of IRF7, which is expressed downstream of both MYD88-dependent and MYD88-independent pathways, was evident following IBV infection in cTECs. This agrees with the previous observation in tracheas of resistant and susceptible lines of chickens following IBV infection [43]. One of the antiviral cytokines enriched during IBV infection in cTECs is IFNβ and this cytokine is up-regulated downstream of TLR3 and IRF7 activation [120,121]. Our data provide evidence that IBV infection also up-regulates TLR3 and IRF7 genes in cTEC.

KEGG pathway analyses at the later time point (18 h) indicating enrichment for the innate immune response, particularly for the TLR signaling pathway following infection with IBV DMV/1639 or IBV Mass41, is not surprising. The replication of IBV in cTECs leads to availability of double-stranded RNA intermediates within cTECs (TLR3 ligand) and the increased TLR3 we observed has been recorded in trachea following IBV infections [38,68]. The increased gene expression of TLR21 following IBV DMV/1639 infection of cTECs at 3 h is difficult to explain since the TLR21 ligand is CpG (cytosine followed by guanine residues) DNA and IBV is an RNA virus [122,123]; however, there is evidence that CpG DNA can activate the innate immune response to suppress IBV replication in ovo [124], which suggests this sensor may play an unknown role during viral infection. In Lee and colleague's IBV work in kidney cells, up-regulation of TLR7 has been recorded at 48 h following infection [51]. However, we did not see TLR7 up-regulation with IBV strains in cTECs and, potentially, this discrepancy may be related to the IBV strain used and differences in host cells and observed time points.

On the other hand, in the trachea, we observed 25 (4 dpi) and 88 (11 dpi) down-regulated mRNAs, and 454 (4 dpi) and 247 (11 dpi) up-regulated mRNAs, for the IBV DMV/1639 group, and 60 (4 dpi) and 53 (11 dpi) down-regulated mRNAs, and 476 (4 dpi) and 57 (11 dpi) up-regulated mRNAs, for the IBV Mass41 group in vivo. Smith and colleagues identified several important DE genes in IBV Mass41-infected tracheal tissues from susceptible and resistant birds, such as TLR3, IRF7, STAT1, IFIH1 (MDA5), MX1, IFIT5, and OASL, which were also up-regulated in our IBV-infected tracheal tissue data [43]. Ghobadian and colleagues indicated that the Iranian variant-2-like IBV strain IS/1494 induced variable host gene expression in different chicken hybrid tracheal tissues but also demonstrated the importance of certain genes such as TLR3, IFIH1 (MDA5), and IRF7 and the enrichment of the TLR signaling pathways [45]. Many of the important genes mentioned in the studies above and found in our DE gene data emphasize the importance of ISGs. For example, in chickens, IFIT5 is expressed downstream of IFNβ expression following IBV infection in kidneys [125] and is known to sequester viral RNA impacting viral replication [126]. In other host–viral models, it has been observed that IFIT5 induces innate responses effective against viral infections [127].

Similar to the results for our cTEC data, KEGG pathway analyses indicated enrichment for the innate immune response. Once again, the enrichment of the cytokine–cytokine interaction pathway for all in vivo treatment groups is not surprising given that the significant involvement of pro-inflammatory cytokines during IBV infection has been well documented [7,128–131].

There is a large interest in understanding IBV immunopathogenesis in reproductive organs due to the detrimental impact of certain strains, including IBV DMV/1639 and IBV Mass-type strains, on the reproductive tracts. The strains used in our study are different in terms of their pathogenesis and specific tissue tropism. Decoding the mechanisms during initial infection may help to explain these differences. Recently, Farooq and colleagues showed that tracheal lesions in IBV Mass-type-infected chickens are more severe than those in IBV DMV/1639-infected chickens, while misshaped eggs or eggs with soft shells were only observed with IBV DMV/1639-infected chickens [59]. The differences in gene expression observed for our different strains may be related to the variable aspects of pathogenicity observed. For example, for cTECs at 3 h, the IBV DMV/1639 group is enriched in a higher number of immune signaling pathways compared to the IBV Mass41 group. Moreover, TGFβ signaling has several roles, including in re-epithelization and inflammation [132] and the enrichment of TGFβ signaling in the IBV Mass41 18 h group, but not the IBV DMV/1639 18 h group, may explain the difference in severity of the tracheal lesions mentioned above. Similarly, for the tracheal tissues at 11 dpi, the IBV DMV/1639 group is associated with more immune signaling pathways compared to the IBV Mass41 group, supporting what was observed in cTECs in vitro. It is important to acknowledge that the differences in enriched KEGG pathways is somewhat dependent on the different number of DE genes between the treatment groups, which may introduce a potential bias, and that the variable number of DE genes may be due small differences in replication kinetics in host cells or tissues. Furthermore, this is the first transcriptomics study evaluating the mRNA expression profiles during IBV DMV/1639 infection and future studies are needed to evaluate the expression profiles in different tissues and at other time points of infection.

While our in vitro and in vivo models for IBV infection provided insights into mRNA host response regulation in their own respect, this study also allows us to have a head-to-head comparison of the infection models for the same strains. Overall, there were 1653 DE mRNA in cTECs and 751 DE mRNA in the trachea for all treatment groups. Although cell culture systems are considered reliable platforms for studying anything from cell behavior to detailed molecular mechanisms, it is not surprising that we see differences between our infection models at different time points. The most evident difference between our models is that the tracheal tissues are a mix of different cells and connective tissues, while the cTEC model is a monolayer of isolated tracheal epithelial cells. It has long been known that the modulation of gene expression in vitro versus in vivo is distinct [133]. In the in vivo model, we reported the down-regulation of ECM components such as collagens and elastin. As the main fibers of the ECM, these components are important for the structural support in cells and tissues [134] and are linked to the regulation of epithelial cell function [135]. The down-regulation of these ECM genes in the trachea may be explained by the IBV-induced epithelial changes in the respiratory tract resulting in a loss of ciliary activity and tracheitis [2]. Furthermore, we observed up-regulated IFN-γ, a type II IFN, in the trachea in vivo. IFN-γ leads to the activation of the antiviral response through the Janus kinase (JAK–STAT signaling pathway [136]. Kameka and colleagues showed an initial IBV-induced down-regulation of IFN-γ in the trachea and lungs of chickens [68] and Ma and colleagues reported that IBV nsp14 targets JAK1 to inhibit JAK-STAT signaling in chicken macrophages, but also highlighted the importance of IFN-γ anti-IBV activity through the induction of ISG expression [137], suggesting that the increase in IFN-γ expression in the trachea may play a role in the antiviral response in the upper respiratory tract.

Furthermore, infection and sample collection time points are vastly different based on the nature of the model systems. These expression profiles can only give us a snapshot in time as the antiviral response against IBV progresses. Nevertheless, 21 down-regulated mRNAs and 141 up-regulated mRNAs are common to both the cTEC and trachea infection models. TLR3, IFIH1 (MDA5), SOCS1, OASL, DDX60, STAT1, MX1, CMPK2, LY96 (MD-2), STAT1, STAT2, TRIM25, IRF7, and IFIT5 are among the up-regulated genes, many of which have been identified as key genes in previous transcriptomic IBV studies mentioned above. In addition, SCNN1D was commonly up-regulated for all treatment groups across the cTEC and trachea data. In multi-ciliated cells, the epithelial sodium channel is located in cilia and plays an essential role in the regulation of epithelial surface liquid volume necessary for cilial transport of mucus [138]. In our study, the up-regulation of SCNN1D potentially contributes to enhanced mucous production in the trachea and the upper respiratory tract following IBV infection [114,139–141]. Finally, MX1 and CMPK2 are up-regulated in all treatment groups across both in vitro and in vivo studies. MX1 is an ISG known to have antiviral activity against a wide range of RNA viruses [142,143]. CMPK2, on the other hand, can act as a host restriction factor to inhibit the replication of coronaviruses, including IBV [144,145].

RNA-seq is a powerful tool and host transcriptomic data can be used to evaluate the effect of pathogen variants on the host mRNA signature to identify key hallmarks of the resulting disease [146]. With IBV, characterizing the expression of specific host antiviral factors may be useful for monitoring the disease and distinct pathogenesis induced by different IBV strains. Additional studies are needed, but the differences in gene expression induced by IBV DMV/1639 and IBV Mass41 in this study could be correlated with the well-documented differences in pathogenesis [24,59,147]. Taken together, these host mRNA expression profiles provide an overview of the response to IBV infection. Furthermore, we identified key genes that may play a role in regulating IBV infection. In future studies, these candidate genes must be verified at the protein expression level by conducting proteomics screening studies, for example. Furthermore, the specific functions of these candidate genes could be assessed by silencing their expression through RNA interference (RNAi) experiments in the context of IBV infection, followed by validation of these results in vivo. This work would help to correlate differential gene expression with strain-specific tissue tropism, virulence, and immune responses observed both in the laboratory and field settings. Overall, this study provides a useful framework for examining IBV infection in tracheal epithelial cells, which could have significant implications for understanding and treating viral respiratory infections.

5. Conclusions

Transcriptomic data revealed important patterns of expression key to uncovering relevant factors in host responses during infection. We reported a total of 248, 1322, 114, and 1093 DE mRNAs for IBV DMV/1639 at 3 h, IBV DMV/1639 at 18 h, IBV Mass41 at 3 h, and IBV Mass41 at 18 h post-infection, respectively, and a total of 479, 335, 536, and 110 DE mRNAs for the IBV DMV/1639 4 dpi, IBV DMV/1639 11 dpi, IBV Mass41 4 dpi, and IBV Mass41 11 dpi groups, respectively. The findings provide insights into strain-specific and temporal-related changes in gene expression, which could be valuable in understanding the molecular mechanisms underlying IBV infection.

We identified important genes DE in both our in vitro and in vivo infection models consistent with previous studies, namely, TLR3, IFIH1 (MDA5), SOCS1, OASL, DDX60, STAT1, MX1, CMPK2, LY96 (MD-2), STAT1, STAT2, TRIM25, IRF7, and IFIT5. Furthermore, we characterized key variations in gene expression in the trachea unique to the in vivo model, such as changes in collagen, elastin, TLR4, TLR7, CCR2, CCL17, and IFN-γ expression. Future studies should confirm expression of these genes at the protein level. Overall, the study highlights the complexity of host–virus interactions and emphasizes the importance of investigating gene expression changes over time to uncover the dynamics of the infection process.

Supplementary Materials: The following supporting information can be downloaded at: https://www.mdpi.com/article/10.3390/v16040605/s1, Figure S1: cTEC_heatmaps; Figure S2: trachea_heatmaps; Table S1: Primers_for_qPCR; Table S2: All_DEGs_mRNA_cTEC_in_vitro; Table S3: Filtered_DEGs_mRNA_cTEC_in_vitro; Table S4: venn_results_cTEC_in_vitro_mRNA; Table S5: GO_KEGG_mRNA_cTEC_in_vitro; Table S6: All_DEGs_mRNA_trachea_in_vivo; Table S7: Filtered_DEGs_mRNA_trachea_in_vivo; Table S8: venn_results_trachea_in_vivo_mRNA; Table S9: GO_KEGG_mRNA_trachea_in_vivo; Table S10: cTEC_trachea_all_mRNA_overlap.

Author Contributions: Conceptualization, M.F.A.-C., N.B., C.A.G., C.M.D. and M.B.; Methodology, M.F.A.-C., N.B., C.A.G., C.M.D., M.B., K.O. and I.M.I.; Formal analysis, M.F.A.-C., N.B., K.O. and I.M.I.; Investigation, M.F.A.-C., N.B., K.O., I.M.I. and S.V.; Resources, M.F.A.-C., N.B., C.A.G., C.M.D. and M.B.; Data curation, K.O., M.F.A.-C. and N.B.; Writing—original draft, K.O., M.F.A.-C. and N.B.; Writing—review and editing, M.F.A.-C., N.B., C.A.G., C.M.D., M.B. and K.O.; Visualization, K.O.; Supervision, Project administration and Funding acquisition, M.F.A.-C., N.B., C.A.G., C.M.D. and M.B. All authors have read and agreed to the published version of the manuscript.

Funding: Kelsey O'Dowd was a recipient of a scholarship from the Swine and Poultry Infectious Diseases Research Centre (CRIPA), a research network financially supported by the Fonds de recherche du Québec (FRQ). Operational funding from Natural Sciences and Engineering Research Council of Canada (NSERC) grant no. 10038035, Livestock Research Innovation Corporation (LRIC) grant no. 10037305, Egg Farmers of Canada (EFC) grant no. 10036252, Canadian Poultry Research Council (CPRC) grant no. 10039973, Ministère de l'Agriculture, des Pêcheries et de l'Alimentation du Québec (MAPAQ) Innov'Action program grant no. IA120588 is acknowledged.

Institutional Review Board Statement: The experimental protocols were approved by the Institutional Animal Care and Use Committee (IACUC) of the Université de Montréal (ethics protocol no. 21-Rech-2120), the Institut national de la recherche scientifique (INRS) (ethics protocol no. 2106-03), and the Veterinary Science Animal Care Committee (VSACC) and the Health Science Animal Care Committee (HSACC) of the University of Calgary (ethics protocol no. AC22-0012).

Data Availability Statement: All relevant data are provided within the paper and the Supplementary Files or available upon request. The datasets generated during this study are available in the Sequence Read Archive (SRA), BioProject PRJNA1088470.

Acknowledgments: We would like to acknowledge Chantale Provost's contribution from the Université de Montréal Diagnostics Laboratory for the whole genome sequencing and annotation of the IBV Mass41 strain. Our appreciation also goes to the animal facilities and their dedicated staff at both the National Experimental Biology Laboratory (NEBL) of the Institut national de la recherche scientifique (INRS) Armand-Frappier Santé Biotechnologie Research Centre and the Veterinary Science Research Station (VSRS), Spyhill Campus, University of Calgary, whose support was essential to our research.

We are grateful to François Lefebvre and Gerardo Zapata at the McGill University Canadian Centre for Computational Genomics (C3G) for their expert assistance in RNA-seq data analysis and insights throughout the project.

Conflicts of Interest: The authors declare no financial or non-financial conflicts of interest related to this work. The current affiliation with Zoetis is provided for transparency.

References

1. Jackwood, M.W.; de Wit, S. Infectious Bronchitis. In *Diseases of Poultry*; Wiley-Blackwell: Hoboken, NJ, USA, 2020; pp. 167–188.
2. Ignjatovic, J.; Sapats, S. Avian infectious bronchitis virus. *Rev. Sci. Tech.* **2000**, *19*, 493–508. [CrossRef] [PubMed]
3. Abdel-Moneim, A.S. Coronaviridae: Infectious Bronchitis Virus. In *Emerging and Re-Emerging Infectious Diseases of Livestock*; Springer International Publishing: Cham, Switzerland, 2017; pp. 133–166.
4. Hofstad, M.S.; Yoder, H.W., Jr. Avian infectious bronchitis: Virus distribution in tissues of chicks. *Avian Dis.* **1966**, *10*, 230–239. [CrossRef] [PubMed]
5. Cavanagh, D. Coronavirus avian infectious bronchitis virus. *Vet. Res.* **2007**, *38*, 281–297. [CrossRef] [PubMed]
6. Najimudeen, S.M.; Hassan, M.S.H.; Cork, S.C.; Abdul-Careem, M.F. Infectious Bronchitis Coronavirus Infection in Chickens: Multiple System Disease with Immune Suppression. *Pathogens* **2020**, *9*, 779. [CrossRef] [PubMed]
7. Najimudeen, S.M.; Abd-Elsalam, R.M.; Ranaweera, H.A.; Isham, I.M.; Hassan, M.S.H.; Farooq, M.; Abdul-Careem, M.F. Replication of infectious bronchitis virus (IBV) Delmarva (DMV)/1639 variant in primary and secondary lymphoid organs leads to immunosuppression in chickens. *Virology* **2023**, *587*, 109852. [CrossRef] [PubMed]
8. Ambali, A.G.; Jones, R.C. Early Pathogenesis in Chicks of Infection with an Enterotropic Strain of Infectious Bronchitis Virus. *Avian Dis.* **1990**, *34*, 809–817. [CrossRef] [PubMed]
9. Fan, W.Q.; Wang, H.N.; Zhang, Y.; Guan, Z.B.; Wang, T.; Xu, C.W.; Zhang, A.Y.; Yang, X. Comparative dynamic distribution of avian infectious bronchitis virus M41, H120, and SAIBK strains by quantitative real-time RT-PCR in SPF chickens. *Biosci. Biotechnol. Biochem.* **2012**, *76*, 2255–2260. [CrossRef] [PubMed]
10. Cook, J.K.A. Duration of Experimental Infectious Bronchitis in Chickens. *Res. Vet. Sci.* **1968**, *9*, 506–514. [CrossRef] [PubMed]
11. Amarasinghe, A.; Abdul-Cader, M.S.; Nazir, S.; De Silva Senapathi, U.; van der Meer, F.; Cork, S.C.; Gomis, S.; Abdul-Careem, M.F. Infectious bronchitis corona virus establishes productive infection in avian macrophages interfering with selected antimicrobial functions. *PLoS ONE* **2017**, *12*, e0181801. [CrossRef] [PubMed]
12. Reddy, V.R.; Trus, I.; Desmarets, L.M.; Li, Y.; Theuns, S.; Nauwynck, H.J. Productive replication of nephropathogenic infectious bronchitis virus in peripheral blood monocytic cells, a strategy for viral dissemination and kidney infection in chickens. *Vet. Res.* **2016**, *47*, 70. [CrossRef] [PubMed]
13. Chong, K.T.; Apostolov, K. The pathogenesis of nephritis in chickens induced by infectious bronchitis virus. *J. Comp. Pathol.* **1982**, *92*, 199–211. [CrossRef] [PubMed]
14. Sevoian, M.; Levine, P.P. Effects of Infectious Bronchitis on the Reproductive Tracts, Egg Production, and Egg Quality of Laying Chickens. *Avian Dis.* **1957**, *1*, 136–164. [CrossRef]
15. McMartin, D.A. The pathogenicity of an infectious bronchitis virus for laying hens, with observations on pathogenesis. *Br. Vet. J.* **1968**, *124*, 576–581. [CrossRef] [PubMed]
16. Cook, J.K.A.; Huggins, M.B. Newly isolated Serotypes of infectious bronchitis virus: Their role in disease. *Avian Pathol.* **1986**, *15*, 129–138. [CrossRef] [PubMed]
17. Sjaak de Wit, J.J.; Cook, J.K.; van der Heijden, H.M. Infectious bronchitis virus variants: A review of the history, current situation and control measures. *Avian Pathol.* **2011**, *40*, 223–235. [CrossRef] [PubMed]
18. Jackwood, M.W.; Hall, D.; Handel, A. Molecular evolution and emergence of avian gammacoronaviruses. *Infect. Genet. Evol.* **2012**, *12*, 1305–1311. [CrossRef] [PubMed]
19. Jordan, B. Vaccination against infectious bronchitis virus: A continuous challenge. *Vet. Microbiol.* **2017**, *206*, 137–143. [CrossRef] [PubMed]
20. Gelb, J., Jr.; Ladman, B.S.; Pope, C.R.; Ruano, J.M.; Brannick, E.M.; Bautista, D.A.; Coughlin, C.M.; Preskenis, L.A. Characterization of nephropathogenic infectious bronchitis virus DMV/1639/11 recovered from Delmarva broiler chickens in 2011. *Avian Dis.* **2013**, *57*, 65–70. [CrossRef]
21. Hassan, M.S.H.; Ojkic, D.; Coffin, C.S.; Cork, S.C.; van der Meer, F.; Abdul-Careem, M.F. Delmarva (DMV/1639) Infectious Bronchitis Virus (IBV) Variants Isolated in Eastern Canada Show Evidence of Recombination. *Viruses* **2019**, *11*, 1054. [CrossRef]
22. Martin, E.; Brash, M.; Stalker, M.; Ojkić, D. Using phylogenetic analysis to examine the changing strains of infectious bronchitis virus infections in Ontario over time. In Proceedings of the 16th Annual Meeting of the Canadian Animal Health Laboratorians Network, Guelph, ON, Canada, 4–7 June 2017.
23. Brochu Morin, M.-E.; Chénier, S.; Bergeron, N. *La Bronchite Infectieuse Aviaire au Québec (Avian Infectious Bronchitis in Quebec). Bulletin Zoosanitaire: Réseau d'alerte et D'information Zoosanitaire (RAIZO)*; Ministère de l'Agriculture, des Pêcheries et de l'Alimentation du Québec: Québec, QC, Canada, 2018.

24. Hassan, M.S.H.; Ali, A.; Buharideen, S.M.; Goldsmith, D.; Coffin, C.S.; Cork, S.C.; van der Meer, F.; Boulianne, M.; Abdul-Careem, M.F. Pathogenicity of the Canadian Delmarva (DMV/1639) Infectious Bronchitis Virus (IBV) on Female Reproductive Tract of Chickens. *Viruses* **2021**, *13*, 2488. [CrossRef]
25. Hassan, M.S.H.; Najimudeen, S.M.; Ali, A.; Altakrouni, D.; Goldsmith, D.; Coffin, C.S.; Cork, S.C.; van der Meer, F.; Abdul-Careem, M.F. Immunopathogenesis of the Canadian Delmarva (DMV/1639) infectious bronchitis virus (IBV): Impact on the reproductive tract in layers. *Microb. Pathog.* **2022**, *166*, 105513. [CrossRef] [PubMed]
26. Mcmartin, D.A.; Macleod, H. Abnormal Oviducts in Laying Hens Following Natural Infection with Infectious Bronchitis at an Early Age. *Brit Vet. J.* **1972**, *128*, xix–xxi.
27. Jones, R.C.; Jordan, F.T. The exposure of day-old chicks to infectious bronchitis and the subsequent development of the oviduct. *Vet. Rec.* **1970**, *87*, 504–505. [CrossRef] [PubMed]
28. Crinion, R.A.P.; Hofstad, M.S. Pathogenicity of Two Embryo-Passage Levels of Avian Infectious Bronchitis Virus for the Oviduct of Young Chickens of Various Ages. *Avian Dis.* **1972**, *16*, 967–973. [CrossRef] [PubMed]
29. Miura, T.A. Respiratory epithelial cells as master communicators during viral infections. *Curr. Clin. Microbiol. Rep.* **2019**, *6*, 10–17. [CrossRef] [PubMed]
30. Hewitt, R.J.; Lloyd, C.M. Regulation of immune responses by the airway epithelial cell landscape. *Nat. Rev. Immunol.* **2021**, *21*, 347–362. [CrossRef] [PubMed]
31. Akira, S.; Takeda, K. Toll-like receptor signalling. *Nat. Rev. Immunol.* **2004**, *4*, 499–511. [CrossRef] [PubMed]
32. Goossens, K.E.; Ward, A.C.; Lowenthal, J.W.; Bean, A.G. Chicken interferons, their receptors and interferon-stimulated genes. *Dev. Comp. Immunol.* **2013**, *41*, 370–376. [CrossRef] [PubMed]
33. Santhakumar, D.; Rubbenstroth, D.; Martinez-Sobrido, L.; Munir, M. Avian Interferons and Their Antiviral Effectors. *Front. Immunol.* **2017**, *8*, 49. [CrossRef] [PubMed]
34. Schneider, W.M.; Chevillotte, M.D.; Rice, C.M. Interferon-stimulated genes: A complex web of host defenses. *Annu. Rev. Immunol.* **2014**, *32*, 513–545. [CrossRef] [PubMed]
35. Yang, E.; Li, M.M.H. All About the RNA: Interferon-Stimulated Genes That Interfere With Viral RNA Processes. *Front. Immunol.* **2020**, *11*, 605024. [CrossRef] [PubMed]
36. Kint, J.; Fernandez-Gutierrez, M.; Maier, H.J.; Britton, P.; Langereis, M.A.; Koumans, J.; Wiegertjes, G.F.; Forlenza, M. Activation of the chicken type I interferon response by infectious bronchitis coronavirus. *J. Virol.* **2015**, *89*, 1156–1167. [CrossRef] [PubMed]
37. Dar, A.; Munir, S.; Vishwanathan, S.; Manuja, A.; Griebel, P.; Tikoo, S.; Townsend, H.; Potter, A.; Kapur, V.; Babiuk, L.A. Transcriptional analysis of avian embryonic tissues following infection with avian infectious bronchitis virus. *Virus Res.* **2005**, *110*, 41–55. [CrossRef] [PubMed]
38. Wang, X.; Rosa, A.J.M.; Oliverira, H.N.; Rosa, G.J.M.; Guo, X.; Travnicek, M.; Girshick, T. Transcriptome of Local Innate and Adaptive Immunity during Early Phase of Infectious Bronchitis Viral Infection. *Viral Immunol.* **2006**, *19*, 768–774. [CrossRef] [PubMed]
39. Guo, X.; Rosa, A.J.; Chen, D.G.; Wang, X. Molecular mechanisms of primary and secondary mucosal immunity using avian infectious bronchitis virus as a model system. *Vet. Immunol. Immunopathol.* **2008**, *121*, 332–343. [CrossRef] [PubMed]
40. Hamzić, E.; Kjaerup, R.B.; Mach, N.; Minozzi, G.; Strozzi, F.; Gualdi, V.; Williams, J.L.; Chen, J.; Wattrang, E.; Buitenhuis, B.; et al. RNA sequencing-based analysis of the spleen transcriptome following infectious bronchitis virus infection of chickens selected for different mannose-binding lectin serum concentrations. *BMC Genom.* **2016**, *17*, 82. [CrossRef] [PubMed]
41. Kemp, V.; Laconi, A.; Cocciolo, G.; Berends, A.J.; Breit, T.M.; Verheije, M.H. miRNA repertoire and host immune factor regulation upon avian coronavirus infection in eggs. *Arch. Virol.* **2020**, *165*, 835–843. [CrossRef] [PubMed]
42. Chuwatthanakhajorn, S.; Chang, C.S.; Ganapathy, K.; Tang, P.C.; Chen, C.F. Comparison of Immune-Related Gene Expression in Two Chicken Breeds Following Infectious Bronchitis Virus Vaccination. *Animals* **2023**, *13*, 1642. [CrossRef]
43. Smith, J.; Sadeyen, J.R.; Cavanagh, D.; Kaiser, P.; Burt, D.W. The early immune response to infection of chickens with Infectious Bronchitis Virus (IBV) in susceptible and resistant birds. *BMC Vet. Res.* **2015**, *11*, 256. [CrossRef] [PubMed]
44. Silva, A.P.D.; Hauck, R.; Kern, C.; Wang, Y.; Zhou, H.; Gallardo, R.A. Effects of Chicken MHC Haplotype on Resistance to Distantly Related Infectious Bronchitis Viruses. *Avian Dis.* **2019**, *63*, 310–317. [CrossRef]
45. Ghobadian Diali, H.; Hosseini, H.; Fallah Mehrabadi, M.H.; Yahyaraeyat, R.; Ghalyanchilangeroudi, A. Evaluation of viral load and transcriptome changes in tracheal tissue of two hybrids of commercial broiler chickens infected with avian infectious bronchitis virus: A comparative study. *Arch. Virol.* **2022**, *167*, 377–391. [CrossRef] [PubMed]
46. Yuan, L.X.; Yang, B.; Fung, T.S.; Chen, R.A.; Liu, D.X. Transcriptomic analysis reveals crucial regulatory roles of immediate-early response genes and related signaling pathways in coronavirus infectious bronchitis virus infection. *Virology* **2022**, *575*, 1–9. [CrossRef] [PubMed]
47. Cong, F.; Liu, X.; Han, Z.; Shao, Y.; Kong, X.; Liu, S. Transcriptome analysis of chicken kidney tissues following coronavirus avian infectious bronchitis virus infection. *BMC Genom.* **2013**, *14*, 743. [CrossRef] [PubMed]
48. Xu, P.; Liu, P.; Zhou, C.; Shi, Y.; Wu, Q.; Yang, Y.; Li, G.; Hu, G.; Guo, X. A Multi-Omics Study of Chicken Infected by Nephropathogenic Infectious Bronchitis Virus. *Viruses* **2019**, *11*, 1070. [CrossRef] [PubMed]
49. Dinan, A.M.; Keep, S.; Bickerton, E.; Britton, P.; Firth, A.E.; Brierley, I. Comparative Analysis of Gene Expression in Virulent and Attenuated Strains of Infectious Bronchitis Virus at Subcodon Resolution. *J. Virol.* **2019**, *93*, 10–1128. [CrossRef] [PubMed]

50. Liu, H.; Yang, X.; Zhang, Z.; Li, J.; Zou, W.; Zeng, F.; Wang, H. Comparative transcriptome analysis reveals induction of apoptosis in chicken kidney cells associated with the virulence of nephropathogenic infectious bronchitis virus. *Microb. Pathog.* **2017**, *113*, 451–459. [CrossRef] [PubMed]
51. Lee, R.; Jung, J.S.; Yeo, J.I.; Kwon, H.M.; Park, J. Transcriptome analysis of primary chicken cells infected with infectious bronchitis virus strain K047-12 isolated in Korea. *Arch. Virol.* **2021**, *166*, 2291–2298. [CrossRef] [PubMed]
52. Lin, J.; Wang, Z.; Wang, J.; Yang, Q. Microarray analysis of infectious bronchitis virus infection of chicken primary dendritic cells. *BMC Genom.* **2019**, *20*, 557. [CrossRef] [PubMed]
53. Zuo, J.; Cao, Y.; Wang, Z.; Shah, A.U.; Wang, W.; Dai, C.; Chen, M.; Lin, J.; Yang, Q. The mechanism of antigen-presentation of avian bone marrowed dendritic cells suppressed by infectious bronchitis virus. *Genomics* **2021**, *113*, 1719–1732. [CrossRef] [PubMed]
54. Li, H.; Cui, P.; Fu, X.; Zhang, L.; Yan, W.; Zhai, Y.; Lei, C.; Wang, H.; Yang, X. Identification and analysis of long non-coding RNAs and mRNAs in chicken macrophages infected with avian infectious bronchitis coronavirus. *BMC Genom.* **2021**, *22*, 67. [CrossRef]
55. Yang, Q.; Gong, H.; Liu, S.; Huang, S.; Yan, W.; Wang, K.; Li, H.; Lei, C.-W.; Wang, H.-N.; Yang, X. Differential analysis of IBV-infected primary chicken embryonic fibroblasts and immortalized DF-1. *Microbiol. Spectr.* **2024**, *12*, e02402–e02423. [CrossRef] [PubMed]
56. Jackwood, M.W.; Jordan, B.J. Molecular Evolution of Infectious Bronchitis Virus and the Emergence of Variant Viruses Circulating in the United States. *Avian Dis.* **2021**, *65*, 631–636. [CrossRef] [PubMed]
57. Abdel-Moneim, A.S.; Zlotowski, P.; Veits, J.; Keil, G.M.; Teifke, J.P. Immunohistochemistry for detection of avian infectious bronchitis virus strain M41 in the proventriculus and nervous system of experimentally infected chicken embryos. *Virol. J.* **2009**, *6*, 15. [CrossRef] [PubMed]
58. Amarasinghe, A.; Abdul-Cader, M.S.; Almatrouk, Z.; van der Meer, F.; Cork, S.C.; Gomis, S.; Abdul-Careem, M.F. Induction of innate host responses characterized by production of interleukin (IL)-1beta and recruitment of macrophages to the respiratory tract of chickens following infection with infectious bronchitis virus (IBV). *Vet. Microbiol.* **2018**, *215*, 1–10. [CrossRef] [PubMed]
59. Farooq, M.; Abd-Elsalam, R.M.; Ratcliff, N.; Hassan, M.S.H.; Najimudeen, S.M.; Cork, S.C.; Checkley, S.; Niu, Y.D.; Abdul-Careem, M.F. Comparative pathogenicity of infectious bronchitis virus Massachusetts and Delmarva (DMV/1639) genotypes in laying hens. *Front. Vet. Sci.* **2023**, *10*, 1329430. [CrossRef] [PubMed]
60. Mueller Slay, A.; Franca, M.; Jackwood, M.; Jordan, B. Infection with IBV DMV/1639 at a Young Age Leads to Increased Incidence of Cystic Oviduct Formation Associated with False Layer Syndrome. *Viruses* **2022**, *14*, 852. [CrossRef] [PubMed]
61. Kint, J.; Maier, H.J.; Jagt, E. Quantification of infectious bronchitis coronavirus by titration in vitro and in ovo. *Methods Mol. Biol.* **2015**, *1282*, 89–98. [CrossRef] [PubMed]
62. Payment, P.; Trudel, M. Isolement et identification des virus. In *Manuel de Techniques Virologiques*, 1st ed.; Presses de l'Université du Québec: Québec, QC, Canada, 1989; pp. 21–44.
63. Reed, L.J.; Muench, H. A Simple Method for Estimating Fifty Per Cent Endpoints. *Am. J. Epidemiol.* **1938**, *27*, 493–497. [CrossRef]
64. Barjesteh, N.; Taha-Abdelaziz, K.; Kulkarni, R.R.; Sharif, S. Innate antiviral responses are induced by TLR3 and TLR4 ligands in chicken tracheal epithelial cells: Communication between epithelial cells and macrophages. *Virology* **2019**, *534*, 132–142. [CrossRef]
65. Shen, C.I.; Wang, C.H.; Liao, J.W.; Hsu, T.W.; Kuo, S.M.; Su, H.L. The infection of primary avian tracheal epithelial cells with infectious bronchitis virus. *Vet. Res.* **2010**, *41*, 6. [CrossRef] [PubMed]
66. Zaffuto, K.M.; Estevez, C.N.; Afonso, C.L. Primary chicken tracheal cell culture system for the study of infection with avian respiratory viruses. *Avian Pathol.* **2008**, *37*, 25–31. [CrossRef] [PubMed]
67. Pajtler, K.; Bohrer, A.; Maurer, J.; Schorle, H.; Schramm, A.; Eggert, A.; Schulte, J.H. Production of chick embryo extract for the cultivation of murine neural crest stem cells. *J. Vis. Exp.* **2010**, *45*, e2380. [CrossRef]
68. Kameka, A.M.; Haddadi, S.; Kim, D.S.; Cork, S.C.; Abdul-Careem, M.F. Induction of innate immune response following infectious bronchitis corona virus infection in the respiratory tract of chickens. *Virology* **2014**, *450–451*, 114–121. [CrossRef] [PubMed]
69. St Paul, M.; Mallick, A.I.; Haq, K.; Orouji, S.; Abdul-Careem, M.F.; Sharif, S. In vivo administration of ligands for chicken toll-like receptors 4 and 21 induces the expression of immune system genes in the spleen. *Vet. Immunol. Immunopathol.* **2011**, *144*, 228–237. [CrossRef] [PubMed]
70. Chen, G.; Yin, Y.; Lin, Z.; Wen, H.; Chen, J.; Luo, W. Transcriptome profile analysis reveals KLHL30 as an essential regulator for myoblast differentiation. *Biochem. Biophys. Res. Commun.* **2021**, *559*, 84–91. [CrossRef] [PubMed]
71. Yin, H.; Cui, C.; Han, S.; Chen, Y.; Zhao, J.; He, H.; Li, D.; Zhu, Q. Fibromodulin Modulates Chicken Skeletal Muscle Development via the Transforming Growth Factor-beta Signaling Pathway. *Animals* **2020**, *10*, 1477. [CrossRef] [PubMed]
72. Villanueva, A.I.; Kulkarni, R.R.; Sharif, S. Synthetic double-stranded RNA oligonucleotides are immunostimulatory for chicken spleen cells. *Dev. Comp. Immunol.* **2011**, *35*, 28–34. [CrossRef] [PubMed]
73. Tan, L.; Huang, M.; Qiu, X.; Zhi, X.; Liang, L.; Sun, Y.; Liao, Y.; Song, C.; Ren, T.; Ding, C. Chicken-derived MERTK protein inhibits Newcastle disease virus replication by increasing STAT1 phosphorylation in DF-1 cells. *Virus Res.* **2023**, *326*, 199065. [CrossRef] [PubMed]
74. Sarson, A.J.; Parvizi, P.; Lepp, D.; Quinton, M.; Sharif, S. Transcriptional analysis of host responses to Marek's disease virus infection in genetically resistant and susceptible chickens. *Anim. Genet.* **2008**, *39*, 232–240. [CrossRef]

75. Giotis, E.S.; Robey, R.C.; Skinner, N.G.; Tomlinson, C.D.; Goodbourn, S.; Skinner, M.A. Chicken interferome: Avian interferon-stimulated genes identified by microarray and RNA-seq of primary chick embryo fibroblasts treated with a chicken type I interferon (IFN-alpha). *Vet. Res.* **2016**, *47*, 75. [CrossRef] [PubMed]
76. Livak, K.J.; Schmittgen, T.D. Analysis of relative gene expression data using real-time quantitative PCR and the 2(-Delta Delta C(T)) Method. *Methods* **2001**, *25*, 402–408. [CrossRef] [PubMed]
77. Bourgey, M.; Dali, R.; Eveleigh, R.; Chen, K.C.; Letourneau, L.; Fillon, J.; Michaud, M.; Caron, M.; Sandoval, J.; Lefebvre, F.; et al. GenPipes: An open-source framework for distributed and scalable genomic analyses. *Gigascience* **2019**, *8*, giz037. [CrossRef] [PubMed]
78. Team, R.C. R: A Language and Environment for Statistical Computing. 2021. Available online: https://www.R-project.org/ (accessed on 4 January 2022).
79. Team, R. RStudio: Integrated Development for R. 2020. Available online: http://www.rstudio.com/ (accessed on 4 January 2022).
80. Xie, Y. knitr: A General-Purpose Package for Dynamic Report Generation in R. 2021. Available online: https://yihui.org/knitr/ (accessed on 4 January 2022).
81. Slowikowski, K. ggrepel: Automatically Position Non-Overlapping Text Labels with 'ggplot2'. 2023. Available online: https://github.com/slowkow/ggrepel (accessed on 26 August 2023).
82. Müller, K.; Wickham, H. tibble: Simple Data Frames. 2023. Available online: https://github.com/tidyverse/tibble (accessed on 26 August 2023).
83. Wickham, H.; Averick, M.; Bryan, J.; Chang, W.; McGowan, L.; François, R.; Grolemund, G.; Hayes, A.; Henry, L.; Hester, J.; et al. Welcome to the Tidyverse. *J. Open Source Softw.* **2019**, *4*, 1686. [CrossRef]
84. Bache, S.; Wickham, H.; Henry, L.; Henry, M.L. magrittr: A Forward-Pipe Operator for R. 2022. Available online: https://magrittr.tidyverse.org (accessed on 26 August 2023).
85. Sjoberg, D. Hablar: Non-Astonishing Results in R. 2023. Available online: https://davidsjoberg.github.io/ (accessed on 26 August 2023).
86. Zhu, H. kableExtra: Construct Complex Table with 'kable' and Pipe Syntax. 2019. Available online: http://haozhu233.github.io/kableExtra/ (accessed on 26 August 2023).
87. DeLuca, D.S.; Levin, J.Z.; Sivachenko, A.; Fennell, T.; Nazaire, M.D.; Williams, C.; Reich, M.; Winckler, W.; Getz, G. RNA-SeQC: RNA-seq metrics for quality control and process optimization. *Bioinformatics* **2012**, *28*, 1530–1532. [CrossRef] [PubMed]
88. Bolger, A.M.; Lohse, M.; Usadel, B. Trimmomatic: A flexible trimmer for Illumina sequence data. *Bioinformatics* **2014**, *30*, 2114–2120. [CrossRef] [PubMed]
89. Dobin, A.; Davis, C.A.; Schlesinger, F.; Drenkow, J.; Zaleski, C.; Jha, S.; Batut, P.; Chaisson, M.; Gingeras, T.R. STAR: Ultrafast universal RNA-seq aligner. *Bioinformatics* **2013**, *29*, 15–21. [CrossRef] [PubMed]
90. Anders, S.; Pyl, P.T.; Huber, W. HTSeq—A Python framework to work with high-throughput sequencing data. *Bioinformatics* **2015**, *31*, 166–169. [CrossRef] [PubMed]
91. Love, M.I.; Huber, W.; Anders, S. Moderated estimation of fold change and dispersion for RNA-seq data with DESeq2. *Genome Biol.* **2014**, *15*, 550. [CrossRef] [PubMed]
92. Stephens, M. False discovery rates: A new deal. *Biostatistics* **2016**, *18*, 275–294. [CrossRef] [PubMed]
93. Gu, Z.; Eils, R.; Schlesner, M. Complex heatmaps reveal patterns and correlations in multidimensional genomic data. *Bioinformatics* **2016**, *32*, 2847–2849. [CrossRef]
94. Mangiola, S.; Papenfuss, A. tidyHeatmap: An R package for modular heatmap production based on tidy principles. *J. Open Source Softw.* **2020**, *5*, 2472. [CrossRef]
95. Blighe, K.; Rana, S.; Lewis, M. EnhancedVolcano: Publication-Ready Volcano Plots with Enhanced Colouring and Labeling. R Package Version 1.18.0. 2023. Available online: https://github.com/kevinblighe/EnhancedVolcano (accessed on 26 August 2023).
96. Venny, J.C.O. An interactive tool for comparing lists with Venn's diagrams. *2007–2015*. Available online: https://bioinfogp.cnb.csic.es/tools/venny/index.html (accessed on 9 January 2024).
97. Kolberg, L.; Raudvere, U.; Kuzmin, I.; Vilo, J.; Peterson, H. gprofiler2—An R package for gene list functional enrichment analysis and namespace conversion toolset g:Profiler. *F1000Res* **2020**, *9*, ELIXIR-709. [CrossRef] [PubMed]
98. Kolberg, L.; Raudvere, U.; Kuzmin, I.; Adler, P.; Vilo, J.; Peterson, H. g:Profiler-interoperable web service for functional enrichment analysis and gene identifier mapping (2023 update). *Nucleic Acids Res.* **2023**, *51*, W207–W212. [CrossRef]
99. Yu, G. Enrichplot: Visualization of Functional Enrichment Result. R Package Version 1.21.3. 2023. Available online: https://bioconductor.org/packages/enrichplot (accessed on 26 August 2023).
100. Yu, G.; Wang, L.G.; Yan, G.R.; He, Q.Y. DOSE: An R/Bioconductor package for disease ontology semantic and enrichment analysis. *Bioinformatics* **2015**, *31*, 608–609. [CrossRef] [PubMed]
101. Wickham, H. *ggplot2: Elegant Graphics for Data Analysis*; Springer International Publishing: Berlin/Heidelberg, Germany, 2016.
102. Grote, S. GOfuncR: Gene ontology enrichment using FUNC. R package version 1.20.0. 2023. Available online: https://bioconductor.org/packages/release/bioc/html/GOfuncR.html (accessed on 26 August 2023).
103. Kanehisa, M.; Sato, Y.; Kawashima, M. KEGG mapping tools for uncovering hidden features in biological data. *Protein Sci.* **2022**, *31*, 47–53. [CrossRef] [PubMed]

104. Luo, W.; Brouwer, C. Pathview: An R/Bioconductor package for pathway-based data integration and visualization. *Bioinformatics* **2013**, *29*, 1830–1831. [CrossRef] [PubMed]
105. Carlson, M. org.Gg.eg.db: Genome wide annotation for Chicken. R package version 3.8.2. 2019. Available online: https://bioconductor.org/packages/release/data/annotation/html/org.Gg.eg.db.html (accessed on 26 August 2023).
106. Cook, J.K.; Darbyshire, J.H.; Peters, R.W. The use of chicken tracheal organ cultures for the isolation and assay of avian infectious bronchitis virus. *Arch. Virol.* **1976**, *50*, 109–118. [CrossRef] [PubMed]
107. Cook, J.K.; Darbyshire, J.H.; Peters, R.W. Growth kinetic studies of avian infectious bronchitis virus in tracheal organ cultures. *Res. Vet. Sci.* **1976**, *20*, 348–349. [CrossRef] [PubMed]
108. Holmes, H.C. The resistance to reinfection of tracheal organ cultures from chickens previously infected with avian infections bronchitis virus. *Res. Vet. Sci.* **1978**, *25*, 122–124. [CrossRef] [PubMed]
109. Colwell, W.M.; Lukert, P.D. Effects of Avian Infectious Bronchitis Virus (IBV) on Tracheal Organ Cultures. *Avian Dis.* **1969**, *13*, 888–894. [CrossRef] [PubMed]
110. Weerts, E.; Bouwman, K.M.; Paerels, L.; Grone, A.; Jan Boelm, G.; Verheije, M.H. Interference between avian corona and influenza viruses: The role of the epithelial architecture of the chicken trachea. *Vet. Microbiol.* **2022**, *272*, 109499. [CrossRef] [PubMed]
111. Steyn, A.; Keep, S.; Bickerton, E.; Fife, M. The Characterization of chIFITMs in Avian Coronavirus Infection In Vivo, Ex Vivo and In Vitro. *Genes* **2020**, *11*, 918. [CrossRef] [PubMed]
112. Zhang, H.; Cai, H.; Li, Q.; Fang, C.; Peng, L.; Lan, J.; Zhou, J.; Liao, M. Identification of Host Proteins Interacting with IBV S1 Based on Tracheal Organ Culture. *Viruses* **2023**, *15*, 1216. [CrossRef] [PubMed]
113. Chandra, M. Comparative nephropathogenicity of different strains of infectious bronchitis virus in chickens. *Poult. Sci.* **1987**, *66*, 954–959. [CrossRef] [PubMed]
114. Cheng, J.; Huo, C.; Zhao, J.; Liu, T.; Li, X.; Yan, S.; Wang, Z.; Hu, Y.; Zhang, G. Pathogenicity differences between QX-like and Mass-type infectious bronchitis viruses. *Vet. Microbiol.* **2018**, *213*, 129–135. [CrossRef] [PubMed]
115. De Wit, J.J. Detection of infectious bronchitis virus. *Avian Pathol.* **2000**, *29*, 71–93. [CrossRef] [PubMed]
116. Barjesteh, N.; Alkie, T.N.; Hodgins, D.C.; Nagy, E.; Sharif, S. Local Innate Responses to TLR Ligands in the Chicken Trachea. *Viruses* **2016**, *8*, 207. [CrossRef]
117. Carty, M.; Guy, C.; Bowie, A.G. Detection of Viral Infections by Innate Immunity. *Biochem. Pharmacol.* **2021**, *183*, 114316. [CrossRef] [PubMed]
118. Barjesteh, N.; O'Dowd, K.; Vahedi, S.M. Antiviral responses against chicken respiratory infections: Focus on avian influenza virus and infectious bronchitis virus. *Cytokine* **2020**, *127*, 154961. [CrossRef] [PubMed]
119. Keestra, A.M.; de Zoete, M.R.; Bouwman, L.I.; Vaezirad, M.M.; van Putten, J.P. Unique features of chicken Toll-like receptors. *Dev. Comp. Immunol.* **2013**, *41*, 316–323. [CrossRef] [PubMed]
120. Karpala, A.J.; Lowenthal, J.W.; Bean, A.G. Activation of the TLR3 pathway regulates IFNbeta production in chickens. *Dev. Comp. Immunol.* **2008**, *32*, 435–444. [CrossRef] [PubMed]
121. Lee, S.B.; Park, Y.H.; Chungu, K.; Woo, S.J.; Han, S.T.; Choi, H.J.; Rengaraj, D.; Han, J.Y. Targeted Knockout of MDA5 and TLR3 in the DF-1 Chicken Fibroblast Cell Line Impairs Innate Immune Response Against RNA Ligands. *Front. Immunol.* **2020**, *11*, 678. [CrossRef]
122. Keestra, A.M.; de Zoete, M.R.; Bouwman, L.I.; van Putten, J.P. Chicken TLR21 is an innate CpG DNA receptor distinct from mammalian TLR9. *J. Immunol.* **2010**, *185*, 460–467. [CrossRef]
123. Brownlie, R.; Zhu, J.; Allan, B.; Mutwiri, G.K.; Babiuk, L.A.; Potter, A.; Griebel, P. Chicken TLR21 acts as a functional homologue to mammalian TLR9 in the recognition of CpG oligodeoxynucleotides. *Mol. Immunol.* **2009**, *46*, 3163–3170. [CrossRef] [PubMed]
124. Dar, A.; Potter, A.; Tikoo, S.; Gerdts, V.; Lai, K.; Babiuk, L.A.; Mutwiri, G. CpG oligodeoxynucleotides activate innate immune response that suppresses infectious bronchitis virus replication in chicken embryos. *Avian Dis.* **2009**, *53*, 261–267. [CrossRef] [PubMed]
125. Huang, M.; Zheng, X.; Zhang, Y.; Wang, R.; Wei, X. Comparative proteomics analysis of kidney in chicken infected by infectious bronchitis virus. *Poult. Sci.* **2023**, *103*, 103259. [CrossRef] [PubMed]
126. Santhakumar, D.; Rohaim, M.; Hussein, H.A.; Hawes, P.; Ferreira, H.L.; Behboudi, S.; Iqbal, M.; Nair, V.; Arns, C.W.; Munir, M. Chicken Interferon-induced Protein with Tetratricopeptide Repeats 5 Antagonizes Replication of RNA Viruses. *Sci. Rep.* **2018**, *8*, 6794. [CrossRef] [PubMed]
127. Zhang, B.; Liu, X.; Chen, W.; Chen, L. IFIT5 potentiates anti-viral response through enhancing innate immune signaling pathways. *Acta Biochim. Biophys. Sin.* **2013**, *45*, 867–874. [CrossRef]
128. Jang, H.; Koo, B.S.; Jeon, E.O.; Lee, H.R.; Lee, S.M.; Mo, I.P. Altered pro-inflammatory cytokine mRNA levels in chickens infected with infectious bronchitis virus. *Poult. Sci.* **2013**, *92*, 2290–2298. [CrossRef] [PubMed]
129. Tang, X.; Qi, J.; Sun, L.; Zhao, J.; Zhang, G.; Zhao, Y. Pathological effect of different avian infectious bronchitis virus strains on the bursa of Fabricius of chickens. *Avian Pathol.* **2022**, *51*, 339–348. [CrossRef] [PubMed]
130. Najimudeen, S.M.; Barboza-Solis, C.; Ali, A.; Buharideen, S.M.; Isham, I.M.; Hassan, M.S.; Ojkic, D.; Van Marle, G.; Cork, S.C.; van der Meer, F.; et al. Pathogenesis and host responses in lungs and kidneys following Canadian 4/91 infectious bronchitis virus (IBV) infection in chickens. *Virology* **2022**, *566*, 75–88. [CrossRef] [PubMed]
131. Zhang, T.; Li, D.; Jia, Z.; Chang, J.; Hou, X. Cellular immune response in chickens infected with avian infectious bronchitis virus (IBV). *Eur. J. Inflamm.* **2017**, *15*, 35–41. [CrossRef]

132. Ramirez, H.; Patel, S.B.; Pastar, I. The Role of TGFbeta Signaling in Wound Epithelialization. *Adv. Wound Care* **2014**, *3*, 482–491. [CrossRef] [PubMed]
133. Kitsis, R.N.; Leinwand, L.A. Discordance between gene regulation in vitro and in vivo. *Gene Expr.* **1992**, *2*, 313–318. [PubMed]
134. McMahon, M.; Ye, S.; Pedrina, J.; Dlugolenski, D.; Stambas, J. Extracellular Matrix Enzymes and Immune Cell Biology. *Front. Mol. Biosci.* **2021**, *8*, 703868. [CrossRef] [PubMed]
135. Kozyrina, A.N.; Piskova, T.; Di Russo, J. Mechanobiology of Epithelia From the Perspective of Extracellular Matrix Heterogeneity. *Front. Bioeng. Biotechnol.* **2020**, *8*, 596599. [CrossRef] [PubMed]
136. Bhat, M.Y.; Solanki, H.S.; Advani, J.; Khan, A.A.; Keshava Prasad, T.S.; Gowda, H.; Thiyagarajan, S.; Chatterjee, A. Comprehensive network map of interferon gamma signaling. *J. Cell Commun. Signal* **2018**, *12*, 745–751. [CrossRef] [PubMed]
137. Ma, P.; Gu, K.; Li, H.; Zhao, Y.; Li, C.; Wen, R.; Zhou, C.; Lei, C.; Yang, X.; Wang, H. Infectious Bronchitis Virus Nsp14 Degrades JAK1 to Inhibit the JAK-STAT Signaling Pathway in HD11 Cells. *Viruses* **2022**, *14*, 1045. [CrossRef] [PubMed]
138. Hanukoglu, I.; Hanukoglu, A. Epithelial sodium channel (ENaC) family: Phylogeny, structure-function, tissue distribution, and associated inherited diseases. *Gene* **2016**, *579*, 95–132. [CrossRef]
139. Hoerr, F.J. The Pathology of Infectious Bronchitis. *Avian Dis.* **2021**, *65*, 600–611. [CrossRef] [PubMed]
140. Stannard, W.; O'Callaghan, C. Ciliary Function and the Role of Cilia in Clearance. *J. Aerosol Med.* **2006**, *19*, 110–115. [CrossRef] [PubMed]
141. Di Matteo, A.M.; Soñez, M.C.; Plano, C.M.; von Lawzewitsch, I. Morphologic Observations on Respiratory Tracts of Chickens after after Hatchery Infectious Bronchitis Vaccination and Formaldehyde Fumigation. *Avian Dis.* **2000**, *44*, 507–518. [CrossRef] [PubMed]
142. Verhelst, J.; Parthoens, E.; Schepens, B.; Fiers, W.; Saelens, X. Interferon-inducible protein Mx1 inhibits influenza virus by interfering with functional viral ribonucleoprotein complex assembly. *J. Virol.* **2012**, *86*, 13445–13455. [CrossRef] [PubMed]
143. Haller, O.; Stertz, S.; Kochs, G. The Mx GTPase family of interferon-induced antiviral proteins. *Microbes Infect.* **2007**, *9*, 1636–1643. [CrossRef] [PubMed]
144. Li, X.; Feng, Y.; Liu, W.; Tan, L.; Sun, Y.; Song, C.; Liao, Y.; Xu, C.; Ren, T.; Ding, C.; et al. A Role for the Chicken Interferon-Stimulated Gene CMPK2 in the Host Response Against Virus Infection. *Front. Microbiol.* **2022**, *13*, 874331. [CrossRef] [PubMed]
145. Zhu, M.; Lv, J.; Wang, W.; Guo, R.; Zhong, C.; Antia, A.; Zeng, Q.; Li, J.; Liu, Q.; Zhou, J.; et al. CMPK2 is a host restriction factor that inhibits infection of multiple coronaviruses in a cell-intrinsic manner. *PLoS Biol.* **2023**, *21*, e3002039. [CrossRef] [PubMed]
146. Byron, S.A.; Van Keuren-Jensen, K.R.; Engelthaler, D.M.; Carpten, J.D.; Craig, D.W. Translating RNA sequencing into clinical diagnostics: Opportunities and challenges. *Nat. Rev. Genet.* **2016**, *17*, 257–271. [CrossRef] [PubMed]
147. Amarasinghe, A.; Popowich, S.; De Silva Senapathi, U.; Abdul-Cader, M.S.; Marshall, F.; van der Meer, F.; Cork, S.C.; Gomis, S.; Abdul-Careem, M.F. Shell-Less Egg Syndrome (SES) Widespread in Western Canadian Layer Operations Is Linked to a Massachusetts (Mass) Type Infectious Bronchitis Virus (IBV) Isolate. *Viruses* **2018**, *10*, 437. [CrossRef] [PubMed]

viruses MDPI

Review

Antiviral Chemotherapy in Avian Medicine—A Review

Ines Szotowska * and Aleksandra Ledwoń

Department of Pathology and Veterinary Diagnostics, Warsaw University of Life Sciences, 02-776 Warsaw, Poland; aleksandra_ledwon@sggw.edu.pl
* Correspondence: ines_daszkowska@sggw.edu.pl

Abstract: This review article describes the current knowledge about the use of antiviral chemotherapeutics in avian species, such as farm poultry and companion birds. Specific therapeutics are described in alphabetical order including classic antiviral drugs, such as acyclovir, abacavir, adefovir, amantadine, didanosine, entecavir, ganciclovir, interferon, lamivudine, penciclovir, famciclovir, oseltamivir, ribavirin, and zidovudine, repurposed drugs, such as ivermectin and nitazoxanide, which were originally used as antiparasitic drugs, and some others substances showing antiviral activity, such as ampligen, azo derivates, docosanol, fluoroarabinosylpyrimidine nucleosides, and novel peptides. Most of them have only been used for research purposes and are not widely used in clinical practice because of a lack of essential pharmacokinetic and safety data. Suggested future research directions are also highlighted.

Keywords: antiviral; birds; avian medicine; viruses; viral infection; therapy

Citation: Szotowska, I.; Ledwoń, A. Antiviral Chemotherapy in Avian Medicine—A Review. *Viruses* **2024**, *16*, 593. https://doi.org/10.3390/v16040593

Academic Editor: Chi-Young Wang

Received: 16 February 2024
Revised: 6 April 2024
Accepted: 10 April 2024
Published: 12 April 2024

1. Introduction

Viral diseases are a serious problem in avian species, both poultry and companion birds. Scientists actively look for methods of prevention and eradication of infectious diseases caused by viral pathogens, especially those considered emerging diseases, such as avian influenza, West Nile disease, Newcastle disease, and proventricular dilatation disease (caused by avian bornaviruses). Different approaches focus on immunoprophylaxis, biosecurity, and supportive care, and antiviral therapy is possible. Despite the fact that there is no antiviral drug licensed for use in any avian species, experimental studies mainly include the efficacy of antiviral drugs in specific viral infections and, to a lesser extent, safety profiles of these drugs and pharmacokinetics. Some antivirals licensed for use in human medicine are currently used with the prescribing cascade in therapy for avian viral diseases. Drugs mentioned in the literature to be used in clinical practice include acyclovir in psittacines [1], pigeons [1], backyard poultry [2], and birds of prey [1]. For herpesvirus infections, they include interferon-alpha-2 in psittacines and pigeons for circovirus infections [1], famciclovir in ducklings for duck hepatitis B virus infections [2], and penciclovir in ducks for herpesvirus and duck hepatitis B virus infections [2].

At present, only three antiviral compounds have been licensed for use in veterinary medicine in some countries, including feline interferon-omega (IFN-ω), which is used to reduce mortality and clinical signs of parvovirosis in dogs and to treat cats infected with feline leukemia virus (FeLV) or feline immunodeficiency virus (FIV) in cats [3], and remdesivir and GS-441524, which are both used to treat feline infectious peritonitis (FIP) [4]. There are many local regulations aimed at limiting the use of antiviral drugs, e.g., in the UE, where the use of amantadine, baloxavir marboxil, celgosivir, favipiravir, galidesivir, laktimidomycin, laninamivir, metisazone, molnupiravir, nitazoxanide, oseltamivir, peramivir, ribavirin, rimantadine, tizoxanide, triazavirin, umifenovir, and zanamivir is prohibited in veterinary medicine since 9 February 2023 [5]. To avoid the development of resistance to the antiviral drugs that are listed above, they are reserved for the treatment of certain infections in humans. However, in the 1990s, several reasons for the low use of antiviral chemotherapy in veterinary medicine [6–8] were given, including the high cost of development of new substances, particularly for use in animal production, use restricted to a single virus and a specific animal species, difficulties encountered in the development of broad-spectrum antivirals with low cytotoxicity, and a lack of rapid diagnostic techniques, allowing for prompt use of a specific antiviral agent in the course of an acute infection. In avian medicine, two different approaches to antiviral therapy should be considered as diagnostic and therapeutic possibilities, and their aims are different. One is the treatment of species used for food production (mainly poultry) and the second is the treatment of other species kept as pets, such as psittacines and passerines, or for other reasons, like birds of prey. Also, the most commonly diagnosed viral infections vary between different species. Nowadays, drug resistance is becoming a serious threat to public health (noted especially in viruses with zoonotic potential, such as influenza virus) and is monitored by investigators from the whole world because of the ease with which mutations occur in many viruses [9–11]. Taking all mentioned above factors into consideration, a review of the literature to assess current knowledge about antiviral chemotherapy in avian species and indicate the possible direction of further research in this field was made.

2. Acyclovir

Acycloguanosine (acyclovir [ACV]) is a synthetic acyclic purine nucleoside analog with an antiviral spectrum essentially limited to herpesviruses [12]. Acyclovir triphosphate acts as both a substrate for and an inhibitor of viral DNA polymerase, thus blocking DNA synthesis [13]. The reason for this herpesviruse specificity is that ACV is a substrate for herpesvirus-encoded thymidine kinase, and production occurs in infected cells. Thymidine kinase converts ACV to ACV monophosphate, which is subsequently converted to ACV diphosphate and ACV triphosphate by cellular enzymes. ACV triphosphate is a potent inhibitor of DNA polymerase, as it competes with d-guanosine triphosphate, which is the natural substrate for the viral DNA polymerase. ACV triphosphate has a higher affinity for the enzyme and is preferentially incorporated into the ends of growing DNA chains. Following the incorporation of acyclovir triphosphate into the growing DNA chain, DNA synthesis ceases because ACV lacks the necessary 3′-hydroxyl group to react with incoming nucleotides [12–14]. Because ACV triphosphate has a higher affinity for viral polymerase than host cellular polymerases, it has limited toxicity for the host cell. Mutations leading to the development of herpesvirus-resistant strains remain a problem, and ACV does not prevent nor treat latent infections [15].

Most of the avian veterinary interest in ACV as an antiviral agent has been in its use to treat herpesviral infections in different bird species. During an outbreak of Pacheco's disease, ACV was administered intramuscularly (IM) to potentially infected birds at 25 mg/kg body weight (BW) and was administered in drinking water at 1 g/L and in food (seed mixture) at 400 mg/kg BW for 7 days [16]. Although the majority of treated birds survived, and all untreated birds died; it was not confirmed by any tests that the treated birds were infected by Pacheco's disease herpesvirus. In monk parakeets (*Myiopsitta monachus*), the pharmacokinetics in healthy specimens and an efficacy in experimentally infected with Pacheco's disease herpesvirus of ACV administered orally and intramuscularly [17,18]. The oral form of ACV administered by gavage was most effective, and clinical signs and death occurred only after the discontinuation of ACV. At the next step of the experiment, surviving monk parakeets were transferred to cages with seronegative monk parakeets with no known exposure to herpesvirus. There have been no deaths caused by herpesvirus infection in a period exceeding 2 years, which suggests that surviving parakeets did not shed the virus during the time of observation [17]. In a pharmacokinetic study, acyclovir was administered in single doses (20 mg/kg BW intravenously (IV) at 40 mg/kg BW IM and 80 mg/kg BW orally (PO) by crop gavage as a sodium salt for intravenous administration and oral capsule), multiple doses (40 mg/kg BW IM at 8h intervals (q8h) for 7 days, 80 mg/kg BW PO by crop gavage q8h for 4 days), in food (400 mg in 2 qt parrot seed), and water (1 mg of sodium salt for intravenous administration/mL). Results showed that acyclovir reaches therapeutic plasma levels greater than 0.01 pg/mL when administered PO by gavage to the crop, IM, IV, and in the medicated food and water. No evidence of drug accumulation or side effects were noted with any route of administration [18].

Acyclovir was administered towards the end of the outbreak of respiratory disease caused by herpesvirus in a flock of Bourke's parrots (*Neopsephotus bourkii*), but it was too late for its efficacy to be evaluated [19].

The efficacy of ACV was assessed in pigeons (*Columbia livia*) and budgerigars (*Melopsittacus undulatus*) experimentally infected with pigeon herpesvirus [20]. Intramuscular injections of ACV at 33 mg/kg BW three times daily did not prevent the appearance of clinical disease in infected pigeons and did not reduce viral shedding. The same treatment before infection protected most of the budgerigars for the duration of treatment, but most of them died soon after treatment was stopped.

The effect of acyclovir on poultry herpesviruses was also investigated [21]. ACV used in doses below 12.5 micrograms/mL proved to be non-toxic for chick embryo fibroblast culture and inhibited in vitro replication of turkey herpesvirus and Marek's disease virus. It has also been shown to diminish the development of tumors in birds infected with Marek's disease virus.

Another study showed that intramuscular administration of ACV at a dose of 10 mg/kg BW q24h prevents the development of clinical signs in chickens experimentally infected with Marek's disease virus if given for 5 days since day 3 after the challenge, which considerably reduces the mortality rate if given for 9 days starting 14 days after the challenge [22].

Plaque reduction assays were used to evaluate possible inhibitory effects of ACV, phosphonoacetate (PAA), and phosphonoformate (PFA) with a plaque-purified isolate of anatid herpesvirus-1 (duck plague virus) [23]. Whereas the interaction between PFA and PAA was additive, synergism occurred with ACV and either PAA or PFA. Drug-resistant mutants of the virus were isolated.

Results of an ACV pharmacokinetics study in hybrid tragopans (*Tragopan caboti x Tragopan temminckii*) where ACV was administered to five healthy adult birds, three males and two females, in a single dose of 40, 80, or 120 mg/kg BW PO suggest that a dosage of 120 mg/kg BW PO q12h in tragopans may achieve effective plasma concentrations (1.0 μg/mL) for potential treatment and prevention of herpesviral infections [24]. Although the nonlinearity of acyclovir pharmacokinetics in this species makes dose extrapolation difficult, this suggestion is based on maintaining plasma acyclovir concentrations above the accepted effective acyclovir plasma level (1.0 μg/mL) for 12 h after administration of the 120 mg/kg dose. Throughout all treatments, all birds appeared clinically healthy based on clinical examination and hematologic testing.

3. Abacavir and Its Derivates

Abacavir and its derivates are widely used in human medicine, especially HIV type 1, in combination with other antiviral drugs to enhance efficacy against HIV [25,26]. Because of low solubility, high cytotoxicity, low bioavailability, and a lack of target specificity of many antiviral chemotherapeutics [27], phosphorylation was proposed to increase the bioavailability and decrease the cytotoxicity of the activated nucleoside analogs in virus-infected cells [28]. As these phosphorylated nucleosides have high permeability and bioavailability, the focus is on producing nucleotide prodrugs, which finally release parent nucleosides at a specific site [25,29–31]. The mechanism proposed for abacavir [32–34] involves its conversion by cytosolic enzymes to carbovir monophosphate (CBV-MP), which is subsequently phosphorylated by host cellular kinases to carbovir triphosphate (CBVTP). Triphosphate is a potent and selective inhibitor of HIV reverse transcriptase by competing with dGTP for incorporation into viral DNA [32].

There is evidence that abacavir and its derivates showed antiviral activity against Newcastle disease virus (NDV), which is the cause of Newcastle disease (ND) [25,35]. Due to its high mortality and morbidity, NDV is a devastating virus and causes huge economic loss to the poultry industry. One study showed that abacavir and its phosphorylated compounds exhibit binding affinity to a fusion protein of Newcastle disease virus, suggesting that these compounds can be considered potent anti-NDV compounds or NDV inhibitors [25]. Because of the better binding affinity of three compounds, these three compounds were chosen for the synthesis of phosphorylated compounds and further in vitro studies on DF-1 cells. One of them (ABC-1) showed marked anti-NDV activity compared to two other compounds and has been further studied [25,35]. The antiviral activity of ABC-1 was also better than the parent compound, abacavir, which has been evidenced by its significant decrease in HA titer and lipid peroxidation and increase in antioxidant enzyme levels. Further studies of ABC-1 showed that tissue oxidative stress has been reduced and the expression of fusion protein caused by NDV infection has been inhibited in the NDV-infected chickens treated with ABC-1 in a dose of 2 mg/kg BW PO from the fourth day post-infection [35]. Immunolocalization, PCR, and flow cytometry analysis also showed that the novel phosphorylated compounds are effective in inhibiting the fusion protein expression, which is important in the replication of NDV.

4. Adefovir and Its Derivates

Adefovir and its derivates, such as adefovir dipivoxil, are antiviral drugs used in human medicine to treat HIV, hepatitis B, and cytomegalovirus infection [36]. The expression of the antiviral efficacy of adefovir requires phosphorylation to the active adefovir diphosphate moiety [37,38]. The diphosphate competitively inhibits deoxyadenosine triphosphate as a substrate for reverse transcriptase [39,40] and/or causes chain termination when incorporated into the growing DNA chain [37].

Duck hepatitis B virus (DHBV) is a model for research on the treatment of hepatitis B virus because of a similar characteristic of both viruses [41,42]. Research on adefovir antiviral activity against DHBV was performed when given as a single drug [43–45] or in combination with other therapeutics [46] and vaccines [47]. Both studies conducted by Heijtink et al. [43,44] showed that adefovir and its derivates have antiviral activity against DHBV both in vitro (in DHBV-infected duck hepatocytes) and in vivo given to Pekin ducks at a dose of 30 mg/kg BW q24h. Another study [45] showed that adefovir at a dosage of 15 mg/kg BW q24h has potent activity against DHBV without any hepatological, hematological, or biochemical evidence of systemic toxicity at this dose. However, a rebound of viral replication was observed after drug withdrawal when adefovir was given as a single drug [43–47]. It has been confirmed that at clinically achievable concentrations, the antiviral effects of all two-drug combinations containing adefovir, penciclovir, and lamivudine against DHBV in vitro are additive or synergistic [46]. Also, the anti-DHBV effect of combinations containing all three drugs is approximately additive, as measured by the inhibition of intracellular DHBV replication, although this is not consistently reflected by comparable inhibition of virus-specific protein synthesis. Results obtained by Guerhier et al. [47] suggest the presence of an additive effect of adefovir and DNA vaccine and a sustained decrease in intrahepatic DHBV DNA observed 12 weeks after the end of therapy.

5. Amantadine

Amantadine is a water-soluble tricyclic amine used as an antiviral agent for the prophylaxis and treatment of influenza A virus in human medicine [48]. Amantadines' antiviral mechanism of action is based on interference with the release of infectious viral nucleic acid into the host cell through interaction with the transmembrane domain of the M2 protein of the influenza A virus [49]. Amantadine by an indirect dopamine-releasing action and direct stimulation of dopamine receptors is also widely used in the treatment of Parkinson's disease [50].

In veterinary medicine, amantadine is used mainly to reduce nociception associated with chronic pain [51,52]. The use of amantadine in antiviral therapy in veterinary medicine is not common, but the irresponsible use of amantadine in commercial poultry in China [53] and Egypt [54] allowed for the emergence of drug-resistant mutants among lethal influenza strains, rendering this drug ineffective for treating human infections [55,56]. Analysis of global H5N1 sequencing data (isolated from both human and avian hosts) showed that the frequency of L26I/V27A mutation in M2, which is the response to resistance to amantadine, is linearly correlated with the mortality rates of human H5N1 infections [55]. Also, analysis of avian influenza isolates from poultry in Vietnam [10], Southeast Asia, and North America [57] showed that resistance to amantadine is a real problem. Results of a study conducted by scientists at the Friedrich–Loeffler–Institut in Germany indicated that the resistance to amantadine conferred by the presence of the amantadine resistance marker at position 31 (Ser31Asn) of the M2 protein evolved rapidly after the application of amantadine in commercial poultry [58]. Asn31 increased virus entry into the cells and cell-to-cell spread and was genetically stable for several passages in cell culture. The co-infection of cell culture with resistant and sensitive strains resulted in the dominance of resistant strains over sensitive viruses, even in the absence of selection by amantadine. Researchers concluded that the rapid emergence, stability, and domination of amantadine-resistant variants over sensitive strains limit the efficacy of amantadine in poultry.

However, some attempts to use amantadine in poultry [56,58–63] and pet birds were made [64–66].

The first study of the prophylactic use of amantadine in poultry was described in 1970 [59]. The optimum prophylactic dosage regimen included the administration of amantadine (10 mg/kg BW orally once daily or 0.025–0.05% amantadine incorporated into feed pellets) at least 2 days pre-infection to 23 days post-infection in turkeys experimentally infected with HPAIV H5N9.

A comprehensive study performed in the 1980s showed that both amantadine and rimantadine administered in water at a concentration of 0.01% were well accepted by chickens, were characterized by good pharmacokinetic properties, and prevented infection with H5N2 influenza virus when given concomitantly with the inoculation with the virus [60]. Further parts of this study demonstrated that amantadine administered in water at a concentration of 0.01% is effective in the treatment of chickens experimentally infected with the virulent H5N2 influenza virus, but it did not prevent virus shedding. Moreover, the majority of contact birds (which were also given amantadine 0.01% in water) died, and the virus recovered from these birds was resistant to amantadine in the plaque assay. The last experiment showed that the vaccine administered at the time of contact did not reduce mortality in the contact birds, but when vaccine and amantadine treatment were administered simultaneously, none of the contact birds died and they all developed antibodies.

Another study also showed rapid development of resistance to amantadine in the H5N2 avian influenza virus during an experiment that simulated layer flock treatment [61].

A few studies showed that amantadine-resistant strains of the avian influenza virus were irreversible, stable, and transmissible with pathogenic potential comparable to the wild-type virus and, even more, amantadine-resistant strains replaced the wild-type virus and became dominant [56,62,63].

Based on anecdotal reports [64], a group of clinically healthy, seropositive, avian bornavirus-shedding African gray parrots (*Psittacus erithacus*) were treated with amantadine for 6 weeks, with no apparent effect on fecal viral shedding [65].

A pharmacokinetic study showed that once-daily oral administration of amantadine at 5 mg/kg BW to orange-winged amazon parrots (*Amazona amazonica*) maintained plasma concentrations above those considered to be therapeutic for chronic pain in dogs without any observed adverse effects [66].

6. Ampligen

Ampligen is an immunomodulator and interferon inducer, which in one study was used alone and in combination with ganciclovir and coumermycin A1 to treat ducks congenitally infected with duck hepatitis B virus [67]. When used alone, ampligen decreased the amount of serum and liver viral DNA. In combination with ganciclovir, the antiviral effect was additive with a greater inhibition of viral DNA replication within the liver. The combination of ampligen with coumermycin A1 also resulted in the inhibition of viral replication but to a lesser extent than ampligen alone. When all three agents were used together, viral DNA replication was again inhibited. During all used treatment regimens, the level of circulating duck hepatitis B surface antigen (DHBsAg) measured in serum remained unchanged. At the end of the treatment period for all regimes, analysis of viral DNA forms in the liver showed that the viral relaxed circular and supercoiled DNA forms had persisted. Within 1 week of cessation of therapy, viral replication had returned to levels recorded before treatment. Interferon-like activity was detected in the sera of the majority of the treated ducks during ampligen therapy.

7. Azo Derivates

Azo dyes (-N=N-) are a class of compounds that are used as dyes and pigments and biomedical applications [68]. Azo derivates show antiviral [69–72], antibacterial [73], antifungal [74], antitumor [75], hypotensive, anti-inflammatory, and antioxidant effects [76].

In one study, embryonated eggs were inoculated with a Newcastle disease virus and an avian influenza virus [77]. The results of the hemagglutination (HA) test in the case of anti-NDV and anti-AIV potential of azo compounds revealed that three of five tested azo compounds actively inhibited NDV growth at a concentration of 0.1 mg/100 μL, and two of five compounds were able to inhibit AIV replication.

8. Baloxavir Marboxil

Baloxavir marboxil (BXM) is a prodrug of baloxavir acid used to treat influenza in human medicine [78]. Baloxavir acid inhibits cap-dependent endonuclease, an essential protein involved in the initiation of viral transcription by cleaving capped mRNA bound to basic polymerase 2.

BXM shows antiviral activity against H5 highly pathogenic avian influenza strains [9,79]. In chickens infected with the H5N6 HPAI virus, a single administration of 2.5 mg/kg BW of BXM immediately after inoculation was determined as the minimum dose required to fully protect chickens from the HPAI virus [80]. The concentration of baloxavir acid, the active form of BXM, in chicken blood at this dose was sufficient for a 48 h antiviral effect post-administration. In a further experiment, when BXM was given at a dose of 20 mg/kg BW q12h PO for 5 days from the moment when clinical signs were noticed at 24 h post-infection to mimic the field situation of an HPAI outbreak, all eight treated birds died. One chicken survived up to 6 days post-infection.

9. Didanosine

Didanosine (2,3-dideoxyinosine, DDI) is a dideoxy analog of purine nucleoside inosine that is a reverse transcriptase enzyme inhibitor and inhibits the replication of HIV [81]. Didanosine is metabolized intracellularly by a sequence of cellular enzymes to its active part dideoxyadenosine triphosphate, which inhibits reverse transcriptase competitively [82]. Phosphorylated didanosine derivates are designed [29,31,83] to overcome the disadvantages of didanosine, such as a short plasma half-life, low bioavailability, and dose-dependent cellular toxicities; it is unstable in its acidic conditions [84] and has poor permeability through intestinal epithelium and low oral bioavailability [85]. In one study, phosphorylated didanosine derivate DDI-10 was chosen from a series of designed derivates and showed antiviral activity against NDV in vitro, as evidenced by a significant reduction in plaque formation and cytopathic effects [86].

In vivo, in NDV-infected chicken, it was shown that superoxide dismutase and catalase were significantly raised, and lipid peroxidation and HA titer levels were decreased upon treatment with 1.5 mg/kg BW of DDI-10 compared to 3 mg/kg BW of DDI [86]. Histopathological alterations in NDV-infected tissues were restored in chickens treated with DDI-10. Another study showed that in NDV-infected chickens treated with DDI-10 glutathione-dependent enzymes, GPx, GST, and GR significantly increased and oxidation and nitration levels decreased compared to NDV-infected chickens [87].

10. Docosanol

n-Docosanol is a long-chain (C-22) saturated fatty alcohol with antiviral activity against herpes simplex virus (HSV), cytomegalovirus, human immunodeficiency virus (HIV), respiratory syncytial virus (RSV), influenza A virus, and murine Friend leukemia virus [88,89]. Some studies showed that n-docosanol has no direct antiviral effect [90], but a metabolic intracellular conversion prevents virus entry and, consequently, allows the cells to abort the infectious cycle of many enveloped viruses [88,91].

n-Doconasol given for 4 successive days at a dose of 40 and 60 mg/kg BW showed therapeutic activity against velogenic Newcastle disease virus (NDV) in domestic chickens [92]. NDV shedding was also reduced in treated birds.

11. Entecavir

Entecavir (ETV) is a deoxyguanosine analog with activity against hepatitis B virus (HBV) [93]. ETV inhibits reverse transcription, DNA replication, and transcription in the viral replication process [94].

Studies showed that ETV is a potent, safe, rapid-acting, and long-term suppressor of DHBV replication but is not able to eliminate the virus from infected duck organisms [94]. The treatment protocol consists of a DNA vaccine given 50 days post-infection, and ETV treatment that started 14 days post-infection at a dose of 0.1 mg/kg BW/day for 244 days did not result in any additional reduction in viral load compared to ETV used alone [95]. A higher dose (1 mg/kg/day) of ETV and different vaccination protocols lead to the clearance of DHBV-infected hepatocytes in ~50% of ETV-treated ducks [96]. In this treatment regimen, ducks were given ETV for 14 days starting from the day when the animals were inoculated and vaccinated at day "0", day 7, and day 14 post-infection.

12. Fluoroarabinosylpyrimidine Nucleosides

Three fluoronucleosides, 1-(2-fluro-2-deoxy-13-D-arabinofuranosyl)-5-iodocytosine (FIAC), 1-(2-fluoro-2-deoxy- [3-D-arabinofuranosyl)-5-iodouracil (FIAU), and its thymine analog (FMAU) have been shown to have potent anti-herpes simplex virus activity in vitro and in vivo [97–101].

It was demonstrated that all three fluoroarabinosylpyrimidine nucleosides (FIAC, FIAU, and FMAU) were potent inhibitors of MDV and HVT in chick kidney cells (CKCs), but only two of them (FMAU and FIAU) were active against these viruses in chick embryo fibroblasts (CEFs) and splenic lymphocyte cultures [102].

13. Ganciclovir

Ganciclovir (9-[(1,3-dihydroxy-2-propoxy)methyl]guanine) is a guanosine analog that is a potent inhibitor of viruses of the family herpesviridae [103] and hepadnaviridae [104]. The primary mechanism of action is inhibition of the replication of viral DNA by ganciclovir-5′-triphosphate (ganciclovir-TP) by chain termination. This inhibition includes a selective and potent inhibition of the viral DNA polymerase [103].

Ganciclovir was tested on a duck hepatitis B infection model to assess its safety and efficacy when given alone [105–109] and with nalidixic acid [109]. In a study conducted by Wang et al. [105], 5-week-old ducks congenitally infected with DHBV were treated with 21-day courses of twice-daily intraperitoneal injections of ganciclovir in a dose of 10 mg/kg BW q24h (alone or with pre-treatment with prednisolone 1 mg/kg once daily IM followed by a 10 mg/kg BW q24h 21-day ganciclovir course) or 30 mg/kg BW q24h without noticing any side effects in clinical observation and laboratory markers of liver, renal, and hematological function. In both protocols with only ganciclovir, the level of viremia rebounded to greater than pre-treatment levels within 2 weeks of cessation of therapy. This rebound phenomenon was not observed in follow-up samples obtained from ducks treated with prednisolone and ganciclovir. In the cited study, ganciclovir treatment failed to produce any consistent or significant reduction in the level of circulating duck hepatitis B surface antigen (DHBsAg). In other studies, when ganciclovir was given at a dose of 10 mg/kg BW q24h for 3 [106] and 4 weeks [107], similar observations were noted. After cessation of treatment, viremia returned to detectable levels within 4 days, despite that the treatment resulted in a substantial reduction in both viremia and liver DHBV DNA replicative intermediates. Also, long-term therapy of congenitally DHBV-infected ducks with ganciclovir at a dose of 10 mg/kg BW q24h for 24 weeks failed to permanently stop DHBV replication [108]. A combination of ganciclovir at a dose of 10 mg/kg BW q24h with nalidixic acid at a dose of 250 mg/kg BW q12h resulted in a substantial decrease in viremia, with DHBV DNA levels becoming undetectable [109]. However, during the follow-up period, the DHBV DNA in serum returned to detectable levels. A pharmacokinetic study showed that ketoprofen given at a dose of 2 mg/kg BW IV at the same time as ganciclovir at a dose of 10 mg/kg BW IV caused increased plasma concentration and prolonged the elimination half-life of ganciclovir in chukar partridges (*Alectoris chukar*) [110].

14. Interferon

Interferons (IFNs) are a class of cytokines elicited on challenge to the host defense and are essential for mobilizing immune responses to pathogens [111]. Divided into three classes, type I, type II, and type III, IFNs do not have direct antiviral activity but affect cells, inducing the synthesis of antiviral agents. Interferons activate a number of enzymes in the cell that allow the degradation of viral genetic material, causing the so-called antiviral status [112]. In human medicine, IFNs have been widely used in the treatment of many diseases, such as hepatitis B, hepatitis C, and multiple sclerosis [112]. IFNs also show anti-cancer effects. In general, the interferon system is species-specific—it will protect cells against viruses only in the same or closely related animal species from which it originates (e.g., interferon produced in rabbit cells will not protect mouse cells, but human interferon can protect monkey cells from some viral attack) [113].

In avian species, the cross-species antiviral activity of goose interferon-gamma against duck plague virus in vitro in duck embryo fibroblasts (DEFs) has been confirmed [114]. Recombinant duck interferon-alpha (rDuIFN-α) inhibits avian influenza (AIV) H5N1 virus in vitro and in vivo [115]. It was demonstrated that the IM administration of 1×10^5 U rDuIFN-α significantly reduces the morbidity and mortality of H5N1 AIV infection in Pekin ducks.

There was an attempt to treat circovirus infection in gray parrots (*Psittacus erithacus*) with type 1 interferon-alpha of feline origin or avian gamma interferon derived from poultry cell cultures [116]. In the feline-origin interferon-treated group, there was no improvement in clinical observations and hematological parameters (severe leukemia) in all 12 birds, which died or were euthanized within 30 weeks. Avian gamma-interferon seemed to be effective in the treatment of psittacine beak and feather disease caused by circovirus in gray parrots. In the avian gamma-interferon-treated group, seven of ten birds were alive after 30 weeks and exhibited normal total white blood cell counts, and samples of blood and feather pulp taken in week 30 were negative for circovirus by PCR.

It has been demonstrated that the combination of ribavirin with recombinant interferon-alpha shows a synergistic effect against avian bornaviruses in vitro [117].

A comprehensive study focused on the effects of nitric oxide (NO) and chicken interferon-gamma on the replication of MDV showed that the addition of S-nitroso-N-acetylpenicillamine resulted in the production of NO and reduced replication of MDV and turkey herpesvirus (HVT) in a dose-dependent manner in vitro in chicken embryo fibroblasts [118]. Further experiments demonstrated that recombinant chicken interferon-gamma and lipopolysaccharide (LPS) inhibited MDV replication in chicken embryo fibroblasts. The addition of NG-monomethyl L-arginine (NMMA) by blocking the production of NO reversed the inhibition of viral replication. Additionally, LPS and interferon were tested when used alone; LPS did not inhibit MDV replication, and recombinant chicken interferon-gamma caused a nonsignificant inhibition of viral replication.

A few studies demonstrated that chicken interferon-alpha showed an inhibitory effect on avian influenza viruses in vitro [119], in ovo [120], and in vivo [120–122].

15. Ivermectin

Recently, drug repurposing became an option for the treatment of emerging diseases, as developing new effective antiviral drugs against a particular pathogen is very time-consuming, laborious, and expensive. Ivermectin, an antiparasitic drug, is one of the recently tested drugs in Flaviviridae [123,124] and SARS-COV-2 [125–128] treatment.

It was shown that ivermectin is a potent inhibitor of Usutu virus (USUV) replication in vitro [124]. USUV is a mosquito-borne arbovirus within the genus Flavivirus and family Flaviviridae. Similar to the closely related West Nile virus (WNV), USUV infections are capable of causing mass mortality in wild and captive birds, especially blackbirds, and both viruses are able to infect humans [129]. In the last few years, a massive spread of USUV has been noticed in the avian populations, mainly the common blackbird (*Turdus merula*) in Germany and other European countries [130]. Also, some anecdotal reports indicated improved clinical outcomes in cases of West Nile virus and USUV infections in hawks and owls treated with ivermectin [131].

16. Novel Peptides

Peptides with antiviral activity characterize biocompatibility, specificity, and effectiveness, and they also overcome the limitations of existing drugs [132]. Synthetic peptides are designed using virtual screening technology and molecular docking technology, which shorten the research cycle and costs and significantly increase the possibility of screening for desirable results [133,134].

Because hydropericardium hepatitis syndrome (HHS) caused by fowl adenovirus serotype 4 (FAdV-4) is the cause of significant economic losses to the poultry industry [135,136], research on treatment possibilities was conducted [137]. Treatment with one (P15) of eight investigated peptides significantly inhibited virus proliferation in vitro in LMH cells, probably through the binding of the peptide to the C-terminal knob domain of the FAdV-4 Fiber2 protein.

Another study showed that four peptides derived from the Marek disease virus (MDV) glycoprotein gH (gHH1, gHH2, gHH3, and gHH5) and one peptide derived from MDV glycoprotein gB (gBH1) have potent antiviral activity against MDV both in vitro in plaque formation assays in primary chicken embryo fibroblast cells (CEFs) and in vivo in lesion formation assays on a chorioallantoic membrane (CAM) [138].

17. Lamivudine

Lamivudine is a nucleoside derivative antiviral drug with a competitive inhibitory effect on viral DNA synthesis and extension [139]. It has been shown to inhibit reverse transcriptase and, therefore, inhibits the replication of human immunodeficiency virus (HIV) by competition binding with cellular nucleotides both in vitro and in vivo [140–144].

As a type of retrovirus, reverse transcriptase also plays a key role in the life cycle of avian leukosis virus subgroup J (ALV-J). The efficacy of lamivudine against ALV-J was tested in vivo in chickens [145]. It has been shown that lamivudine could inhibit ALV-J replication by competing with normal nucleotides for reverse transcriptase binding and inhibit cDNA transcription and extension with a mechanism similar to that of HIV inhibition, but it cannot kill the virus completely.

Lamivudine was also confirmed to show an antihepadnaviral effect in primary duck hepatocytes infected with DHBV in vitro [146]. It has been also shown that the antiviral activity of lamivudine in combination with adefovir [45] or penciclovir [45,146] against DHBV in vitro is additive or synergistic.

18. Nitazoxanide

Originally developed and commercialized as an antiprotozoal agent, nitazoxanide was later identified as a broad-spectrum antiviral drug [147,148]. Nitazoxanide and its active metabolite tizoxanide show antiviral activity in vitro against influenza A and B [147], hepatitis B virus [149], hepatitis C virus [149], paramyxovirus [150], yellow fever virus [151], HIV [152], and many different mammalian coronaviruses [153].

The efficacy of nitazoxanide against West Nile virus in vitro and in vivo has been demonstrated [154]. Treatment of two-week-old chickens resulted in a significant reduction in NDV replication in the trachea and lungs at 72 h post-infection.

19. Oseltamivir

Oseltamivir is the oral prodrug of GS4071, a selective inhibitor of influenza A and B viral neuraminidase widely used in human medicine [155].

Oseltamivir given at a dose of 120 mg/kg BW q12h from 1 day before inoculation to 7 days post-infection could not prevent HPAI infection of inoculated chickens, but treatment limited morbidity, mortality, and chicken-to-chicken transmission of HPAI virus infection [156]. Another study confirmed that oseltamivir reduces the replication of low pathogenic AIV, significantly in chickens and completely in domestic ducks [157]. Research on the safety of oseltamivir in chicken embryos demonstrated that it is non-toxic at concentrations of 0.1, 1.0, and 10.0 mg/kg BW [158].

None of the few mentioned studies conducted to evaluate the efficacy of oseltamivir in avian species reported the emergence of resistant strains. In contrast to amantadine, oseltamivir-resistant H5N1 avian influenza viruses isolated from domestic and wild birds probably emerged due to spontaneous mutations rather than exposure to oseltamivir [159–162].

20. Penciclovir and Famciclovir

Famciclovir (FCV) is the oral form of the potent and selective antiherpesviral and antihepadnaviral agent penciclovir (PCV) and was developed because of the poor absorption of penciclovir given orally [163–165]. Similarly to acyclovir, guanosine analog penciclovir is a highly selective inhibitor of herpesviruses DNA polymerase because it is phosphorylated and thereby only activated in herpesvirus-infected cells [163–167].

In avian species, antiviral activity against duck hepatitis B virus both in vitro [168] and in vivo [169–173] has been mainly studied. An in vitro study compared the antihepadnavirus activities of penciclovir and ganciclovirin primary duck hepatocyte cultures congenitally infected with the duck hepatitis B virus (DHBV) [168]. Both compounds inhibited DHBV DNA replication to a comparable extent during continuous short-term treatment, but penciclovir was more active both during longer-term continuous treatment and in washout experiments. Based on anti-DHBV activity, it has been demonstrated that young ducklings efficiently metabolize FCV given orally to the parent compound, PCV, which is activated to exert an antiviral effect not only in the liver but also in the nonhepatic tissues (kidney, pancreas, and spleen) [169]. In different studies [170,171], it was demonstrated that penciclovir given to DHBV-infected ducks in different treatment protocols (dose ranges from 10 mg/kg BW q24h for 4 weeks to 20 mg/kg BW q12h and 100 mg/kg BW q12h for 3 weeks) suppress viral replication, but it is not able to completely kill the virus, and DHBV DNA plasma levels increased after the cessation of treatment, which indicated that virus replication had resumed. The same effect has been noticed when giving famciclovir at a dose of 5 mg/kg BW and 25 mg/kg BW q12h for 3 weeks [171]. Long-term therapy of congenitally DHBV-infected ducks with penciclovir at a dose of 10 mg/kg BW q24h for 12 or 24 weeks resulted in similar effects—viral replication was inhibited but during the follow-up period, DHBV DNA returned to pre-treatment levels [172]. Nicoll et al. [173] found that penciclovir given to congenitally DHBV-infected ducklings at a dose of 10 mg/kg BW q24h for 17 days controlled viral replication and reduced viral burden in hepatocytes but not in the bile duct epithelial cells, which might be an important reservoir of the virus that is relatively unaffected by antiviral treatment and may play a role in relapse after cessation of therapy. In all mentioned in vivo studies [169–173], no side effects were observed during and after PCV or ACV therapy.

21. Ribavirin

Ribavirin is a broad-spectrum antiviral drug that is a purine analog and can potentially act on numerous steps of the virus life cycle, such as the inhibition of translation due to a reduction in cellular GTP pools or incorporation as a cap analog, which inhibits translation, the inhibition of genome or transcript capping by suppression of GTP synthesis or direct competition, the inhibition of RNA synthesis directly via active-site binding or a reduction in GTP synthesis, ambiguous incorporation into RNA causing increased mutation and production of non-viable genomes, enhancement of the antiviral immune response, and the prevention of spread and pathogenesis [174]. In human medicine, ribavirin is used mainly to treat hepatitis C virus infections, but there is evidence of a benefit in RSV infection and Lassa fever [174].

Ribavirin toxicity and efficacy against Newcastle disease virus in ovo has been studied [175]. Inoculation of a 0.1 mL solution with the lowest used concentration of 10 μg/mL did not stop the replication of the virus, while inoculation of a 0.1 mL solution with the highest used concentration of 40 μg/mL was toxic, and embryos in eggs died. Inoculation of a 0.1 mL solution with a concentration of 20 μg/mL was non-toxic and had antiviral activity.

Ribavirin was proven to inhibit the replication of parrot bornaviruses in vitro but was not able to eliminate the virus [176,177]. Ribavirin showed synergistic effects against parrot bornaviruses with recombinant IFN-α in avian cells [122]. Avian bornaviruses were discovered in 2008 in parrots suffering from proventricular dilatation disease (PDD), which is a chronic neurologic and gastrointestinal disorder of birds belonging to the order Psittaciformes [178,179]. Recently, evidence that avian bornaviruses also cause the disease in canaries (*Serinus canaria*) was published [180,181]. Bornaviruses that are able to infect other species of birds, such as ducks, geese, swans, and estrildid finches, were also described [182]. However, their pathogenicity is still unclear. Because avian bornaviruses are a common cause of losses in psittacine collections and can be a threat to endangered species conservation programs, they are currently one of the most intensively studied exotic bird viruses in the field of treatment and prevention [182].

22. Zidovudine

Zidovudine is an antiviral drug used in HIV infection treatment in human medicine [183]. Mechanism studies show that zidovudine is phosphorylated by the host cell enzymes. The triphosphate of zidovudine appears to be the active form of the drug and it competes well with thymidine 5′-triphosphate for binding to the HIV reverse transcriptase and also functions as an alternative substrate. The incorporation of zidovudine monophosphate results in chain termination.

Avian leukosis virus (ALV) is an oncogenic virus belonging to alpha retrovirus [184], which is the cause of avian leukosis in poultry [185]. ALV also cause immunosuppression in infected birds, resulting in huge economic losses due to secondary infections [186,187]. One study [188] showed that a combination of zidovudine and short hairpin RNA was able to significantly inhibit ALV subtype J replication in vitro.

23. Conclusions

The main conclusion is that the current knowledge about the use of antiviral drugs in avian species in clinical practice is poor. However, numerous experimental studies showed that many antiviral drugs can effectively inhibit the replication of some avian viruses, depending on the substance and virus species. There are many more in vitro studies than in vivo experiments. Even promising results of these in vitro studies should be confirmed in experimentally infected birds if they have not been performed yet. In some studies, even though they were conducted on birds, the main goal was to determine drug efficacy on animal models to assess its usefulness in human medicine (e.g., ducks infected with duck hepatitis B virus, which are animal models of hepatitis B virus infection in human), not to determine if the drug can be useful in the treatment of disease in birds. There are a few pharmacokinetic studies of specific antiviral substances in avian species. A small number of pharmacokinetic studies makes it difficult to determine dosage and use them in clinical practice. Dose extrapolation from mammals to avian species is hard because of many differences in metabolism (e.g., metabolic rate and specific metabolic processes).

Considering antiviral therapy in birds, the risk of drug-resistance development should also be kept in mind, especially in zoonotic infections, such as HPAI. Antiviral therapy with classic antiviral drugs in poultry is generally useless because of residues of drugs in tissues and eggs, and as mentioned above, a high risk of drug-resistant viral strain development. However, further research on the use of antiviral drugs in birds is warranted because, in some situations, antiviral therapy can be the only way to save endangered bird species. Also, some viral infections in birds kept in a zoo and companion animals could be treated.

Future studies in this field should focus on pharmacokinetics in drugs proven to be effective in specific infections in birds in vitro and in vivo to determine dosage and enable their wider application in clinical practice. Further studies on substances that were not tested in avian viral infections yet are also warranted.

Author Contributions: Conceptualization, I.S. and A.L.; methodology, I.S. and A.L.; writing—original draft preparation, I.S.; writing—review and editing, A.L. All authors have read and agreed to the published version of the manuscript.

Funding: This work received no external funding.

Institutional Review Board Statement: Not applicable.

Informed Consent Statement: Not applicable.

Data Availability Statement: Not applicable.

Conflicts of Interest: The authors declare no conflicts of interest.

References

1. Carpenter, J.W.; Marion, C.J. Chapter 5: Birds. In *Exotic Animal Formulary*, 5th ed; W.B. Saunders: St. Louis, MO, USA, 2018; pp. 291–293.
2. Carpenter, J.W.; Marion, C.J. Chapter 6: Backyard Poultry and Waterfowl. In *Exotic Animal Formulary*, 5th ed; W.B. Saunders: St. Louis, MO, USA, 2018; p. 558.
3. European Medicines Agency. Available online: https://www.ema.europa.eu/en/medicines/veterinary/EPAR/virbagen-omega (accessed on 3 February 2024).
4. Sorrell, S.; Pugalendhi, S.J.; Gunn-Moore, D. Current treatment options for feline infectious peritonitis in the UK. *Companion Anim.* **2022**, *27*, 79–90. [CrossRef]
5. Commission Implementing Regulation (EU). 2022/1255 of 19 July 2022 Designating Antimicrobials or Groups of Antimicrobials Reserved for Treatment of Certain Infections in Humans, in Accordance with Regulation (EU) 2019/6 of the European Parliament and of the Council. Available online: https://eur-lex.europa.eu/eli/reg_impl/2022/1255/oj (accessed on 8 February 2024).
6. Dal Pozzo, F.; Thiry, E. Antiviral chemotherapy in veterinary medicine: Current applications and perspectives. *Rev. Sci. Tech.* **2014**, *33*, 791–801. [CrossRef] [PubMed]
7. Rollinson, E.A. Prospects for antiviral chemotherapy in veterinary medicine. I: Feline virus diseases. *Antivir. Chem. Chemother.* **1992**, *3*, 249–262. [CrossRef]
8. Rollinson, E.A. Prospects for antiviral chemotherapy in veterinary medicine. II: Avian, piscine, canine, porcine, bovine and equine virus diseases. *Antivir. Chem. Chemother.* **1992**, *3*, 311–326. [CrossRef]
9. Nguyen, H.T.; Chesnokov, A.; De La Cruz, J.; Pascua, P.N.Q.; Mishin, V.P.; Jang, Y.; Jones, J.; Di, H.; Ivashchenko, A.A.; Killian, M.L.; et al. Antiviral susceptibility of clade 2.3.4.4b highly pathogenic avian influenza A(H5N1) viruses isolated from birds and mammals in the United States, 2022. *Antivir. Res.* **2023**, *217*, 105679. [CrossRef]
10. Nguyen, H.T.; Nguyen, T.; Mishin, V.P.; Sleeman, K.; Balish, A.; Jones, J.; Creanga, A.; Marjuki, H.; Uyeki, T.M.; Nguyen, D.H.; et al. Antiviral susceptibility of highly pathogenic avian influenza A(H5N1) viruses isolated from poultry, Vietnam, 2009–2011. *Emerg. Infect. Dis.* **2013**, *19*, 1963–1971. [CrossRef] [PubMed]
11. Kayed, A.E.; Kutkat, O.; Kandeil, A.; Moatasim, Y.; El Taweel, A.; El Sayes, M.; El-Shesheny, R.; Aboulhoda, B.E.; Abdeltawab, N.F.; Kayali, G.; et al. Comparative pathogenic potential of avian influenza H7N3 viruses isolated from wild birds in Egypt and their sensitivity to commercial antiviral drugs. *Arch. Virol.* **2023**, *168*, 82. [CrossRef] [PubMed]
12. Cross, G. Antiviral therapy. *Semin. Avian Exot. Pet Med.* **1995**, *4*, 96–102. [CrossRef]
13. Gnann, J.W., Jr.; Barton, N.H.; Whitley, R.J. Acyclovir: Mechanism of action, pharmacokinetics, safety and clinical applications. *Pharmacotherapy* **1983**, *3*, 275–283. [CrossRef] [PubMed]

14. Furman, P.A.; St Clair, M.H.; Spector, T. Acyclovir triphosphate is a suicide inactivator of the herpes simplex virus DNA polymerase. *J. Biol. Chem.* **1984**, *259*, 9575–9579. [CrossRef] [PubMed]
15. Saral, R.; Ambinder, R.F.; Burns, W.H.; Angelopulos, C.M.; Griffin, D.E.; Burke, P.J.; Lietman, P.S. Acyclovir prophylaxis against herpes simplex virus infection in patients with leukemia. A randomized, double-blind, placebo-controlled study. *Ann. Intern. Med.* **1983**, *99*, 773–776. [CrossRef] [PubMed]
16. Smith, C.G. Use of acyclovir in an outbreak of Pacheco's parrot disease. *AAV Today* **1987**, *1*, 55–56. [CrossRef]
17. Norton, T.M.; Gaskin, J.; Kollias, G.V.; Homer, B.; Clark, C.H.; Wilson, R. Efficacy of acyclovir against herpesvirus infection in Quaker parakeets. *Am. J. Vet. Res.* **1991**, *52*, 2007–2009. [CrossRef] [PubMed]
18. Norton, T.M.; Kollias, G.V.; Clark, C.H.; Gaskin, J.; Wilson, R.C.; Coniglario, J. Acyclovir (Zovirax) pharmacokinetics in Quaker parakeets, *Myiopsitta monachus*. *J. Vet. Pharmacol. Ther.* **1992**, *15*, 252–258. [CrossRef] [PubMed]
19. Shivaprasad, H.L.; Phalen, D.N. A novel herpesvirus associated with respiratory disease in Bourke's parrots (*Neopsephotus bourkii*). *Avian Pathol.* **2012**, *41*, 531–539. [CrossRef] [PubMed]
20. Thiry, E.; Vindevogel, H.; Leroy, P.; Pastoret, P.P.; Schwers, A.; Brochier, B.; Anciaux, Y.; Hoyois, P. In vivo and in vitro effect of acyclovir on pseudorabies virus, infectious bovine rhinotracheitis virus and pigeon herpesvirus. *Ann. Rech. Vet.* **1983**, *14*, 239–245. [PubMed]
21. Samorek-Salamonowicz, E.; Cakala, A.; Wijaszka, T. Effect of acyclovir on the replication of turkey herpesvirus and Marek's disease virus. *Res. Vet. Sci.* **1987**, *42*, 334–338. [CrossRef] [PubMed]
22. Samorek, S.E.; Cakala, A. Effects of acyclovir on the replication of virulent and vaccinal herpesvirus in vitro and in vivo. *Zesz. Nauk. Akad. Roln Wroc. Wet.* **1988**, *45*, 109–117.
23. Johnson, J.C.; Attanasio, R. Synergistic inhibition of anatid herpesvirus replication by acyclovir and phosphonocompounds. *Intervirology* **1987**, *28*, 89–99. [CrossRef] [PubMed]
24. Rush, E.M.; Hunter, R.P.; Papich, M.; Raphael, B.L.; Calle, P.P.; Clippinger, T.L.; Cook, R.A. Pharmacokinetics and safety of acyclovir in tragopans (*Tragopan* species). *J. Avian Med. Surg.* **2005**, *19*, 271–276. [CrossRef]
25. Suresh, K.A.; Venkata Subbaiah, K.C.; Lavanya, R.; Chandrasekhar, K.; Chamarti, N.R.; Kumar, M.S.; Wudayagiri, R.; Valluru, L. Design, Synthesis and Biological Evaluation of Novel Phosphorylated Abacavir Derivatives as Antiviral Agents against Newcastle Disease Virus Infection in Chicken. *Appl. Biochem. Biotechnol.* **2016**, *180*, 61–81.
26. Geetha, S.; Emmanuel, F.M.; Rodger, D.M. Abacavir/Lamividine combination in the treatment of HIV: A review. *Ther. Clin. Risk Manag.* **2010**, *6*, 83–94.
27. Kesharwani, R.K.; Srivastava, V.; Singh, P.; Rizvi, S.I.; Adeppa, K.; Misra, K. A novel approach for overcoming drug resistance in breast cancer chemotherapy by targeting new synthetic curcumin analogues against aldehyde dehydrogenase 1 (ALDH1A1) and glycogen synthase kinase-3 β (GSK-3β). *Appl. Biochem. Biotechnol.* **2015**, *176*, 1996–2017. [CrossRef] [PubMed]
28. Balzarini, J.; Stefano, A.; Alshaimaa, H.A.; Susan, M.D.; Carlo-Federico, P.; Chris, M. Improved antiviral activity of the aryloxymethoxyalaninyl phosphoramidate (APA) prodrug of abacavir (ABC) is due to the formation of markedly increased carbovir 50-triphosphate metabolite levels. *FEBS Lett.* **2004**, *573*, 38–44. [CrossRef] [PubMed]
29. Youcef, M.; Jan, B.; Christopher, M. Aryloxy phosphoramidate triesters: A technology for delivering monophosphorylated nucleosides and sugars into cells. *ChemMedChem* **2009**, *4*, 1779–1791.
30. Rao, V.K.; Reddy, S.S.; Krishna, S.B.; Reddy, S.C.; Reddy, P.N.; Reddy, C.M.T.; Raju, C.N.; Ghosh, S.K. Design, synthesis and anti colon cancer activity evaluation of phosphorylated derivatives of Lamivudine (3TC). *Lett. Drug Des. Discov.* **2011**, *8*, 59–64.
31. Sekhar, K.C.; Janardhan, A.; Kumar, Y.N.; Narasimha, G.; Raju, C.N.; Ghosh, S.K. Amino acid esters substituted phosphorylated emtricitabine and didanosine derivatives as antiviral and anticancer agents. *Appl. Biochem. Biotechnol.* **2014**, *173*, 1303–1318. [CrossRef] [PubMed]
32. Faletto, M.B.; Miller, W.H.; Garvey, E.P.; St. Clair, M.H.; Daluge, S.M.; Good, S.S. Unique Intracellular Activation of a New Anit-HIV Agent (1592U89) in the Human T-Lymphoblastoid Cell Line CEM-T4. *Antimicrob. Agents Chemother.* **1997**, *41*, 1099–1107. [CrossRef]
33. Daluge, S.M.; Good, S.S.; Faletto, M.B. A novel carbocyclic nucleoside analog with potent, selective antihuman immunodeficiency virus activity. *Antimicrob. Agents Chemother.* **1997**, *41*, 1082–1093. [CrossRef] [PubMed]
34. Foster, R.H.; Faulds, D. Abacavir. *Drugs* **1998**, *55*, 729–736. [CrossRef] [PubMed]
35. Suresh, K.A.; Venkata Subbaiah, K.C.; Thirunavukkarasu, C.; Chennakesavulu, S.; Rachamallu, A.; Chamarti, N.R.; Wudayagiri, R.; Valluru, L. Phosphorylated abacavir analogue (ABC-1) has ameliorative action against Newcastle disease virus induced pathogenesis in chicken. *Biotechnol. Appl. Biochem.* **2019**, *66*, 977–989. [CrossRef] [PubMed]
36. Noble, S.; Goa, K.L. Adefovir Dipivoxil. *Drugs* **1999**, *58*, 479–487. [CrossRef] [PubMed]
37. Balzarini, J. Metabolism and mechanism of antiretroviral action of purine and pyrimidine derivatives. *Pharm. World Sci.* **1993**, *16*, 113–126. [CrossRef] [PubMed]
38. Naesens, L.; Snoeck, R.; Andrei, G.; Balzarini, J.; Neyts, J.; De Clercq, E. HPMPC (cidofovir), PMEA (adefovir) and related acyclic nucleoside phosphonate analogues: A review of their pharmacology and clinical potential in the treatment of viral infections. *Antivir. Chem. Chemother.* **1997**, *8*, 1–23. [CrossRef]
39. Holy, A.; Votruba, I.; Merta, A.; Cerný, J.; Veselý, J.; Vlach, J.; Sedivá, K.; Rosenberg, I.; Otmar, M.; Hrebabecký, H.; et al. Acyclic nucleotide analogues: Synthesis, antiviral activity and inhibitory effects on some cellular and virus-encoded enzymes in vitro. *Antivir. Res.* **1990**, *13*, 295–311. [CrossRef] [PubMed]

40. Balzarini, J.; Hao, Z.; Herdewijn, P.; Johns, D.G.; De Clercq, E. Intracellular metabolism and mechanism of anti-retrovirus action of 9-(2-phosphonylmethoxyethyl)adenine, a potent anti-human immunodeficiency virus compound. *Proc. Natl. Acad. Sci. USA* **1991**, *88*, 1499–1503. [CrossRef] [PubMed]
41. Chassot, S.; Lambert, V.; Kay, A.; Trépo, C.; Cova, L. Duck hepatitis B virus (DHBV) as a model for understanding hepadnavirus neutralization. *Arch. Virol. Suppl.* **1993**, *8*, 133–139. [PubMed]
42. Schultz, U.; Grgacic, E.; Nassal, M. Duck hepatitis B virus: An invaluable model system for HBV infection. *Adv. Virus Res.* **2004**, *63*, 1–70. [PubMed]
43. Heijtink, R.A.; Kruining, J.; De Wilde, G.A.; Balzarini, J.; De Clercq, E.; Schalm, S.W. Inhibitory effects of acyclic nucleoside phosphonates on human hepatitis B virus and duck hepatitis B virus infections in tissue culture. *Antimicrob. Agents Chemother.* **1994**, *38*, 2180–2182. [CrossRef] [PubMed]
44. Heijtink, R.A.; De Wilde, G.A.; Kruining, J.; Berk, L.; Balzarini, J.; De Clercq, E.; Holy, A.; Schalm, S.W. Inhibitory effect of 9-(2-phosphonylmethoxyethyl)-adenine (PMEA) on human and duck hepatitis B virus infection. *Antivir. Res.* **1993**, *21*, 141–153. [CrossRef] [PubMed]
45. Nicoll, A.J.; Colledge, D.L.; Toole, J.J.; Angus, P.W.; Smallwood, R.A.; Locarnini, S.A. Inhibition of duck hepatitis B virus replication by 9-(2-phosphonylmethoxyethyl)adenine, an acyclic phosphonate nucleoside analogue. *Antimicrob. Agents Chemother.* **1998**, *42*, 3130–3135. [CrossRef] [PubMed]
46. Colledge, D.; Civitico, G.; Locarnini, S.; Shaw, T. In vitro antihepadnaviral activities of combinations of penciclovir, lamivudine, and adefovir. *Antimicrob. Agents Chemother.* **2000**, *44*, 551–560. [CrossRef] [PubMed]
47. Le Guerhier, F.; Thermet, A.; Guerret, S.; Chevallier, M.; Jamard, C.; Gibbs, C.S.; Trépo, C.; Cova, L.; Zoulim, F. Antiviral effect of adefovir in combination with a DNA vaccine in the duck hepatitis B virus infection model. *J. Hepatol.* **2003**, *38*, 328–334. [CrossRef] [PubMed]
48. Mondal, D. Amantadine. In *xPharm: The Comprehensive Pharmacology Reference*; Enna, S.J., Bylund, D.B., Eds.; Elsevier: Amsterdam, The Netherlands, 2007; pp. 1–4.
49. Hay, A.J.; Wolstenholme, A.J.; Skehel, J.J.; Smith, M.H. The molecular basis of the specific anti-influenza action of amantadine. *EMBO J.* **1985**, *4*, 3021–3024. [CrossRef] [PubMed]
50. Bailey, E.V.; Stone, T.W. The mechanism of action of amantadine in Parkinsonism: A review. *Arch. Int. Pharmacodyn. Ther.* **1975**, *216*, 246–262. [PubMed]
51. Rychel, J.K. Diagnosis and treatment of osteoarthritis. *Top. Companion Anim. Med.* **2010**, *25*, 20–25. [CrossRef] [PubMed]
52. KuKanich, B. Outpatient oral analgesics in dogs and cats beyond nonsteroidal anti-inflammatory drugs: An evidencebased approach. *Vet. Clin. N. Am. Small Anim. Pract.* **2013**, *43*, 1109–1125. [CrossRef] [PubMed]
53. Cyranoski, D. China's chicken farmers under fire for antiviral abuse. *Nature* **2005**, *435*, 1009. [CrossRef] [PubMed]
54. Hussein, I.; Abdelwhab, E. *Why the Veterinary Use of Antivirals in Egypt Should Stop?* Nature Middle East: Dubai, United Arab Emirates, 2016.
55. Yuan, S.; Jiang, S.C.; Zhang, Z.W.; Fu, Y.F.; Zhu, F.; Li, Z.L.; Hu, J. Abuse of amantadine in poultry may be associated with higher fatality rate of H5N1 infections in humans. *J. Med. Virol.* **2022**, *94*, 2588–2597. [CrossRef] [PubMed]
56. Bean, W.J.; Threlkeld, S.C.; Webster, R.G. Biologic potential of amantadine-resistant influenza A virus in an avian model. *J. Infect. Dis.* **1989**, *159*, 1050–1056. [CrossRef] [PubMed]
57. Ilyushina, N.A.; Govorkova, E.A.; Webster, R.G. Detection of amantadine-resistant variants among avian influenza viruses isolated in North America and Asia. *Virology* **2005**, *341*, 102–106. [CrossRef] [PubMed]
58. Abdelwhab, E.M.; Veits, J.; Mettenleiter, T.C. Biological fitness and natural selection of amantadine resistant variants of avian influenza H5N1 viruses. *Virus Res.* **2017**, *228*, 109–113. [CrossRef] [PubMed]
59. Lang, G.; Narayan, O.; Rouse, B.T. Prevention of malignant avian influenza by 1-adamantanamine hydrochloride. *Arch. Gesamte Virusforsch.* **1970**, *32*, 171–184. [CrossRef] [PubMed]
60. Webster, R.G.; Kawaoka, Y.; Bean, W.J. Vaccination as a strategy to reduce the emergence of amantadine- and rimantadine-resistant strains of A/Chick/Pennsylvania/83 (H5N2) influenza virus. *J. Antimicrob. Chemother.* **1986**, *18* (Suppl. B), 157–164. [CrossRef] [PubMed]
61. Beard, C.W.; Brugh, M.; Webster, R.G. Emergence of amantadine-resistant H5N2 avian influenza virus during a simulated layer flock treatment program. *Avian Dis.* **1987**, *31*, 533–537. [CrossRef] [PubMed]
62. Bean, W.J.; Webster, R.G. Biological properties of amantadine-resistant influenza-virus mutants. *Antivir. Res.* **1988**, *9*, 128.
63. Scholtissek, C.; Faulkner, G.P. Amantadine-resistant and -sensitive influenza A strains and recombinants. *J. Gen. Virol.* **1979**, *44*, 807–815. [CrossRef] [PubMed]
64. Clubb, S.L.; Meyer, M.J. Clinical management of psittacine birds affected with proventricular dilatation disease. In Proceeding of the Annual Conference Association of Avian Veterinarians, Wellington, New Zealand, 2–6 September 2006; pp. 85–90.
65. Hoppes, S.; Gray, P.L.; Payne, S.; Shivaprasad, H.L.; Tizard, I. The isolation, pathogenesis, diagnosis, transmission, and control of avian bornavirus and proventricular dilatation disease. *Vet. Clin. N. Am. Exot. Anim. Pract.* **2010**, *13*, 495–508. [CrossRef] [PubMed]
66. Berg, K.J.; Sanchez-Migallon Guzman, D.; Knych, H.K.; Drazenovich, T.L.; Paul-Murphy, J.R. Pharmacokinetics of amantadine after oral administration of single and multiple doses to orange-winged Amazon parrots (*Amazona amazonica*). *Am. J. Vet. Res.* **2020**, *81*, 651–655. [CrossRef] [PubMed]

170. Lin, E.; Luscombe, C.; Wang, Y.Y.; Shaw, T.; Locarnini, S. The guanine nucleoside analog penciclovir is active against chronic duck hepatitis B virus infection in vivo. *Antimicrob. Agents Chemother.* **1996**, *40*, 413–418. [CrossRef] [PubMed]
171. Tsiquaye, K.N.; Sutton, D.; Maung, M.; Boyd, M.R. Antiviral Activities and Pharmacokinetics of Penciclovir and Famciclovir in Pekin Ducks Chronically Infected with Duck Hepatitis B Virus. *Antivir. Chem. Chemother.* **1996**, *7*, 153–159. [CrossRef]
172. Lin, E.; Luscombe, C.; Colledge, D.; Wang, Y.Y.; Locarnini, S. Long-Term Therapy with the Guanine Nucleoside Analog Penciclovir Controls Chronic Duck Hepatitis B Virus Infection In Vivo. *Antimicrob. Agents Chemother.* **1998**, *42*, 2132–2137. [CrossRef] [PubMed]
173. Nicoll, A.; Locarnini, S.; Chou, S.T.; Smallwood, R.; Angus, P. Effect of nucleoside analogue therapy on duck hepatitis B viral replication in hepatocytes and bile duct epithelial cells in vivo. *J. Gastroenterol. Hepatol.* **2000**, *15*, 304–310. [CrossRef] [PubMed]
174. Graci, J.D.; Cameron, C.E. Mechanisms of action of ribavirin against distinct viruses. *Rev. Med. Virol.* **2006**, *16*, 37–48. [CrossRef] [PubMed]
175. Omer, M.O.; Almalki, W.H.; Shahid, I.; Khuram, S.; Altaf, I.; Imran, S. Comparative study to evaluate the anti-viral efficacy of Glycyrrhiza glabra extract and ribavirin against the Newcastle disease virus. *Pharmacogn. Res.* **2014**, *6*, 6–11.
176. Ramírez-Olivencia, G.; Estébanez, M.; Membrillo, F.J.; Ybarra, M.C. Uso de ribavirina en virus distintos de la hepatitis C. Una revisión de la evidencia. *Enfermedades Infecc. Y Microbiol. Clin.* **2019**, *37*, 602–608. [CrossRef] [PubMed]
177. Musser, J.M.; Heatley, J.J.; Koinis, A.V.; Suchodolski, P.F.; Guo, J.; Escandon, P.; Tizard, I.R. Ribavirin Inhibits Parrot Bornavirus 4 Replication in Cell Culture. *PLoS ONE* **2015**, *10*, e0134080. [CrossRef] [PubMed]
178. Honkavuori, K.S.; Shivaprasad, H.L.; Williams, B.L.; Quan, P.-L.; Hornig, M.; Street, C.; Palacios, G.; Hutchison, S.K.; Franca, M.; Egholm, M.; et al. Novel borna virus in psittacine birds with proventricular dilatation disease. *Emerg. Infect. Dis.* **2008**, *14*, 1883–1886. [CrossRef] [PubMed]
179. Kistler, A.L.; Gancz, A.; Clubb, S.; Skewes-Cox, P.; Fischer, K.; Sorber, K.; Chiu, C.Y.; Lublin, A.; Mechani, S.; Farnoushi, Y.; et al. Recovery of divergent avian bornaviruses from cases of proventricular dilatation disease: Identification of a candidate etiologic agent. *Virol. J.* **2008**, *5*, 88. [CrossRef] [PubMed]
180. Rinder, M.; Baas, N.; Hagen, E.; Drasch, K.; Korbel, R. Canary Bornavirus (*Orthobornavirus serini*) Infections Are Associated with Clinical Symptoms in Common Canaries (*Serinus canaria* dom.). *Viruses* **2022**, *14*, 2187. [CrossRef] [PubMed]
181. Szotowska, I.; Ledwoń, A.; Dolka, I.; Bonecka, J.; Szeleszczuk, P. Bornaviral infections in Atlantic canaries (*Serinus canaria*) in Poland. *Avian Pathol.* **2023**, *52*, 242–250. [CrossRef] [PubMed]
182. Rubbenstroth, D. Avian Bornavirus Research-A Comprehensive Review. *Viruses* **2022**, *14*, 1513. [CrossRef] [PubMed]
183. Furman, P.A.; Barry, D.W. Spectrum of antiviral activity and mechanism of action of zidovudine. An overview. *Am. J. Med.* **1988**, *85*, 176–181. [PubMed]
184. Nair, V.; Fadly, A. Leukosis/sarcoma group. In *Diseases of Poultry*, 13th ed.; Swayne, D.E., Glisson, J.R., McDougald, L.R., Nolan, L.K., Suarez, D.L., Nair, V., Eds.; Wiley-Blackwell: Hoboken, NJ, USA, 2013; pp. 553–592.
185. Payne, L.N.; Nair, V. The long view: 40 years of avian leukosis research. *Avian Pathol.* **2012**, *41*, 11–19. [CrossRef] [PubMed]
186. Su, Q.; Zhang, Y.; Li, Y.; Cui, Z.; Chang, S.; Zhao, P. Epidemiological investigation of the novel genotype avian hepatitis E virus and co-infected immunosuppressive viruses in farms with hepatic rupture haemorrhage syndrome, recently emerged in China. *Transbound. Emerg. Dis.* **2019**, *66*, 776–784. [CrossRef] [PubMed]
187. Wang, P.; Lin, L.; Shi, M.; Li, H.; Gu, Z.; Li, M.; Gao, Y.; Teng, H.; Mo, M.; Wei, T.; et al. Vertical transmission of ALV from ALV-J positive parents caused severe immunosuppression and significantly reduced marek's disease vaccine efficacy in three-yellow chickens. *Vet. Microbiol.* **2020**, *244*, 108683. [CrossRef] [PubMed]
188. Wang, Q.; Su, Q.; Liu, B.; Li, Y.; Sun, W.; Liu, Y.; Xue, R.; Chang, S.; Wang, Y.; Zhao, P. Enhanced Antiviral Ability by a Combination of Zidovudine and Short Hairpin RNA Targeting Avian Leukosis Virus. *Front. Microbiol.* **2022**, *12*, 808982. [CrossRef] [PubMed]

viruses

MDPI

Communication

An Amplicon-Based Application for the Whole-Genome Sequencing of GI-19 Lineage Infectious Bronchitis Virus Directly from Clinical Samples

Hoang Duc Le [1,2], Tuyet Ngan Thai [1], Jae-Kyeom Kim [1], Hye-Soon Song [1], Moon Her [1], Xuan Thach Tran [2], Ji-Ye Kim [1,*] and Hye-Ryoung Kim [1,*]

[1] Avian Disease Division, Animal and Plant Quarantine Agency, Gimcheon 39660, Gyeongsangbuk-do, Republic of Korea; lh.duc@ibt.ac.vn (H.D.L.); ttn267@korea.kr (T.N.T.); jaekum42@korea.kr (J.-K.K.); hssong1217@korea.kr (H.-S.S.); herm@korea.kr (M.H.)

[2] Institute of Biotechnology, Vietnam Academy of Science and Technology, Cau Giay, Hanoi 11300, Vietnam; tranthach90@gmail.com

[*] Correspondence: jiyekim@korea.kr (J.-Y.K.); dvmkim77@korea.kr (H.-R.K.); Tel.: +82-54-912-0817 (J.-Y.K.); +82-54-912-0814 (H.-R.K.)

Abstract: Infectious bronchitis virus (IBV) causes a highly contagious respiratory disease in chickens, leading to significant economic losses in the poultry industry worldwide. IBV exhibits a high mutation rate, resulting in the continuous emergence of new variants and strains. A complete genome analysis of IBV is crucial for understanding its characteristics. However, it is challenging to obtain whole-genome sequences from IBV-infected clinical samples due to the low abundance of IBV relative to the host genome. Here, we present a novel approach employing next-generation sequencing (NGS) to directly sequence the complete genome of IBV. Through in silico analysis, six primer pairs were designed to match various genotypes, including the GI-19 lineage of IBV. The primer sets successfully amplified six overlapping fragments by long-range PCR and the size of the amplicons ranged from 3.7 to 6.4 kb, resulting in full coverage of the IBV genome. Furthermore, utilizing Illumina sequencing, we obtained the complete genome sequences of two strains belonging to the GI-19 lineage (QX genotype) from clinical samples, with 100% coverage rates, over 1000 × mean depth coverage, and a high percentage of mapped reads to the reference genomes (96.63% and 97.66%). The reported method significantly improves the whole-genome sequencing of IBVs from clinical samples; thus, it can improve understanding of the epidemiology and evolution of IBVs.

Keywords: infectious bronchitis virus; avian coronavirus; GI-19 lineage; whole-genome sequencing; amplicon-based genome sequencing; next-generation sequencing

check for updates

Citation: Le, H.D.; Thai, T.N.; Kim, J.-K.; Song, H.-S.; Her, M.; Tran, X.T.; Kim, J.-Y.; Kim, H.-R. An Amplicon-Based Application for the Whole-Genome Sequencing of GI-19 Lineage Infectious Bronchitis Virus Directly from Clinical Samples. *Viruses* **2024**, *16*, 515. https://doi.org/10.3390/v16040515

Academic Editor: Chi-Young Wang

Received: 28 February 2024
Revised: 15 March 2024
Accepted: 23 March 2024
Published: 27 March 2024

1. Introduction

The infectious bronchitis virus (IBV) is the primary cause of infectious bronchitis (IB), an acute and contagious disease in chickens. The rapid transmission and frequent occurrence of the disease have led to huge economic losses for the poultry industry worldwide [1]. IBV belongs to the genus *Gammacoronavirus*, family *Coronaviridae*, which is characterized by viruses possessing a positive single-stranded RNA genome. The IBV genome has a length of approximately 27.6 kilobases (kb) and comprises 5′ and 3′ untranslated regions and about 10 open reading frames (ORFs) coding for 4 structural proteins (spike glycoprotein (S), envelope protein (E), membrane protein (M), and nucleocapsid protein (N)) and other non-structural proteins [2,3]. The S glycoprotein is cleaved into subunits S1 and S2. The S1 subunit is responsible for host cell attachment and contains a receptor binding domain and hypervariable regions (HVR) [4–6]. Thus, the S1 gene has been widely used to classify IBV genotypes and serotypes [7]. Mutations caused by the high error rates of the viral RNA polymerase and recombination within the S1 unit have led to various strains or genotypes of IBV worldwide [2].

According to the most recent classification based on the S1 gene [7], IBVs can be divided into 6 genotypes (GI–GVI) and 32 distinct lineages. More genotypes (GVII–GIX) have been found in China and Mexico [8]. Most IBV genotypes are specific to a geographic region, and some countries have domestic lineages. In particular, the GI-19 lineage, known as the QX type, is one of the major genotypes worldwide and is the dominant lineage in Korea [9–11]. In 1991, nephropathogenic IBV of the KM91 type belonging to the GI-19 lineage emerged [12]. Since then, the QX type of the GI-19 lineage has predominated, and the K40/09 type, a recombinant of the KM91-type and QX-type strains, emerged in 2005 [13]. Previous studies have demonstrated that QX-type IBVs have recombined with various field strains, including vaccine strains, resulting in the emergence of novel variants and changes in the antigenic properties of IBV [14–17]. These mutations and recombinations continually lead to the emergence of new IBV strains, making the virus extremely difficult to identify and characterize [16,18].

Recently, it was reported that not only the S1 gene but also non-structural proteins may play critical roles in the replication and pathogenicity of IBV [19,20], suggesting that whole-genome sequencing is required to fully characterize IBV viruses and understand their epidemiology, including their antigenicity, tissue tropism, and pathogenicity [21]. Current advances in metagenomic next-generation sequencing (mNGS) technologies combined with Sequence-Independent, Single-Primer Amplification (SISPA) have provided a useful tool for uncovering the entire genome of IBV [22–25]. Generally, these methods have been applied to IBV isolates amplified by serial passage in embryonated chicken eggs [26–28]. However, despite the need for the mNGS of viruses in clinical tissue samples, variations in amplification due to the low viral genetic load in tissue samples can pose challenges for metagenomic sequencing [29,30]. To circumvent this difficulty, different enrichment techniques employing specific primers targeting the whole genome of the virus have been developed. Specific amplicon-based sequencing approaches have proven successful since they can generate sufficient amounts of genetic material for whole-genome sequencing [22,31].

In this study, we developed an amplicon-based sequencing method for the direct sequencing of the entire genome of IBV in clinical samples. Additionally, we evaluated whether the method was performant when used with the non-targeted SISPA approach with Illumina sequencing technology.

2. Materials and Methods

2.1. Virus Isolation and Propagation

The clinical samples, designated as AD04 and AQ10, were collected from the cecal tonsils of 23-day-old and 29-day-old broiler chicken carcasses, respectively, which were suspected of harboring IBV in South Korea in 2023. The chicken carcasses from two different farms were submitted for IBV diagnostic work-up at the Avian Disease Division, Animal and Plant Quarantine Agency. The chickens displayed evident respiratory symptoms and depression before death. Subsequently, IBVs were isolated from the clinical samples by injecting 0.2 mL of 10% tissue homogenates into the allantoic cavity of 10-day-old specific pathogen-free chicken embryonated eggs and incubating them at 37 °C for 72 h. The allantoic fluid from the inoculated eggs was collected for RNA extraction and stored at −70 °C for further use. The isolated samples were designated as AD04-CE1 and AQ10-CE1, respectively.

2.2. RNA Extraction and IBV Real-Time RT-PCR Assay

The total RNA was extracted from the clinical samples and allantoic fluid using the TANBead Nucleic Acid Extraction Kit on an automated TANBead Maelstrom™ 4800 (Taiwan Advanced Nanotech Inc., Taoyuan, Taiwan) according to the manufacturer's instructions. Additionally, the genomic DNA was removed from the extracted RNA using a DNA-free™ Kit (Thermo Fisher Scientific, Waltham, MA, USA) according to the manufacturer's guidelines.

The IBV detection and quantification in the RNA samples were performed using real-time RT-PCR targeting the 5′-UTR region of IBV, as previously described [32]. The reaction mixture consisted of 10 μL RealMOD™ Probe M^2 2X qRT-PCR mix (iNtRON Biotechnology Inc., Gyeonggi, Republic of Korea), 0.5 μL forward primer, 0.5 μL reverse primer, 0.5 μL probe, 3 μL RNA, and nuclease-free water in a final volume of 20 μL. Real-time RT-PCR was performed on a LightCycler®96 Instrument (Roche, Basel, Switzerland) under the following conditions: reverse transcription at 50 °C for 10 min and initial denaturation at 95 °C for 10 min, followed by 40 cycles of 95 °C for 15 s and 60 °C for 1 min. The fluorescence intensities were acquired during the 60 °C step of each cycle, and the cycle threshold (Ct) value was analyzed using the LightCycler®96 SW 1.1 software.

2.3. In Silico Design of the Primer Sets

Full-length sequences of IBV (n = 55) available in the National Center for Biotechnology Information (NCBI) GenBank (up until November 2023) were downloaded to design the universal primers (Table S1). The alignment of the genome sequences was performed to evaluate the nucleotide conservation across the IBV genomes with CLC Main Workbench software version 20.0.4 (Qiagen, Hilden, Germany) using a very accurate alignment algorithm. Six universal primer sets covering the entire genome (Table 1) were designed from conservative regions of the IBV genomes. The criteria for the primers were as follows: amplicon length, 3.7–6.4 kb; primer length, 19–24 nucleotides; number of degenerate bases < 4; and overlaps between amplicons > 140 bp. The primers were synthesized by Macrogen Inc. (Seoul, South Korea). The stock concentration was 100 pmol/μL, and working primer concentrations of 10 pmol/μL were obtained by diluting the stock solution in nuclease-free water (Table 1).

Table 1. List of primers used to amplify six fragments of IBV.

Name	Primer Name	Sequence (5′ to 3′)	Position *	Product Size (bp)
Amplicon 1	IBF1	CTTAACAAAACGGACTTAAATACC	57	6429
	IBR1	GCAACYTCRGGAGACATAAATG	6485	
Amplicon 2	IBF2	GCAGGDTTYTATTTCTGGC	6226	6165
	IBR2	GTATCAGCCGAGCCTCACTG	12390	
Amplicon 3	IBF3	GAYCCACCATGTAARTTTGG	11749	5589
	IBR3	CRGGCTCRAAATTATTRCC	17337	
Amplicon 4	IBF4	GTATGTTRACCAAYTAYGAATTG	16264	3969
	IBR4	GTAAATARTTACWATTCCKCC	20232	
Amplicon 5	IBF5	GGTGGACAMTGTTYTGTACWG	20083	5719
	IBR5	CGMGCTTTTCKYGCTATTGC	25801	
Amplicon 6	IBF6	GACCTAARAARTCTGTTTAATG	23849	3721
	IBR6	CCCTCGATCGTACTCCGCG	27569	

* Nucleotide positions are relative to those of the YX10 strain (NCBI accession no. JX840411).

2.4. cDNA Synthesis and Amplicon Analysis

For the cDNA synthesis, 5 μL total RNA from each sample, together with an IBV gene-specific primer (5′-TACCGTTCGTTTCCA-3′), was subjected to reverse transcription using SuperScript IV Reverse Transcriptase (Thermo Fisher Scientific, Waltham, MA, USA) according to the manufacturer's guidelines. Six individual amplicons were amplified using the following mixture: 10 μL LongAmp®Taq 2X Master Mix (New England Biolabs, Ipswich, MA, USA), 0.5 μL forward primer (10 pmol/μL), 0.5 μL reverse primer (10 pmol/μL), and 2 μL of cDNA in a final volume of 20 μL. The cycling conditions were as follows: 95 °C for 5 s, followed by 35 cycles of 95 °C for 45 s, 53 °C for 45 s, and 65 °C for 5 min, with a final extension at 65 °C for 10 min. The PCR products were run on a 1% agarose gel to confirm the presence of amplicons. The amplicons generated for each primer pair were pooled (in equal volumes) into a single mixture for library preparation and Illumina sequencing. The pooled mixture was purified/cleaned up using AMPure XP beads (Beckman Coulter, Brea, CA, USA) following the manufacturer's instructions.

2.5. SISPA

The total RNA extracted from the clinical samples and isolated samples was used for SISPA, as previously described [25]. The dsDNA generated by SISPA was quantified using the Qubit dsDNA HS assay (Thermo Fisher Scientific, Waltham, MA, USA) according to the manufacturer's guidelines.

2.6. Amplicon and Metagenome Sequencing Libraries Preparation

Libraries were prepared using the NEXTFLEX®rapid XP DNA-seq 2.0 kit for Illumina platforms (PerqkinElmer, Waltham, MA, USA). The quantification of the libraries was carried out using the Qubit dsDNA HS assay kit (Thermo Fisher Scientific, Waltham, MA, USA), and the size of the libraries was measured using the Agilent TapeStation 4200 (Agilent Technologies, Santa Clara, CA, USA). High-quality libraries were pooled to achieve equimolar concentrations, 1% PhiX Control v3 Library (Illumina, San Diego, CA, USA) was added, and then next-generation paired-end sequencing (2 × 150 bp) was performed on an Illumina MiniSeq instrument using the 300-cycle MiniSeq Mid Output Reagent Cartridge (Illumina, San Diego, CA, USA).

2.7. Bioinformatic Analysis

The quality of the raw Illumina sequencing reads was assessed by fastp [33]. Adapter trimming was performed using Cutadapt and Trimmomatic with the default parameters [34]. The filtered reads were then aligned to the reference genome (IBV strain YX10, NCBI accession no. JX840411) using BWA-MEM [35] with the default settings. Subsequently, the mapped reads were retrieved using the Bamtofastq tool and subjected to de novo assembly using MEGAHIT software (v. 1.2.9) [36]. To evaluate the quality of the assembly, the Quality Assessment Tool for Genome Assembly (QUAST, v.5.0.2) was employed to compare the relative quality of each strain. The average coverage was calculated using Qualimap (v. 2.2.1) while examining the mapping of the raw sequence reads to the reference genome using BWA-MEM and Samtools.

For the genome annotation, the GATU program was utilized with the reference genome of the YX10 strain (accession no. JX840411) [37]. The pairwise identities were determined using CLC Main Workbench software version 20.0.4 (Qiagen, Hilden, Germany).

2.8. Phylogenetic Analysis and Sanger Sequencing

The alignments of both the full genome and the S1 gene were conducted utilizing prototype strains from various lineages and reference strains. These alignments were executed using MAFFT version 7.467 software [38]. Phylogenetic trees were then generated by the neighbor-joining method, with 1000 bootstrap replications, using MEGA 11 software [39]. The nucleotide differences between the clinical and isolated samples based on NGS were verified by custom Sanger sequencing (Cosmo Genetech, Seoul, Republic of Korea).

3. Results

3.1. RT-qPCR and Generation of Amplicons

The RT-qPCR results showed that all the samples were IBV positive. The range of Ct values of the four samples ranged from 19.1 to 23.17. The six primer sets were designed to target highly conserved regions of the IBV genomes (Table 1). The presence of amplicons of the expected size was confirmed using 1% agarose gel electrophoresis. Six overlapping fragments were successfully obtained via long PCR amplification from both the clinical and isolated samples (Figure 1).

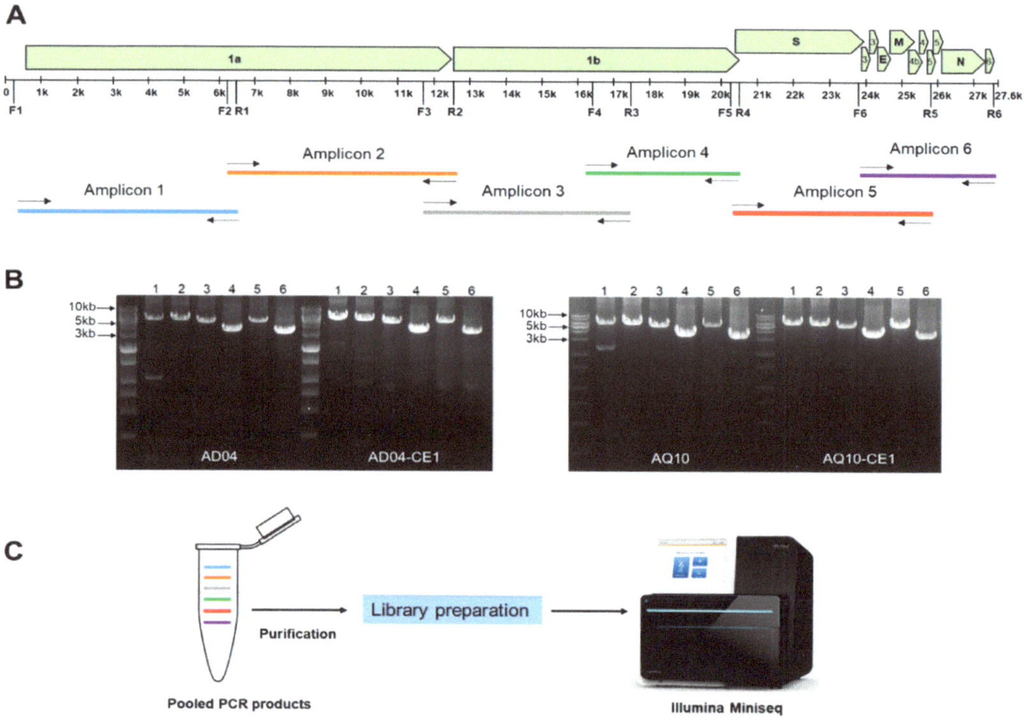

Figure 1. Overview of amplicon-based sequencing. (**A**) The locations of the six primer pairs on the IBV genome and their positions relative to those of the IBV genes. The regions amplified by each primer set and the overlap between the PCR products are also illustrated. (**B**) PCR results of the IBV genome amplification from the clinical and isolated samples. (**C**) PCR products were pooled in equal amounts, purified, and subjected to library preparation for Illumina sequencing.

3.2. Complete Genome Characterization by Amplicon Sequencing

The full-length IBV genomes of both the clinical samples and their respective isolates were successfully obtained using amplicon-based Illumina sequencing. The coverage rates of the IBV were 100% in all four amplicon sequencing samples. There were 13 ORFs (5′-UTR-1a-1ab-S-3a-3b-E-M-4b-4c-5a-5b-N-6-3′-UTR) identified within the IBV genomes. The mean depth of coverage of AD04 and AD04-CE1 was 1239 and 2629, respectively. Similarly, the AQ010 and AQ010-CE1 samples had mean coverage depths of 1069 and 2385, respectively. The coverage depth across the reference genome of the sequencing samples is shown in Figure 2.

Phylogenetic analysis of the four amplicon sequencing samples and IBV reference strains was performed using the full-length S1 gene and full-length IBV genomes, respectively. The results showed that the sequences of AD04, AD04-CE1, AQ10, and AQ10-CE1 were of the GI-19 genotype (Figure 3).

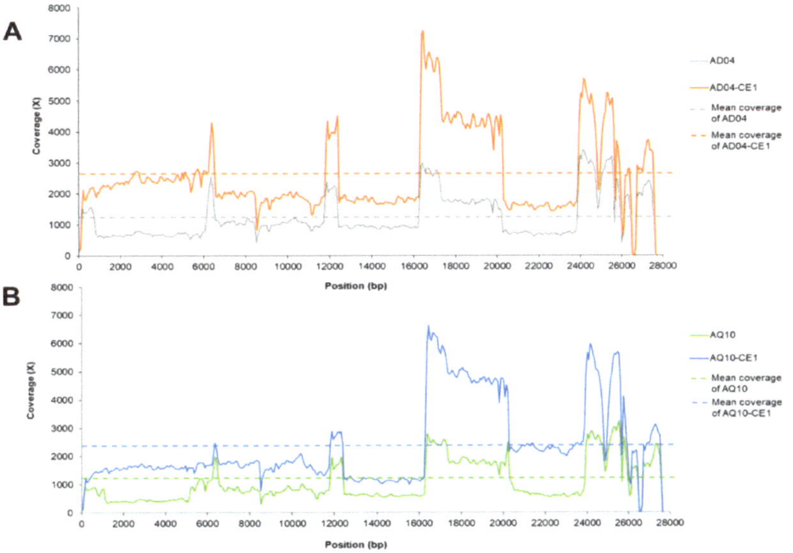

Figure 2. Coverage across the reference genome by the amplicon sequences from the AD04 and AD04-CE1 samples (**A**) and AQ10 and AQ10-CE1 samples (**B**). The *x*-axis represents the length of the reference genome YX10 (accession no. JX840411; 27,674 nucleotides). The *y*-axis represents the coverage (X).

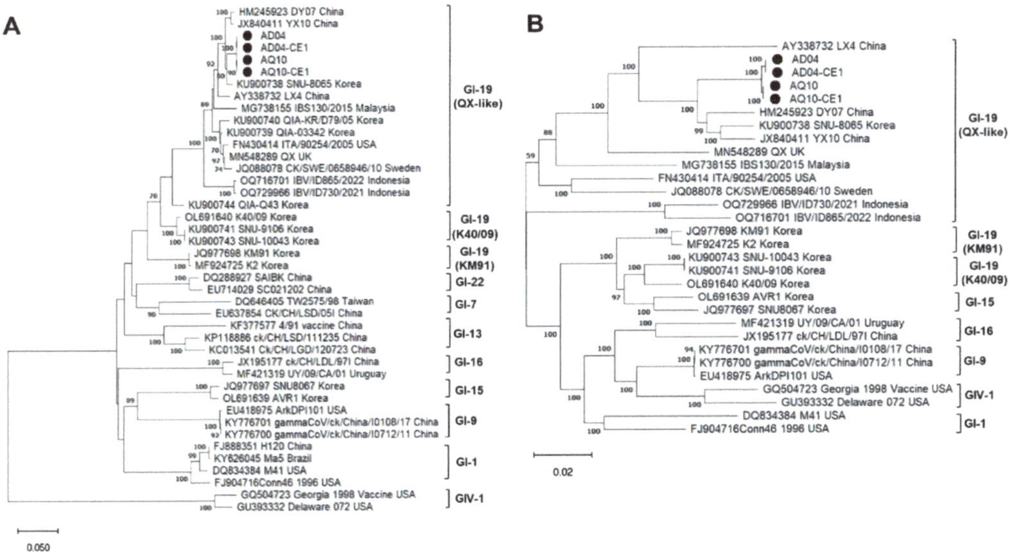

Figure 3. Phylogenetic analyses based on the S1 (**A**) and full-genome (**B**) sequences of AD04, AD04-CE1, AQ10, and AQ10-CE1 obtained by amplicon sequencing, and the reference IBV strains. The maximum likelihood method in Mega 11 software was used, with 1000 bootstrap replicates.

The full-genome sequences of AD04 and AQ10 shared a 99.58% identity. The S1 genes of AD04 and AQ10 had high nucleotide and amino acid identities of 99.88% and 99.81%, respectively. The nucleotide and amino acid sequence identities of the S1 gene between the AD04 and 18 IBV isolates in the GI-19 branch of the phylogenetic tree (Figure 3) were

84.75–98.02% and 85–97.59%, respectively, while those between the AD10 and GI-19 IBVs were 84.69–98.02% and 85.19–97.78%, respectively.

3.3. Comparison of Amplicon Sequencing and Metagenome Sequencing Approaches for IBV

Next, we conducted a comparison between the results of the amplicon sequencing and metagenome sequencing. Among the four metagenome sequencing samples, the full-length sequence of IBV was successfully obtained from only the AD04-CE1 and AQ10-CE1 samples. All the isolated samples used for the sequencing showed 100% coverage rates for the IBV full genome. The sequences of AD04-CE1 and AQ10-CE1 obtained by metagenomic sequencing were annotated, with the IBV genome structure comprising 13 ORFs, similar to that of the amplicon-based sequencing samples. The mean coverage depths of AD04-CE1 and AQ010-CE1 were 864 and 4525, respectively. However, we were unsuccessful in acquiring the complete genome of IBV from the clinical samples using the SISPA approach. AD04 (with a Ct value of 22.3) showed a genome coverage of 22.58%, with a mean depth coverage of 14. The AQ10 (with a Ct value of 19.1) exhibited a genome coverage of 95.37%, with a mean depth coverage of 1148 (Table 2).

Table 2. Comparison between the amplicon-based sequencing and metagenome sequencing.

	Sample Name	Number of Read	Mapped Reads to Reference Sequence (%) [a]	Coverage (%) [b]	Mean of Depth Coverage [c]	SD
Amplicon-based sequencing	**AD04**	271,693	265,341 (97.66%)	100	1239	711
	AD04-CE1	577,061	551,186 (95.52%)	100	2629	1313
	AQ10	258,588	249,866 (96.63%)	100	1069	714
	AQ10-CE1	482,990	470,782 (97.47%)	100	2385	1455
Metagenome sequencing	**AD04**	339,616	2,901 (0.85%)	22.58 [d]	14	98
	AD04-CE1	578,112	193,793 (33.52%)	100	864	2170
	AQ10	552,618	246,618 (44.63%)	95.37 [e]	1148	8406
	AQ10-CE1	1,218,715	989,833 (81.22%)	100	4525	24,717

[a] Mapped reads to a reference sequence were calculated using the IBV reference strain YX10 (accession no. JX840411). [b] Coverage rate was calculated using the following formula: assembly contigs/reference genome. [c] Sequencing depth was calculated using the following formula: average read length × number of reads matching the reference/reference genome size. [d] Gaps at nucleotide positions: 1–32; 719–2387; 3486–7466; 7914–8436; 9398–11,769; 12,513–15,290; 16,312–20,627; 20,946–26,083; 27,061–27,674. [e] Gaps at nucleotide positions: 1–58; 16,933–17,152; 23,347–23,814; 24,106–24,617; 27,652–27,674.

A pairwise comparison of the IBV genome between AQ10 and AQ10-CE1 showed 100% similarity. However, there was a single nucleotide difference. Specific primer pairs were designed to confirm the substitution by Sanger sequencing. The Sanger sequencing results confirmed the presence of a single nucleotide substitution of T for C at position 5673 in the ORF1b between AD04 and AD04-CE1. However, this substitution did not lead to an amino acid change in the 1b polyprotein (Figure 4).

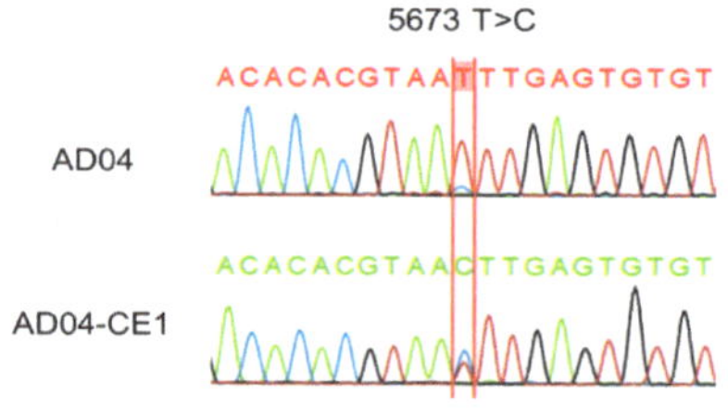

Figure 4. Sanger sequencing confirmation of a single nucleotide difference between the AD04 and AD04-CE1 samples.

4. Discussion

Whole-genome sequencing, combined with various NGS protocols, is a powerful tool for investigating genome epidemiology and understanding the evolutionary dynamics of viruses [21–25]. Nonspecific amplification of purified nucleic acids in combination with mNGS allows all the genetic material directly recovered from a sample to be sequenced and analyzed, and SISPA represents one such metagenomic approach [23–25]. This method involves random priming and avoids the selection of specific RNA sequences, thus minimizing the biases associated with amplicon-based sequencing and allowing the detection of multiple pathogens [22,23]. However, in clinical samples, the low viral genetic loads and the overwhelming proportion of sequencing reads from the host DNA pose challenges to achieving the complete genome sequences of viruses by metagenomic sequencing [29,30,40,41]. In this study, the clinical samples, AD04 and AQ10, exhibited relatively low proportions of mapped reads to the reference genome, at 0.85% and 44.63%, respectively, demonstrating the limitation in obtaining the complete genome sequences of IBV directly from clinical samples using SISPA-mNGS.

To overcome these difficulties, the targeted enrichment of viral genomes from clinical samples using PCR has been used to reduce the nonspecific reads, streamline the bioinformatics analysis, and allow greater accuracy compared with metagenomics [31]. Recent studies have demonstrated that amplicon-based approaches offer greater genome coverage and higher sensitivity than mNGS [40–43]. These protocols are designed to amplify short and overlapping amplicons (about 1000 bp or less) across the genome and have been used to sequence the Zika virus, Crimean–Congo hemorrhagic fever virus, and SARS-CoV-2 from clinical samples [40,41,44,45]. However, they have not been successful in sequencing coronaviruses because these viruses have a high mutation rate that makes it difficult to design multiple primer pairs that do not result in primer mismatches [44,45].

In this study, we developed a protocol based on long-amplicon PCR to reduce the number of reactions. Six primer sets for amplicon sizes of 3.7–6.4 kb were designed to cover the whole IBV genome across various lineages, including GI-19. The primer sets successfully amplified bands of the correct size from two IBV strains, and sequencing of the amplicons using the Illumina MiniSeq platform resulted in high read accuracy and high levels of sequencing depth. These results indicate that the targeted long-amplicon PCR method provides high genomic coverage, with a mean depth of genome coverage of more than 1000-fold and high read mapping percentages ranging from 95.52% to 97.66%, in clinical and isolate samples.

Until now, mNGS for IBV whole-genome sequencing was usually performed on IBV isolates amplified by egg inoculation [26–28]. However, it is also important to conduct mNGS on IBV-infected clinical samples to detect co-infection with various IBV strains [46]. Moreover, there is a concern that viral passage through eggs or cell cultures can introduce single nucleotide substitutions, insertions, deletions, and recombination not initially present in the original clinical sample, potentially complicating the analysis [46,47]. The results of this study also revealed a single nucleotide difference between the genomes of IBV in the AD04 and AD04-CE1 samples, confirming that genetic variation during egg serial passage is a real possibility. This suggests that the introduction of a method to directly analyze the whole-genome sequence of the IBV from clinical samples using the long-amplicon-based approach would be useful for studying IBV mutations and evolution.

Among the IBVs, the QX-type subgroup belonging to the lineage GI-19 is widely prevalent in chicken flocks globally and currently predominant in South Korea [9–11]. In recent years, a variety of distinct QX-like IBVs (QX-I to IV) have been reported, as well as various recombinants [16,18]. Previous studies have demonstrated that recombination breakpoints were detected not only in the S1 gene but also in other parts of the IBV genome [15–18]. The construction of phylogenetic trees and sequence analysis suggested potential recombinant strains genetically distinct from others, and then the putative recombination events were identified using specialized software [16,17]. In this study, sequence comparisons of the S1 gene and phylogenetic analysis of both the S1 gene and the whole-genome of AD04 and AQ10 demonstrated that these strains belonged to the QX-type.

We found that the six primer pairs developed in this study are sufficient for the efficient amplification of viral DNA for whole-genome sequencing analysis of the GI-19 lineage. In the future, it is expected that this protocol will be applied to the genomes of other subgroups of the GI-19 lineage. Additionally, the protocol may be applicable to various IBV lineages, such as GI-1 (Mass type), GI-13 (4/91 type), and GVI-1 (TC07-2 type), since the primer sets were designed for the purpose of detecting various lineages by in silico analysis. Further evaluations with serial dilutions of viral RNA and clinical samples exhibiting higher Ct values will also be necessary to assess the sensitivity of the protocol.

In conclusion, we developed a novel method based on long-amplicon-based Illumina sequencing for high-accuracy whole-genome sequencing of the GI-19 lineage. The results indicate that this method can be applied for the direct sequencing of the full genomes of IBV in clinical samples, allowing accurate identification of IBV prevalence patterns. Also, it could facilitate metagenomic sequencing of an IBV vaccine and/or field strains in multiple co-infected samples. Additionally, the method is efficient in that it reduces the time and cost by enabling whole-genome sequencing without the need for a virus isolation procedure, and it can be used in a wide range of areas, such as diagnosis, study of virus characteristics, and effective vaccine programs on poultry farms.

Supplementary Materials: The following supporting information can be downloaded at https://www.mdpi.com/article/10.3390/v16040515/s1, Table S1: IBV reference strains used to design the primers in this study.

Author Contributions: Conceptualization, H.D.L.; methodology, H.D.L. and T.N.T., investigation, H.D.L., T.N.T., H.-S.S. and J.-K.K.; formal analysis, H.D.L. and X.T.T.; project administration, J.-Y.K.; funding acquisition, J.-Y.K.; supervision, M.H. and H.-R.K.; writing—original draft, H.D.L., X.T.T. and T.N.T.; writing—review and editing, H.D.L., T.N.T., H.-R.K. and J.-Y.K. All authors have read and agreed to the published version of the manuscript.

Funding: This work was supported by grants from the Animal and Plant Quarantine Agency (Grant No. B-1543084-2022-24-01) of the Ministry of Agriculture, Food and Rural Affairs of the Republic of Korea.

Institutional Review Board Statement: The samples were collected from chicken carcasses in commercial broiler farms under field conditions and did not involve the use of experimental animals. Therefore, there was no need for ethical approval for the study.

Informed Consent Statement: Not applicable.

Data Availability Statement: The sequences of the IBV strains in this study are available in the GenBank database under accession number PP374733 for AD04 and PP374734 for AQ10.

Acknowledgments: We thank the members of the Avian Disease Division for the technical assistance and the curation of clinical samples used in this study.

Conflicts of Interest: The authors declare no conflicts of interest.

References

1. Cavanagh, D. Coronavirus avian infectious bronchitis virus. *Vet. Res.* **2007**, *38*, 281–297. [CrossRef] [PubMed]
2. Jackwood, M.W.; de Wit, S. Infectious Bronchitis. In *Diseases of Poultry*, 14th ed.; Swayne, D.E., Ed.; Wiley-Blackwell: Hoboken, NJ, USA, 2020; pp. 167–188.
3. Leghari, R.A.; Fan, B.; Wang, H.; Bai, J.; Zhang, L.; Abro, S.H.; Jiang, P. Full-length genome sequencing analysis of avian infectious bronchitis virus isolate associated with nephropathogenic infection. *Poult. Sci.* **2016**, *95*, 2921–2929. [CrossRef] [PubMed]
4. Cavanagh, D.; Davis, P.J.; Cook, J.K.; Li, D.; Kant, A.; Koch, G. Location of the amino acid differences in the S1 spike glycoprotein subunit of closely related serotypes of infectious bronchitis virus. *Avian Pathol.* **1992**, *21*, 33–43. [CrossRef] [PubMed]
5. Koch, G.; Hartog, L.; Kant, A.; van Roozelaar, D.J. Antigenic domains on the peplomer protein of avian infectious bronchitis virus: Correlation with biological functions. *J. Gen. Virol.* **1990**, *71 Pt 9*, 1929–1935. [CrossRef]

6. Hong, S.M.; Kim, S.J.; An, S.H.; Kim, J.; Ha, E.J.; Kim, H.; Kwon, H.J.; Choi, K.S. Receptor binding motif surrounding sites in the spike 1 protein of infectious bronchitis virus have high susceptibility to mutation related to selective pressure. *J. Vet. Sci.* **2023**, *24*, e51. [CrossRef] [PubMed]
7. Valastro, V.; Holmes, E.C.; Britton, P.; Fusaro, A.; Jackwood, M.W.; Cattoli, G.; Monne, I. S1 gene-based phylogeny of infectious bronchitis virus: An attempt to harmonize virus classification. *Infect. Genet. Evol.* **2016**, *39*, 349–364. [CrossRef] [PubMed]
8. Mendoza-González, L.; Marandino, A.; Panzera, Y.; Tomás, G.; Williman, J.; Techera, C.; Gayosso-Vázquez, A.; Ramírez-Andoney, V.; Alonso-Morales, R.; Realpe-Quintero, M.; et al. Research Note: High genetic diversity of infectious bronchitis virus from Mexico. *Poult Sci.* **2022**, *101*, 102076. [CrossRef] [PubMed]
9. Jang, I.; Thai, T.N.; Lee, J.I.; Kwon, Y.K.; Kim, H.R. Nationwide Surveillance for Infectious Bronchitis Virus in South Korea from 2020 to 2021. *Avian Dis.* **2022**, *66*, 135–140. [CrossRef] [PubMed]
10. Lee, H.C.; Jeong, S.; Cho, A.Y.; Kim, K.J.; Kim, J.Y.; Park, D.H.; Kim, H.J.; Kwon, J.H.; Song, C.S. Genomic Analysis of Avian Infectious Bronchitis Viruses Recently Isolated in South Korea Reveals Multiple Introductions of GI-19 Lineage (QX Genotype). *Viruses* **2021**, *13*, 1045. [CrossRef]
11. Lee, E.K.; Jeon, W.J.; Lee, Y.J.; Jeong, O.M.; Choi, J.G.; Kwon, J.H.; Choi, K.S. Genetic diversity of avian infectious bronchitis virus isolates in Korea between 2003 and 2006. *Avian Dis.* **2008**, *52*, 332–337. [CrossRef]
12. Lee, S.K.; Sung, H.W.; Kwon, H.M. S1 glycoprotein gene analysis of infectious bronchitis viruses isolated in Korea. *Arch. Virol.* **2004**, *149*, 481–494. [CrossRef] [PubMed]
13. Lim, T.H.; Lee, H.J.; Lee, D.H.; Lee, Y.N.; Park, J.K.; Youn, H.N.; Kim, M.S.; Lee, J.B.; Park, S.Y.; Choi, I.S.; et al. An emerging recombinant cluster of nephropathogenic strains of avian infectious bronchitis virus in Korea. *Infect. Genet. Evol.* **2011**, *11*, 678–685. [CrossRef] [PubMed]
14. Legnardi, M.; Tucciarone, C.M.; Franzo, G.; Cecchinato, M. Infectious Bronchitis Virus Evolution, Diagnosis and Control. *Vet. Sci.* **2020**, *7*, 79. [CrossRef] [PubMed]
15. Gong, H.; Ni, R.; Qiu, R.; Wang, F.; Yan, W.; Wang, K.; Li, H.; Fu, X.; Chen, L.; Lei, C.; et al. Evaluation of a novel recombinant strain of infectious bronchitis virus emerged from three attenuated live vaccine strains. *Microb. Pathog.* **2022**, *164*, 105437. [CrossRef] [PubMed]
16. Kim, H.J.; Lee, H.C.; Cho, A.Y.; Choi, Y.J.; Lee, H.; Lee, D.H.; Song, C.S. Novel recombinant avian infectious bronchitis viruses from chickens in Korea, 2019-2021. *Front. Vet. Sci.* **2023**, *10*, 1107059. [CrossRef] [PubMed]
17. Yan, W.; Qiu, R.; Wang, F.; Fu, X.; Li, H.; Cui, P.; Zhai, Y.; Li, C.; Zhang, L.; Gu, K.; et al. Genetic and pathogenic characterization of a novel recombinant avian infectious bronchitis virus derived from GI-1, GI-13, GI-28, and GI-19 strains in Southwestern China. *Poult. Sci.* **2021**, *100*, 101210. [CrossRef] [PubMed]
18. Youn, S.-Y.; Lee, J.-Y.; Bae, Y.-C.; Kwon, Y.-K.; Kim, H.-R. Genetic and Pathogenic Characterization of QX(GI-19)-Recombinant Infectious Bronchitis Viruses in South Korea. *Viruses* **2021**, *13*, 1163. [CrossRef] [PubMed]
19. Armesto, M.; Cavanagh, D.; Britton, P. The replicase gene of avian coronavirus infectious bronchitis virus is a determinant of pathogenicity. *PLoS ONE* **2009**, *4*, e7384. [CrossRef] [PubMed]
20. Zhao, J.; Zhang, K.; Cheng, J.; Jia, W.; Zhao, Y.; Zhang, G. Replicase 1a gene plays a critical role in pathogenesis of avian coronavirus infectious bronchitis virus. *Virology* **2020**, *550*, 1–7. [CrossRef]
21. Ramirez-Nieto, G.; Mir, D.; Almansa-Villa, D.; Cordoba-Argotti, G.; Beltran-Leon, M.; Rodriguez-Osorio, N.; Garai, J.; Zabaleta, J.; Gomez, A.P. New Insights into Avian Infectious Bronchitis Virus in Colombia from Whole-Genome Analysis. *Viruses* **2022**, *14*, 2562. [CrossRef]
22. Butt, S.L.; Erwood, E.C.; Zhang, J.; Sellers, H.S.; Young, K.; Lahmers, K.K.; Stanton, J.B. Real-time, MinION-based, amplicon sequencing for lineage typing of infectious bronchitis virus from upper respiratory samples. *J. Vet. Diagn. Investig.* **2021**, *33*, 179–190. [CrossRef]
23. Kariithi, H.M.; Volkening, J.D.; Leyson, C.M.; Afonso, C.L.; Christy, N.; Decanini, E.L.; Lemiere, S.; Suarez, D.L. Genome Sequence Variations of Infectious Bronchitis Virus Serotypes From Commercial Chickens in Mexico. *Front. Vet. Sci.* **2022**, *9*, 931272. [CrossRef]
24. Brinkmann, A.; Uddin, S.; Krause, E.; Surtees, R.; Dinçer, E.; Kar, S.; Hacıoğlu, S.; Özkul, A.; Ergünay, K.; Nitsche, A. Utility of a Sequence-Independent, Single-Primer-Amplification (SISPA) and Nanopore Sequencing Approach for Detection and Characterization of Tick-Borne Viral Pathogens. *Viruses* **2021**, *13*, 203. [CrossRef]
25. Chrzastek, K.; Lee, D.H.; Smith, D.; Sharma, P.; Suarez, D.L.; Pantin-Jackwood, M.; Kapczynski, D.R. Use of Sequence-Independent, Single-Primer-Amplification (SISPA) for rapid detection, identification, and characterization of avian RNA viruses. *Virology* **2017**, *509*, 159–166. [CrossRef] [PubMed]
26. Mase, M.; Hiramatsu, K.; Watanabe, S.; Iseki, H. Complete Genome Sequences of Infectious Bronchitis Virus Genotype JP-II (GI-7) and JP-III (GI-19) Strains Isolated in Japan. *Microbiol. Resour. Announc.* **2023**, *12*, e0067022. [CrossRef]
27. Bali, K.; Bálint, Á.; Farsang, A.; Marton, S.; Nagy, B.; Kaszab, E.; Belák, S.; Palya, V.; Bányai, K. Recombination Events Shape the Genomic Evolution of Infectious Bronchitis Virus in Europe. *Viruses* **2021**, *13*, 535. [CrossRef] [PubMed]
28. Jude, R.; da Silva, A.P.; Rejmanek, D.; Crossley, B.; Jerry, C.; Stoute, S.; Gallardo, R. Whole-genome sequence of a genotype VIII infectious bronchitis virus isolated from California layer chickens in 2021. *Microbiol. Resour. Announc.* **2023**, *12*, e0095922. [CrossRef]

29. Van Borm, S.; Steensels, M.; Mathijs, E.; Vandenbussche, F.; van den Berg, T.; Lambrecht, B. Metagenomic sequencing determines complete infectious bronchitis virus (avian Gammacoronavirus) vaccine strain genomes and associated viromes in chicken clinical samples. *Virus Genes* **2021**, *57*, 529–540. [CrossRef] [PubMed]
30. Houldcroft, C.J.; Beale, M.A.; Breuer, J. Clinical and biological insights from viral genome sequencing. *Nat. Rev. Microbiol.* **2017**, *15*, 183–192. [CrossRef]
31. Grubaugh, N.D.; Gangavarapu, K.; Quick, J.; Matteson, N.L.; De Jesus, J.G.; Main, B.J.; Tan, A.L.; Paul, L.M.; Brackney, D.E.; Grewal, S.; et al. An amplicon-based sequencing framework for accurately measuring intrahost virus diversity using PrimalSeq and iVar. *Genome Biol.* **2019**, *20*, 8. [CrossRef]
32. Callison, S.A.; Hilt, D.A.; Boynton, T.O.; Sample, B.F.; Robison, R.; Swayne, D.E.; Jackwood, M.W. Development and evaluation of a real-time Taqman RT-PCR assay for the detection of infectious bronchitis virus from infected chickens. *J. Virol. Methods* **2006**, *138*, 60–65. [CrossRef] [PubMed]
33. Chen, S.; Zhou, Y.; Chen, Y.; Gu, J. fastp: An ultra-fast all-in-one FASTQ preprocessor. *Bioinformatics* **2018**, *34*, i884–i890. [CrossRef] [PubMed]
34. Bolger, A.M.; Lohse, M.; Usadel, B. Trimmomatic: A flexible trimmer for Illumina sequence data. *Bioinformatics* **2014**, *30*, 2114–2120. [CrossRef] [PubMed]
35. Li, H.; Durbin, R. Fast and accurate long-read alignment with Burrows-Wheeler transform. *Bioinformatics* **2010**, *26*, 589–595. [CrossRef] [PubMed]
36. Li, D.; Liu, C.M.; Luo, R.; Sadakane, K.; Lam, T.W. MEGAHIT: An ultra-fast single-node solution for large and complex metagenomics assembly via succinct de Bruijn graph. *Bioinformatics* **2015**, *31*, 1674–1676. [CrossRef]
37. Tcherepanov, V.; Ehlers, A.; Upton, C. Genome Annotation Transfer Utility (GATU): Rapid annotation of viral genomes using a closely related reference genome. *BMC Genomics* **2006**, *7*, 150. [CrossRef] [PubMed]
38. Katoh, K.; Rozewicki, J.; Yamada, K.D. MAFFT online service: Multiple sequence alignment, interactive sequence choice and visualization. *Brief. Bioinform.* **2019**, *20*, 1160–1166. [CrossRef] [PubMed]
39. Tamura, K.; Stecher, G.; Kumar, S. MEGA11: Molecular Evolutionary Genetics Analysis Version 11. *Mol. Biol. Evol.* **2021**, *38*, 3022–3027. [CrossRef] [PubMed]
40. Quick, J.; Grubaugh, N.D.; Pullan, S.T.; Claro, I.M.; Smith, A.D.; Gangavarapu, K.; Oliveira, G.; Robles-Sikisaka, R.; Rogers, T.F.; Beutler, N.A.; et al. Multiplex PCR method for MinION and Illumina sequencing of Zika and other virus genomes directly from clinical samples. *Nat. Protoc.* **2017**, *12*, 1261–1276. [CrossRef]
41. D'Addiego, J.; Wand, N.; Afrough, B.; Fletcher, T.; Kurosaki, Y.; Leblebicioglu, H.; Hewson, R. Recovery of complete genome sequences of Crimean-Congo haemorrhagic fever virus (CCHFV) directly from clinical samples: A comparative study between targeted enrichment and metagenomic approaches. *J. Virol. Methods* **2024**, *323*, 114833. [CrossRef]
42. Zakotnik, S.; Knap, N.; Bogovič, P.; Zorec, T.M.; Poljak, M.; Strle, F.; Avšič-Županc, T.; Korva, M. Complete Genome Sequencing of Tick-Borne Encephalitis Virus Directly from Clinical Samples: Comparison of Shotgun Metagenomic and Targeted Amplicon-Based Sequencing. *Viruses* **2022**, *14*, 1267. [CrossRef] [PubMed]
43. Chen, N.F.G.; Chaguza, C.; Gagne, L.; Doucette, M.; Smole, S.; Buzby, E.; Hall, J.; Ash, S.; Harrington, R.; Cofsky, S.; et al. Development of an amplicon-based sequencing approach in response to the global emergence of mpox. *PLoS Biol.* **2023**, *21*, e3002151. [CrossRef] [PubMed]
44. Hourdel, V.; Kwasiborski, A.; Balière, C.; Matheus, S.; Batéjat, C.F.; Manuguerra, J.C.; Vanhomwegen, J.; Caro, V. Rapid Genomic Characterization of SARS-CoV-2 by Direct Amplicon-Based Sequencing Through Comparison of MinION and Illumina iSeq100(TM) System. *Front. Microbiol.* **2020**, *11*, 571328. [CrossRef] [PubMed]
45. Park, C.; Kim, K.W.; Park, D.; Hassan, Z.U.; Park, E.C.; Lee, C.S.; Rahman, M.T.; Yi, H.; Kim, S. Rapid and sensitive amplicon-based genome sequencing of SARS-CoV-2. *Front. Microbiol.* **2022**, *13*, 876085. [CrossRef] [PubMed]
46. Oade, M.S.; Keep, S.; Freimanis, G.L.; Orton, R.J.; Britton, P.; Hammond, J.A.; Bickerton, E. Attenuation of Infectious Bronchitis Virus in Eggs Results in Different Patterns of Genomic Variation across Multiple Replicates. *J. Virol.* **2019**, *93*, e00492-19. [CrossRef]
47. Tsai, C.T.; Wu, H.Y.; Wang, C.H. Genetic sequence changes related to the attenuation of avian infectious bronchitis virus strain TW2575/98. *Virus Genes* **2020**, *56*, 369–379. [CrossRef]

viruses

MDPI

Article

Analysis of Chicken IFITM3 Gene Expression and Its Effect on Avian Reovirus Replication

Hongyu Ren [1,2,†], Sheng Wang [1,2,†], Zhixun Xie [1,2,*], Lijun Wan [1,2], Liji Xie [1,2], Sisi Luo [1,2], Meng Li [1,2], Zhiqin Xie [1,2], Qing Fan [1,2], Tingting Zeng [1,2], Yanfang Zhang [1,2], Minxiu Zhang [1,2], Jiaoling Huang [1,2] and You Wei [1,2]

1 Guangxi Key Laboratory of Veterinary Biotechnology, Guangxi Veterinary Research Institute, Nanning 530000, China; renhongyu328@126.com (H.R.); wangsheng1021@126.com (S.W.); wanlijun0529@163.com (L.W.); xie3120371@163.com (L.X.); 2004-luosisi@163.com (S.L.); mengli4836@163.com (M.L.); xzqman2002@sina.com (Z.X.); fanqing1224@126.com (Q.F.); tingtingzeng1986@163.com (T.Z.); zhangyanfang409@126.com (Y.Z.); zhminxiu2010@163.com (M.Z.); huangjiaoling728@126.com (J.H.); weiyou0909@163.com (Y.W.)

2 Key Laboratory of China (Guangxi)-ASEAN Cross-Border Animal Disease Prevention and Control, Ministry of Agriculture and Rural Affairs of China, Nanning 530000, China

* Correspondence: xiezhixun@126.com

† These authors contributed equally to this work.

Abstract: Interferon-inducible transmembrane protein 3 (IFITM3) is an antiviral factor that plays an important role in the host innate immune response against viruses. Previous studies have shown that IFITM3 is upregulated in various tissues and organs after avian reovirus (ARV) infection, which suggests that IFITM3 may be involved in the antiviral response after ARV infection. In this study, the chicken IFITM3 gene was cloned and analyzed bioinformatically. Then, the role of chicken IFITM3 in ARV infection was further explored. The results showed that the molecular weight of the chicken IFITM3 protein was approximately 13 kDa. This protein was found to be localized mainly in the cytoplasm, and its protein structure contained the CD225 domain. The homology analysis and phylogenetic tree analysis showed that the IFITM3 genes of different species exhibited great variation during genetic evolution, and chicken IFITM3 shared the highest homology with that of *Anas platyrhynchos* and displayed relatively low homology with those of birds such as *Anser cygnoides* and *Serinus canaria*. An analysis of the distribution of chicken IFITM3 in tissues and organs revealed that the IFITM3 gene was expressed at its highest level in the intestine and in large quantities in immune organs, such as the bursa of Fabricius, thymus and spleen. Further studies showed that the overexpression of IFITM3 in chicken embryo fibroblasts (DF-1) could inhibit the replication of ARV, whereas the inhibition of IFITM3 expression in DF-1 cells promoted ARV replication. In addition, chicken IFITM3 may exert negative feedback regulatory effects on the expression of TBK1, IFN-γ and IRF1 during ARV infection, and it is speculated that IFITM3 may participate in the innate immune response after ARV infection by negatively regulating the expression of TBK1, IFN-γ and IRF1. The results of this study further enrich the understanding of the role and function of chicken IFITM3 in ARV infection and provide a theoretical basis for an in-depth understanding of the antiviral mechanism of host resistance to ARV infection.

Keywords: IFITM3; avian reovirus; bioinformatics analysis; antiviral; innate immunity

check for updates

Citation: Ren, H.; Wang, S.; Xie, Z.; Wan, L.; Xie, L.; Luo, S.; Li, M.; Xie, Z.; Fan, Q.; Zeng, T.; et al. Analysis of Chicken IFITM3 Gene Expression and Its Effect on Avian Reovirus Replication. *Viruses* **2024**, *16*, 330. https://doi.org/10.3390/v16030330

Academic Editor: Chi-Young Wang

Received: 9 January 2024
Revised: 18 February 2024
Accepted: 18 February 2024
Published: 21 February 2024

1. Introduction

Avian reovirus (ARV) is a pathogen that circulates widely in poultry and can cause viral arthritis, tenosynovitis and malabsorption syndrome. This virus can also induce severe immunosuppression, which can easily lead to complications or secondary infection with other diseases. These effects lead to reduced production performance and increased mortality in chickens [1–3], resulting in major economic losses in the poultry industry. At present, the prevention and control of ARV mainly involve vaccination, but due to continuous mutation of the strain, the expected immune protection effect is not achieved [4–6]. Therefore, in-depth study of the innate immune regulatory mechanism of ARV infection is highly important for its prevention and control.

Innate immunity is the body's first line of defense against viral infections. After viral invasion, the pattern recognition receptor of the host cell specifically recognizes the molecular pattern associated with the pathogen and thereby activates specific signaling pathways and induces the production of antiviral cytokines such as interferon (IFN) and interleukin, which causes the body to enter an antiviral state [7,8]. Among these, the interferon-mediated antiviral effect is an important part of the host antiviral response [9]. IFN induces the production of many interferon-stimulated genes (ISGs) by activating the JAK/STAT signaling pathway [10], and ISGs are the main executors of IFN antiviral functions [11]. Studies have shown that ARV infection can induce the transcriptional expression of IFN-α, IFN-β and ISGs such as IFITM1, IFITM3, IFIT5, Mx, ISG12 and other cytokines in various tissues and organs; at the early stage of ARV infection, IFITM3 is significantly upregulated in peripheral blood lymphocytes, joints, the thymus and the bursa of Fabricius and shows a consistent trend with the viral load of ARV in these tissues and organs, which suggests that IFITM3 plays a crucial role in ARV infection [12–14].

The IFITM is an important ISG. Different species have different varieties of IFITM proteins. The human IFITMs include IFITM1-3, IFITM5 and IFITM10. Similar to humans, chickens also have five IFITM genes. IFITMs play a significant role in biological activities such as tumorigenesis, cell adhesion and immune signal transduction [15,16]. According to previous research findings, IFITM1, IFITM2 and IFITM3 are related to immune regulatory processes in the body, and the expression of IFITM3 exerts a certain limiting effect on the replication of a variety of highly pathogenic viruses [17–19]. IFITM3 is expressed in fish, amphibians, poultry and mammals, and its antiviral activity is relatively conserved from prokaryotes to vertebrates [20,21]. Early studies have found that IFITM3 can effectively inhibit the replication of a variety of enveloped viruses, such as influenza A viruses (IAVs), dengue virus (DENV) and Ebola virus (EBOV) [21–23], mainly by affecting the fusion of the virus to the endosomal membrane to prevent the virus from entering cells [24,25]. Additional studies in this research area revealed that IFITM3 effectively inhibits nonenveloped viruses, such as foot-and-mouth disease virus (FMDV), norovirus (NoV) and mammalian orthoreoviruses [18,26,27]. Although nonenveloped viruses cannot mediate membrane fusion via proteins on the envelope as do enveloped viruses, they still need to enter cells through endosomes. IFITM3 inhibits viral replication by inhibiting the process of virus entry from endosomes into the cytoplasm. The antiviral mechanism of IFITM3 in mammalian orthoreovirus infection has been well described, and IFITM3 restricts the entry of the virus into host cells by altering the acidic environment of endosomes and reducing protease activity [18]. However, the mechanism of action of chicken IFITM3 has been relatively poorly studied, and the role of IFITM3 in ARV infection has not been reported.

Therefore, in this study, we conducted further investigations on the biological role of chicken IFITM3 in preventing ARV infection. First, we cloned the chicken IFITM3 gene and performed bioinformatic analysis and analyses of its subcellular localization and tissue-organ distribution. Subsequently, the effect of IFITM3 on ARV replication and the regulatory effect of IFITM3 on the expression of correlated molecules in the innate immune signaling pathway were analyzed via overexpression or RNA inhibition assays. The results of this study will provide new ideas for further exploration of the mechanism of the innate immune response to host resistance during ARV infection.

2. Materials and Methods

2.1. Ethics Statement

This study was approved by the Animal Ethics Committee of Guangxi Veterinary Research Institute. The animal experiments and sample collection were conducted in accordance with the guidance of protocol #2019C0408 issued by the Animal Ethics Committee of Guangxi Veterinary Research Institute.

2.2. Animals, Virus and Cells

The "white leghorn" specific-pathogen-free (SPF) chicken embryos used in this study were purchased from Beijing Boehringer Ingelheim Vital Biotechnology Co., Ltd. (Beijing, China). The ARV S1133 strain was purchased from the China Institute of Veterinary Drug Control. DF-1 cells were preserved in our laboratory and cultured in DMEM (Gibco, Grand Island, NY, USA) supplemented with 10% fetal bovine serum (Gibco).

2.3. Cloning and Bioinformatics Analysis of the IFITM3 Gene

The nucleotide sequences of IFITM3 genes were downloaded from the National Center for Biotechnology Information (NCBI) database. Sequence alignment analysis was performed with DNAStar software (DNAstar 7.1) to design primers (Table 1). Total RNA was extracted from DF-1 cells and reverse-transcribed into cDNA, and the resulting cDNA was subsequently used as a template for the amplification of the IFITM3 gene.

Table 1. PCR primers used in this study.

Primers	Primer Sequences (5′-3′)	Usage
IFITM3-1	F: GCGTCGACCATGCAGAGCTACCCTCAGCAC R: GCGCGGCCGCTCAGGGCCTCACAGTGTACAA	RT–PCR
IFITM3-2	F: GGAGTCCCACCGTATGAAC R: GGCGTCTCCACCGTCACCA	RT–qPCR
ARV σC	F: CCACGGGAAATCTCACGGTCACT R: TACGCACGGTCAAGGAACGAATGT	RT–qPCR
MAVS	F: CCTGACTCAAACAAGGGAAG R: AATCAGAGCGATGCCAACAG	RT–qPCR
IRF1	F: GCTACACCGCTCACGA R: TCAGCCATGGCGATTT	RT–qPCR
IRF7	F: CAGTGCTTCTCCAGCACAAA R: TGCATGTGGTATTGCTCGAT	RT–qPCR
STING	F: TGACCGAGAGCTCCAAGAAG R: CGTGGCAGAACTACTTTCAG	RT–qPCR
TBK1	F: AAGAAGGCACACATCCGAGA R: GGTAGCGTGCAAATACAGC	RT–qPCR
NF-κB	F: CATTGCCAGCATGGCTACTAT R: TTCCAGTTCCCGTTTCTTCAC	RT–qPCR
MDA5	F: CAGCCAGTTGCCCTCGCCTCA R: AACAGCTCCCTTGCACCGTCT	RT–qPCR
LGP2	F: CCAGAATGAGCAGCAGGAC R: AATGTTGCACTCAGGGATGT	RT–qPCR
IFN-α	F: ATGCCACCTTCTCTCACGAC R: AGGCGCTGTAATCGTTGTCT	RT–qPCR
IFN-β	F: ACCAGGATGCCAACTTCT R: TCACTGGGTGTTGAGACG	RT–qPCR
IFN-γ	F: ATCATACTGAGCCAGATTGTTTCG R: TCTTTCACCTTCTTCACGCCAT	RT–qPCR
GAPDH	F: GCACTGTCAAGGCTGAGAACG R: GATGATAACACGCTTAGCACCAC	RT–qPCR

The conserved domain was predicted based on the NCBI CD-Search database. SOPMA software (http://npsa-pbil.ibcp.fr/cgi-bin/npsa_automat.pl?page=npsa_sopma.html, accessed on 17 February 2024) was used for secondary structure prediction analysis of the chicken IFITM3 protein. SWISS-MODEL (https://swissmodel.expasy.org/interactive#alignment, accessed on 17 February 2024) was used to predict the tertiary structure of the protein. DNAstar 7.1 and MEGA 11 were used for homology analysis and phylogenetic tree construction. The GenBank accession numbers of the IFITM3 genes from different species are shown in Table 2.

Table 2. GenBank accession numbers of the IFITM3 genes used in this study.

Name of Species	GenBank Accession Number
Homo sapiens	BC070243.1
Gorilla gorilla gorilla	KU570011.1
Capra hircus	KM236557.1
Gallus gallus	KC876032.1
Serinus canaria	XM_009102512.1
Anas platyrhynchos	KJ739866.1
Mus musculus	BC010291.1
Anser cygnoides	KX594327.1
Sus scrofa	JQ315416.1

2.4. Overexpression of the IFITM3 Protein

The recombinant plasmid pEF1α-Myc-IFITM3 was constructed and transfected into DF-1 cells using Lipofectamine^{TM} 3000 (Invitrogen, Carlsbad, CA, USA) to overexpress the IFITM3 protein. Twenty-four hours after transfection, the cells were infected with ARV S1133 (MOI = 1), and cell samples and culture medium supernatant were collected 24 h later. RNA from cell samples was extracted and reverse-transcribed into cDNA. The changes in the expression of ARV σC gene and innate immune signaling pathway-correlated molecules were detected by real-time fluorescence quantitative PCR (RT–qPCR). The utilized primers [12,14,28] were described previously (Table 1). In addition, the above-mentioned culture medium was diluted for the infection of DF-1 cells. The lesions of the cells were observed and recorded, and the $TCID_{50}$ of the virus was calculated by the Reed–Muench method.

2.5. IFITM3 RNA Interference Assay

Three small interfering RNAs (siRNAs) for the chicken IFITM3 gene were designed (Table 3), and the utilized primers were synthesized by GenePharma (Suzhou, China). siRNAs or siNCs (30 pmol) were transfected separately into DF-1 cells using LipofectamineTM RNAiMAX (Invitrogen) to inhibit the expression of IFITM3 protein. Twenty-four hours after transfection, the cells were infected with the ARV S1133 strain, and cell samples and culture medium supernatant were collected 24 h later. The cell samples were used to detect the changes in the expression of ARV σC gene and innate immune signaling pathway-correlated molecules, and the culture supernatant was used for the detection of viral replication.

Table 3. siRNA sequences targeting the IFITM3 gene.

siRNA	Sequences	Sequences
siIFITM3-35	GCAUCAACAUGCCUUCUUATT	UAAGAAGGCAUGUUGAUGCTT
siIFITM3-200	GGAUCAUCGCCAAGGACUUTT	AAGUCCUUGGCGAUGAUCCTT
siIFITM3-242	GGACAGCGAAGAUCUUUAATT	UUAAAGAUCUUCGCUGUCCTT
siNC	UUCUCCGAACGUGUCACGUTT	ACGUGACACGUUCGGAGAATT

2.6. RNA Extraction and RT–qPCR

Total RNA was extracted from the samples using a TRIzol kit (Invitrogen). The RNA was reverse-transcribed to cDNA using Maxima™ H Minus cDNA Synthesis Master Mix (Thermo Fisher Scientific, Boston, MA, USA) and stored at −80 °C for subsequent assays.

Based on the gene sequence information in GenBank, primers for ARV σC, IFITM3 and innate immune signaling pathway-related molecules were designed and synthesized (Table 1). RT–qPCR was performed using PowerUp SYBR Green Master Mix (Thermo Fisher Scientific), and the GAPDH gene served as an internal control. The reaction program was as follows: 94 °C for 2 min and 40 cycles of 94 °C for 15 s and 60 °C for 30 s. The detection results were analyzed by the $2^{-\Delta\Delta Ct}$ method.

2.7. Confocal Microscopy Analysis of the Subcellular Localization of the IFITM3 Protein

The cells were transfected with the recombinant plasmids pEF1α-Myc-IFITM3 and pEF1α-Myc, respectively. After 24 h of incubation, the culture medium was discarded. The cells were subsequently washed three times with phosphate-buffered saline (PBS) (Solarbio, Beijing, China) and fixed with 4% paraformaldehyde (Solarbio) for 30 min at room temperature. After three washes with PBS, the cells were infiltrated with 0.1% Triton X-100 (Solarbio) for 15 min and blocked with 5% BSA (Solarbio) for 1 h at room temperature. The cells were incubated with mouse anti-Myc monoclonal antibody (Invitrogen) as the primary antibody at 37 °C for 2 h and then with Alexa Fluor 488-labeled goat anti-mouse IgG (Invitrogen) as the secondary antibody at 37 °C while protected from light for 1 h. The nuclei were then stained with DAPI (Solarbio) for 10 min at room temperature while protected from light. After washing with PBS, 50% glycerol was added to the cell plates, and the results were observed by laser confocal microscopy.

2.8. Western Blotting

The cells transfected with the recombinant plasmids were washed with PBS and lysed on ice for 30 min using lysis buffer supplemented with protease inhibitors (Sangon Biotech, Shanghai, China). The lysate was then boiled at 100 °C for 10 min and centrifuged to obtain protein samples. The proteins were separated by SDS–PAGE and then transferred to polyvinylidene difluoride membranes (Millipore, Billerica, MA, USA). The membranes were blocked overnight with 5% skim milk at 4 °C and incubated with primary antibody at 37 °C for 2 h and then with the secondary antibody for 1 h. Mouse anti-Myc monoclonal antibody (Invitrogen) and mouse anti-β-actin antibody (Invitrogen) were used as primary antibodies. AP-labeled goat anti-mouse IgG (H+L) (Beyotime Biotechnology, Beijing, China) was used as the secondary antibody. The proteins were then visualized using a BCIP/NBT alkaline phosphatase color development kit (Beyotime Biotechnology).

2.9. Statistical Analysis

All the data were statistically analyzed using Student's t test and graphed using GraphPad Prism 8. The data were obtained from biological replicates and technical replicates. The results are expressed as the mean ± standard deviation (SD) of three independent experiments. Each sample was measured three times during RT–qPCR. * indicates $p < 0.05$, ** indicates $p < 0.01$, *** indicates $p < 0.001$, and **** indicates $p < 0.0001$.

3. Results

3.1. Cloning, Bioinformatics Analysis and Subcellular Localization of IFITM3

The full-length sequence of chicken IFITM3 (approximately 342 bp) was successfully cloned using the IFITM3-1 primers (Figure 1). The sequence was uploaded to the NCBI-BLAST online website for comparison, and the results confirmed that the cloned sequence was the full-length sequence encoded by the IFITM3 gene of *Gallus gallus*, which consists of 342 bases and encodes a total of 113 amino acids. Based on the NCBI CD-Search, the CD225 conserved domain in the chicken IFITM3 protein was predicted (Figure 2A). The secondary structure analysis of the IFITM3 protein showed that alpha helices accounted for 42.48%, beta turns accounted for 1.77%, random coils accounted for 40.71%, and extended strands accounted for 15.04% (Figure 2B). Tertiary structure prediction showed that the global model quality estimation (GMQE) of the chicken IFITM3 protein and IFITM3 derived from Northern Bobwhite equaled 0.61, and the coverage rate was 80.91% (Figure 2C). Homology analysis revealed that chicken IFITM3 exhibited the highest homology (99.4%) with that of *Anas platyrhynchos*. The homologies between chicken IFITM3 and those of *Anser cygnoides* and *Serinus canaria* were 46% and 45.7%, respectively, and the homologies between chicken IFITM3 and those of *Homo sapiens*, *Gorilla gorilla gorilla*, *Capra hircus*, *Sus scrofa* and *Mus musculus* were 50.4%, 53.5%, 51%, 49% and 46.5%, respectively. We constructed a phylogenetic tree to explore the genetic relationships between chicken IFITM3 and IFITM3s from other species (Figure 3). The results showed that chicken IFITM3 is most closely related to IFITM3 in *A. platyrhynchos*. *A. cygnoides* and *S. canaria* are found in the same group of birds as chickens, but their IFITM3s are distantly related to chicken IFITM3. Chicken IFITM3 is most distantly related to IFITM3s in mammals, such as *H. sapiens* and *G. gorilla gorilla*. These results are consistent with the results of the homology analysis described above. The subcellular localization of the IFITM3 protein in DF-1 cells was analyzed by immunofluorescence and laser confocal microscopy. The nuclei were labeled with blue fluorescence, and the IFITM3 protein was labeled with green fluorescence. As shown in Figure 4, DF-1 cells transfected with the pEF1α-Myc-IFITM3 plasmid exhibit green fluorescence in the cytoplasm, whereas control cells transfected with the pEF1α-Myc vector do not show green fluorescence, indicating that the IFITM3 protein is localized in the cytoplasm of DF-1 cells.

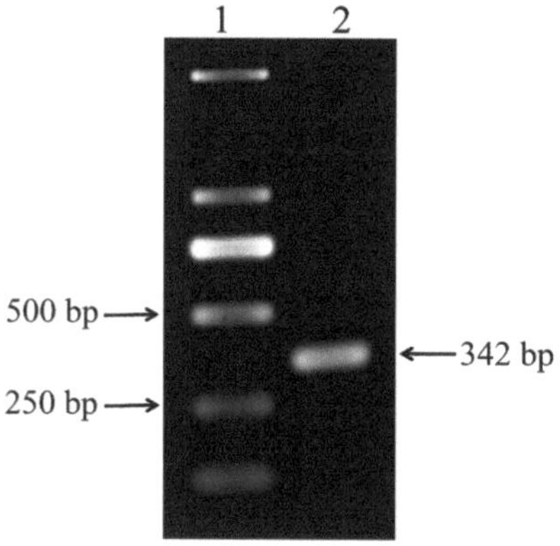

Figure 1. Analysis of the PCR product of the IFITM3 gene via agarose gel electrophoresis. Lane 1: DL2000 DNA marker; Lane 2: Amplification product of the IFITM3 gene. The size of the amplified IFITM3 gene fragment is 342 bp.

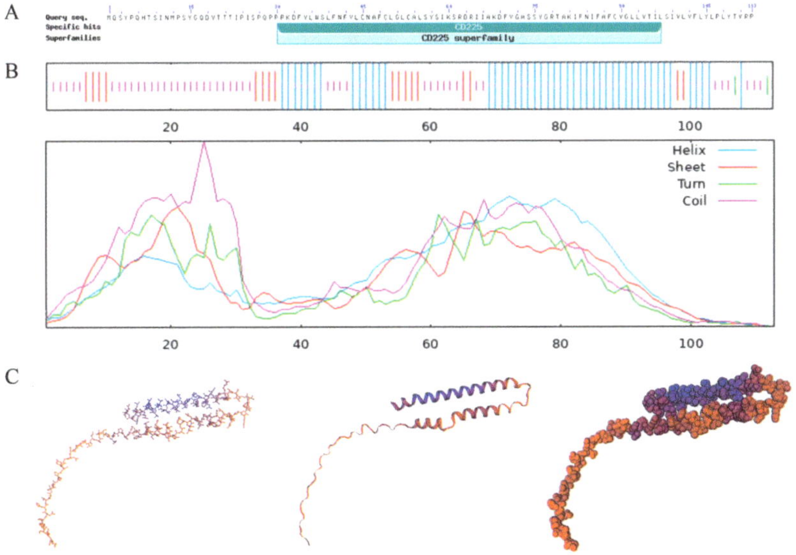

Figure 2. Structural analysis of the IFITM3 protein. (**A**). Schematic diagram of the conserved domain of the IFITM3 protein. The diagram shows the CD225 conserved domain. (**B**). Secondary structure of the IFITM3 protein. The longest lines represent alpha helices (Hh), the second longest lines represent extended strands (Ee), the third longest lines represent beta turns (Tt), and the shortest lines represent random coils (Cc). (**C**). Tertiary structure of the IFITM3 protein. The global model quality estimation (GMQE) of the chicken IFITM3 protein and IFITM3 derived from Northern Bobwhite equaled 0.61, and the coverage rate was 80.91%.

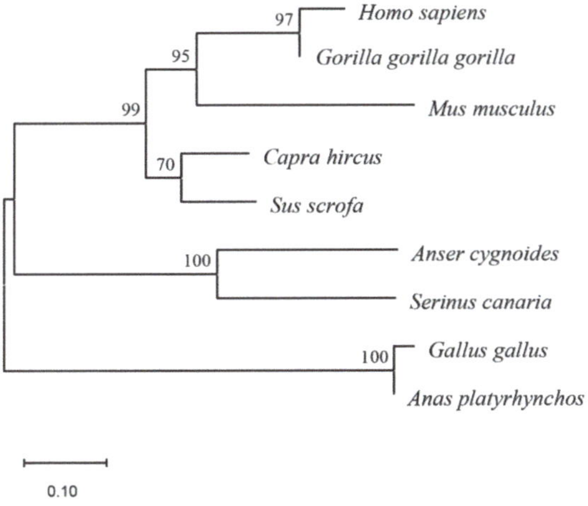

Figure 3. Phylogenetic tree analysis of IFITM3 genes in different species. A phylogenetic tree was constructed using MEGA 11 via the neighbor-joining method. The scale bar indicates the length of the branches, and the bootstrap confidence values are shown on the nodes of the tree.

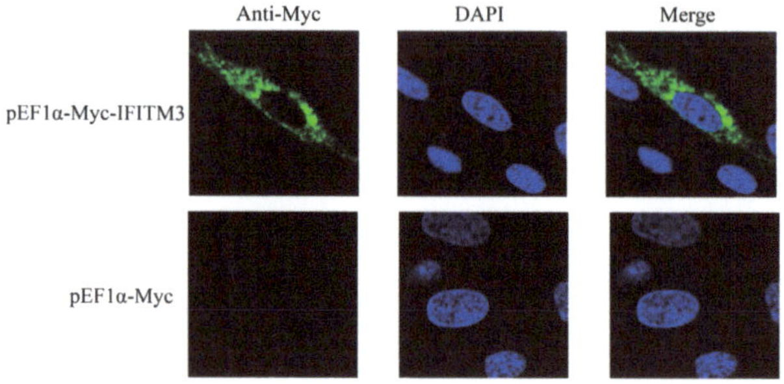

Figure 4. Subcellular localization of the IFITM3 protein (63× magnification). The subcellular localization of the IFITM3 protein in DF-1 cells was observed by laser confocal microscopy. The panels show nuclei stained with DAPI (blue), the IFITM3 protein labeled with Alexa Fluor 488-labeled goat anti-mouse IgG (green) and a merged image.

3.2. Distribution Characteristics of IFITM3 in Chicken Tissues and Organs

The distribution of the IFITM3 gene in different tissues and organs of 14-day-old SPF chickens was determined by RT–qPCR. The results showed that IFITM3 was widely expressed in a variety of tissues and organs of chickens, and its highest expression was found in the intestine, followed by the bursa of Fabricius, blood, lung, pancreas, trachea, thymus and spleen. IFITM3 was expressed at low levels in the liver, skin, heart, glandular stomach, gizzard, joint and kidney, and its relative expression in muscle and brain tissues was extremely low (Figure 5).

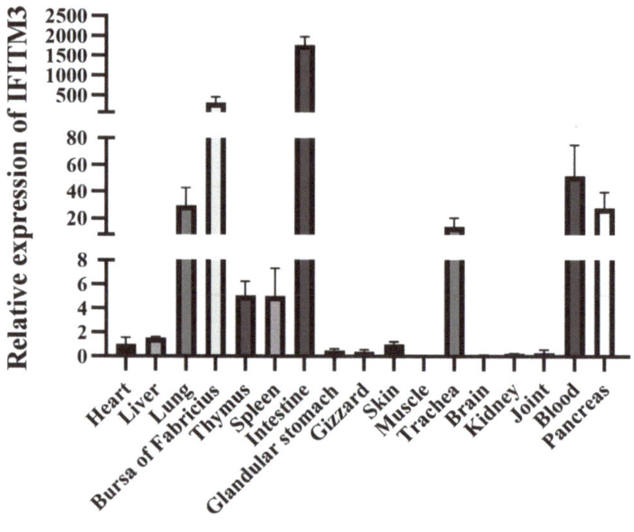

Figure 5. Analysis of the IFITM3 gene expression in different tissues and organs. RT–qPCR was used to measure the IFITM3 mRNA levels in the heart, liver, lung, bursa of Fabricius, thymus, spleen, intestine, glandular stomach, gizzard, skin, muscle, trachea, brain, kidney, joint, blood and pancreas of 14-day-old SPF chickens. The data are presented as the mean ± SD of three independent experiments.

3.3. High-Level Expression of IFITM3 Reduces ARV Replication

The effect of IFITM3 on ARV replication was analyzed via overexpression and interference assays. First, the overexpression of chicken IFITM3 in DF-1 cells was verified by Western blotting and RT–qPCR. Western blot analysis of DF-1 cell samples transfected with pEF1α-Myc-IFITM3 revealed that a specific band of approximately 13 kDa could be detected by Myc-tagged antibody, whereas no specific bands were detected in cell samples transfected with the empty vector (Figure 6A). The RT–qPCR results showed that, compared with that in the control group, the expression of IFITM3 in D-F1 cells transfected with pEF1α-Myc-IFITM3 was significantly upregulated, and its expression increased by approximately 155-fold (Figure 6B). Subsequently, IFITM3 was overexpressed in DF-1 cells, the resulting cells were subsequently infected with ARV, and the mRNA level of the ARV σC gene was then detected by RT–qPCR to determine the changes in the viral load. The results showed that the viral load of ARV was significantly reduced after IFITM3 overexpression (Figure 6C). Moreover, the detection of viral titers in cell culture supernatants also showed that the viral titer of ARV after the overexpression of IFITM3 was significantly lower than that in the control group (Figure 6D). Therefore, we inferred that the overexpression of chicken IFITM3 could effectively inhibit the replication of ARV, and based on this finding, we speculated that inhibition of the expression of IFITM3 may be beneficial for ARV replication. In the following experiments, three siRNAs were designed and synthesized to inhibit the expression of IFITM3. As shown in Figure 6E, si242 exerted the greatest inhibitory effect. The expression of IFITM3 in DF-1 cells was inhibited by transfection with si242, and ARV infection was performed 24 h after transfection. The mRNA level of the ARV σC gene and the viral titer in the cell supernatant were subsequently measured. The results showed that the level of ARV replication increased significantly after inhibition of the expression of IFITM3 (Figure 6F,G). The results were consistent with the expectations.

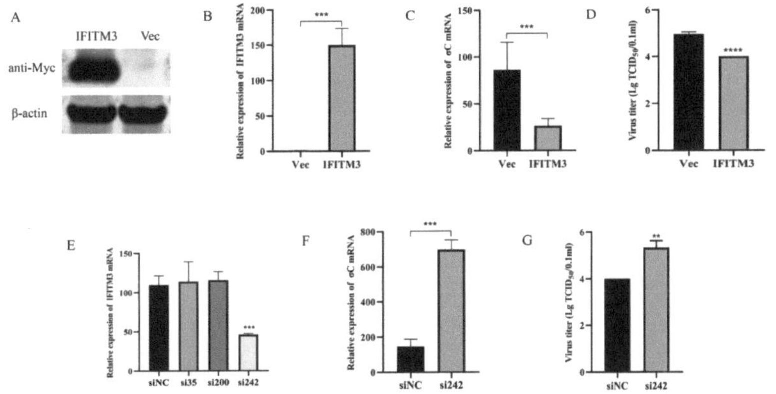

Figure 6. IFITM3 inhibits the replication of ARV in DF-1 cells. DF-1 cells were transfected with pEF1α-Myc-IFITM3 or pEF1α-Myc (Vec), and high levels of IFITM3 expression in DF-1 cells were confirmed by Western blotting (**A**) and RT–qPCR (**B**). DF-1 cells were transfected with pEF1α-Myc-IFITM3 or pEF1α-Myc (Vec) and then infected with the ARV S1133 strain (MOI = 1). After 24 h, the replication of ARV in DF-1 cells was detected by RT–qPCR (**C**) and by determining the viral titer (**D**). The inhibition efficiency of the three siRNAs on IFITM3 was detected by RT–qPCR (**E**). DF-1 cells were transfected with si242 or siNC and then infected with the ARV S1133 strain (MOI = 1). After 24 h, the replication of ARV in DF-1 cells was detected by RT–qPCR (**F**) and by determining the viral titer (**G**). Asterisks indicate significant differences (** $p < 0.01$, *** $p < 0.001$, **** $p < 0.0001$).

3.4. *Effect of IFITM3 on Innate Immune Signaling Pathway-Correlated Molecules during ARV Infection*

The above-described test results showed that chicken IFITM3 exerts an inhibitory effect on the replication of ARV. To further explore the antiviral mechanism of IFITM3 in the process of ARV infection, we studied the regulatory effect of IFITM3 on the innate immune response after ARV infection. IFITM3 was overexpressed or inhibited in DF-1 cells, and 24 h later, the cells were infected with ARV. The changes in the expression of molecules related to the innate immune signaling pathway were then detected by RT–qPCR, and the results are shown in Figure 7. After infection, the expression of MAVS, IRF7, STING,

NF-κB, MAD5, LGP2, IFN-α and IFN-β was upregulated compared with that in the control group, regardless of whether IFITM3 was overexpressed or inhibited. Interestingly, the expression levels of IRF1, TBK1 and IFN-γ were significantly downregulated after IFITM3 overexpression ($p < 0.05$ or $p < 0.01$). However, the expression levels of IRF1, TBK1 and IFN-γ were significantly upregulated after IFITM3 inhibition ($p < 0.05$ or $p < 0.001$). It is speculated that changes in the expression of IFITM3 during ARV infection may affect the expression of IRF1, TBK1 and IFN-γ.

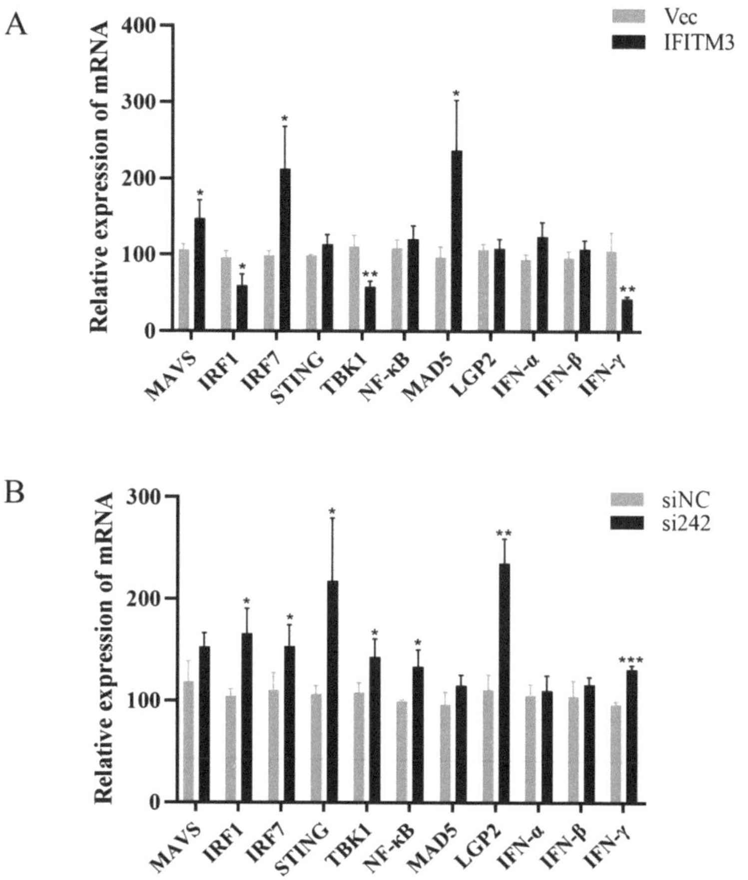

Figure 7. Effect of IFITM3 on the expression of molecules associated with innate immune signaling pathways during ARV infection. DF-1 cells were transfected with pEF1α-Myc-IFITM3 or pEF1α-Myc (Vec) and then infected with the ARV S1133 strain (MOI = 1). After 24 h of infection, RT–qPCR was used to measure the changes in the expression of MAVS, IRF1, IRF7, STING, TBK1, NF-κB, MAD5, LGP2, IFN-α, IFN-β and IFN-γ (**A**). DF-1 cells were transfected with si242 or siNC and then infected with the ARV S1133 strain (MOI = 1). After 24 h of infection, RT–qPCR was used to measure the changes in the expression of MAVS, IRF1, IRF7, STING, TBK1, NF-κB, MAD5, LGP2, IFN-α, IFN-β and IFN-γ (**B**). The data are presented as the mean ± SD of three independent experiments. Asterisks indicate significant differences (* $p < 0.05$, ** $p < 0.01$, *** $p < 0.001$).

4. Discussion

IFITM3 is an important effector of the innate immune system and plays an important role in host resistance to viral infections. Gene structure is often closely related to biological function. In this study, we cloned the chicken IFITM3 gene and analyzed this gene via bioinformatic approaches. Multiple comparison analyses revealed that the homology between chicken IFITM3 and *A. platyrhynchos* was as high as 99.4%. Furthermore, chicken IFITM3 did not exhibit more than 50% homology with that of *A. cygnoides* or *S. canaria*. The homologies of chicken IFITM3 with those of other mammals did not exceed 55%. The same results were obtained via phylogenetic tree analysis, which revealed substantial genetic variation in the IFITM3 genes of different species. The homology between chicken IFITM3 and *A. platyrhynchos* IFITM3 was high, whereas chicken IFITM3 exhibited low homology with bird IFITM3s, such as those of *A. cygnoides* and *S. canaria*. Studies have shown that IFITM proteins belong to the CD225 superfamily, and their members share a highly conserved region of amino acids, the CD225 domain [29]. The CD225 domain was also identified in the protein structure analysis of chicken IFITM3. The CD225 domain consists of an intramembrane domain (IMD), cytoplasmic intracellular loop (CIL) and transmembrane domain (TMD) [30]. Previous studies have shown that the CD225 domain contains multiple key regions associated with antiviral effects, which are also closely correlated with the antiviral effects of IFITM3 [31]. The first intramembrane domain (IM1) contains two critical residues, F75 and F78, which are decisive factors affecting the interaction of the IFITM3 protein with the host [29]. GxxxG is an oligomeric motif in the CD225 domain. The glycine-95 in GxxxG is closely related to the oligomerization of IFITM3 and its antiviral activity [32]. Therefore, the conserved structure of the CD225 superfamily may cause IFITM3 proteins derived from different species to exhibit certain similarities in their biological functions. Additionally, the question of whether IFITM3 proteins from different species have antiviral specificity deserves in-depth study, as do their mechanisms of action.

The antiviral function of proteins is closely related to their subcellular localization in cells and their distribution in tissues and organs. The subcellular localization of the chicken IFITM3 protein in DF-1 cells was analyzed by laser confocal microscopy, and the results showed that IFITM3 was localized in the cytoplasm of DF-1 cells. Some previous analyses have investigated the subcellular localization of the IFITM3 protein. S. E. Smith [33] reported that the IFITM3 protein in chickens localizes to the perinuclear area of DF-1 cells, and the human IFITM3 protein also localizes to the perinuclear area of human-derived A549 cells. The distribution of IFITM3 in chicken tissues and organs was then analyzed, and the highest expression of the IFITM3 gene was found in the chicken intestine. This expression pattern is similar to that of human IFITM3, which is most highly expressed in the ileum and cecum in the human digestive system [34]. Moreover, IFITM3 is significantly upregulated in the intestines of pigs infected with porcine circovirus type 2 (PCV2) and porcine parvovirus virus (PPV) [35]. Zoya Alteber et al. [15] experimented with IFITM3-deficient mice and revealed that the IFITM3 gene is involved in regulating the stability of the intestinal environment. IFITM3 also significantly improves the incidence of colitis and prevents inflammation-associated tumorigenesis. After ARV infection, the virus replicates primarily in the host's gut and subsequently spreads through the fecal-oral route and respiratory tract [1,36,37]. However, whether ARV infection further induces the expression of the IFITM3 gene in the gut is unknown. Furthermore, IFITM3 was found to be abundantly expressed in immune organs such as the bursa of Fabricius, thymus and spleen. Studies have shown that high expression of IFITM3 can be induced in a variety of immune organs after ARV infection, which is generally consistent with the trend found for the expression of ARV [12,14].

Further experimental results showed that overexpression of IFITM3 in DF-1 cells could inhibit the replication of ARV, whereas the inhibition of IFITM3 expression in DF-1 cells could promote the replication of ARV, indicating that IFITM3 is an important antiviral factor against ARV infection. Recent studies have shown that IFITM3 can also inhibit the replication of a variety of avian-derived viruses. Stable expression of the duck IFITM3 protein in DF-1 cells can significantly limit the replication of H6N2 and H11N9 IAV strains [38]. Both chicken and duck IFITM3 can effectively inhibit the replication of avian Tembusu virus (ATMUV) [39].

To date, studies on the antiviral mechanism of IFITM proteins have focused mainly on their ability to block contact between viruses and cells and less on their ability to regulate innate immune signaling pathways. Therefore, in this study, the effect of IFITM3 on the expression of innate immune-related molecules after ARV infection was further investigated. The results showed that the expression of MAVS, IRF7, STING, NF-κB, MAD5, LGP2, IFN-α and IFN-β was upregulated compared with that in the control group, regardless of whether IFITM3 was overexpressed or inhibited after infection. Previous studies have shown that ARV infection induces the upregulation of these cytokines [12]. It is hypothesized that changes in IFITM3 expression during ARV infection may not affect the expression of these molecules. In addition, previous studies revealed that the expression of TBK1 and IFN-γ is significantly upregulated after ARV infection [12]. However, in the present study, the expression of TBK1, IFN-γ and IRF1 was significantly downregulated after the overexpression of IFITM3 and significantly upregulated after the inhibition of IFITM3. This interesting phenomenon deserves more in-depth discussion. Researchers have shown that IFITM3 is induced by type I IFNs and can also negatively regulate the production of type I IFNs [40], indicating that IFITM3 may play a role in innate immunity as a negative feedback regulator. TBK1 is an important linker molecule that connects upstream receptor signaling and downstream gene activation in apoptosis, inflammation and immune responses [41,42]. TBK1 has been found to be involved in lipopolysaccharide (LPS)-induced IFITM3 expression [43]. This finding suggests a potential link between IFITM3 and TBK1 in the body's inflammatory response. Nevertheless, in ARV infection, IFITM3 may exert a negative regulatory effect on TBK1. IFN-γ is a cytokine with antiviral activity and immunomodulatory functions that can act on different types of immune cells to regulate innate and adaptive immunity [44]. IRF1 plays a very important role in the innate immune response induced by IFN-γ [45,46]. IFN-γ mainly regulates transcription factors such as IRF1 through the JAK/STAT signaling pathway and thus drives subsequent transcriptional regulation [47]. In this study, the overexpression of IFITM3 during ARV infection significantly downregulated the expression of IFN-γ and IRF1, whereas the inhibition of IFITM3 significantly upregulated the expression of IFN-γ and IRF1. It is hypothesized that IFITM3 may be involved in the body's innate immune response by negatively regulating IFN-γ and IRF1 during ARV infection.

In this study, the chicken IFITM3 gene was cloned and bioinformatically analyzed, and its role in ARV infection was then further analyzed. The results of this study lay a theoretical foundation for obtaining an in-depth understanding of the antiviral mechanism of host resistance to ARV and provide new ideas for the development of new ARV prevention measures. However, the specific regulatory mechanism of IFITM3 on innate immunity during ARV infection needs to be further studied.

Author Contributions: Z.X. (Zhixun Xie) designed and coordinated the study and helped review the manuscript. H.R. performed the experiments, analyzed the data and wrote the manuscript. S.W. assisted with the experiments and revised the manuscript. L.W., L.X., S.L., M.L., Z.X. (Zhiqin Xie), Q.F., T.Z., Y.Z., M.Z., J.H. and Y.W. assisted with the animal experiments. All authors have read and agreed to the published version of the manuscript.

Funding: This work was supported by Guangxi Science and Technology Projects (AA23062050), the Natural Science Foundation of China (project 31660715), the Natural Science Foundation of China (project 32300148), the Guangxi Basic Research Funds supported by the Special Project (Guike special 23-1), the Guangxi BaGui Scholars Program Foundation (2019A50) and the Guangxi Science Base and Talents Special Program (AD17195083).

Institutional Review Board Statement: The animal study was reviewed and approved by the Animal Ethics Committee of Guangxi Veterinary Research Institute (No. #2019C0408).

Informed Consent Statement: Not applicable.

Data Availability Statement: The original contributions presented in the study are included in the article, and further inquiries can be directed to the corresponding author.

Conflicts of Interest: The authors declare no conflicts of interest.

References

1. Jones, R.C. Avian reovirus infections. *Rev. Sci. Tech.* **2000**, *19*, 614–625. [CrossRef]
2. van der Heide, L. The history of avian reovirus. *Avian Dis.* **2000**, *44*, 638–641. [CrossRef]
3. Teng, L.; Xie, Z.; Xie, L.; Liu, J.; Pang, Y.; Deng, X.; Xie, Z.; Fan, Q.; Luo, S.; Feng, J.; et al. Sequencing and phylogenetic analysis of an avian reovirus genome. *Virus Genes* **2014**, *48*, 381–386. [CrossRef] [PubMed]
4. Souza, S.O.; De Carli, S.; Lunge, V.R.; Ikuta, N.; Canal, C.W.; Pavarini, S.P.; Driemeier, D. Pathological and molecular findings of avian reoviruses from clinical cases of tenosynovitis in poultry flocks from Brazil. *Poult. Sci.* **2018**, *97*, 3550–3555. [CrossRef] [PubMed]
5. Tang, Y.; Lu, H. Whole genome alignment based one-step real-time RT-PCR for universal detection of avian orthoreoviruses of chicken, pheasant and turkey origins. *Infect. Genet. Evol.* **2016**, *39*, 120–126. [CrossRef] [PubMed]
6. Lu, H.; Tang, Y.; Dunn, P.A.; Wallner-Pendleton, E.A.; Lin, L.; Knoll, E.A. Isolation and molecular characterization of newly emerging avian reovirus variants and novel strains in Pennsylvania, USA, 2011–2014. *Sci. Rep.* **2015**, *5*, 14727. [CrossRef] [PubMed]
7. Iwasaki, A.; Pillai, P.S. Innate immunity to influenza virus infection. *Nat. Rev. Immunol.* **2014**, *14*, 315–328. [CrossRef] [PubMed]
8. Green, A.M.; Beatty, P.R.; Hadjilaou, A.; Harris, E. Innate immunity to dengue virus infection and subversion of antiviral responses. *J. Mol. Biol.* **2014**, *426*, 1148–1160. [CrossRef] [PubMed]
9. Haller, O.; Weber, F. The interferon response circuit in antiviral host defense. *Verh.-K. Acad. Voor Geneeskd. Van Belg.* **2009**, *71*, 73–86.
10. Takeuchi, O.; Akira, S. Pattern recognition receptors and inflammation. *Cell* **2010**, *140*, 805–820. [CrossRef]
11. Secombes, C.J.; Zou, J. Evolution of Interferons and Interferon Receptors. *Front. Immunol.* **2017**, *8*, 209. [CrossRef]
12. Xie, L.; Xie, Z.; Wang, S.; Huang, J.; Deng, X.; Xie, Z.; Luo, S.; Zeng, T.; Zhang, Y.; Zhang, M. Altered gene expression profiles of the MDA5 signaling pathway in peripheral blood lymphocytes of chickens infected with avian reovirus. *Arch. Virol.* **2019**, *164*, 2451–2458. [CrossRef]
13. Wang, S.; Xie, L.; Xie, Z.; Wan, L.; Huang, J.; Deng, X.; Xie, Z.Q.; Luo, S.; Zeng, T.; Zhang, Y.; et al. Dynamic Changes in the Expression of Interferon-Stimulated Genes in Joints of SPF Chickens Infected With Avian Reovirus. *Front. Vet. Sci.* **2021**, *8*, 618124. [CrossRef]
14. Wang, S.; Wan, L.; Ren, H.; Xie, Z.; Xie, L.; Huang, J.; Deng, X.; Xie, Z.; Luo, S.; Li, M.; et al. Screening of interferon-stimulated genes against avian reovirus infection and mechanistic exploration of the antiviral activity of IFIT5. *Front. Microbiol.* **2022**, *13*, 998505. [CrossRef] [PubMed]
15. Alteber, Z.; Sharbi-Yunger, A.; Pevsner-Fischer, M.; Blat, D.; Roitman, L.; Tzehoval, E.; Elinav, E.; Eisenbach, L. The anti-inflammatory IFITM genes ameliorate colitis and partially protect from tumorigenesis by changing immunity and microbiota. *Immunol. Cell Biol.* **2018**, *96*, 284–297. [CrossRef]
16. Ranjbar, S.; Haridas, V.; Jasenosky, L.D.; Falvo, J.V.; Goldfeld, A.E. A Role for IFITM Proteins in Restriction of Mycobacterium tuberculosis Infection. *Cell Rep.* **2015**, *13*, 874–883. [CrossRef] [PubMed]
17. Huang, I.C.; Bailey, C.C.; Weyer, J.L.; Radoshitzky, S.R.; Becker, M.M.; Chiang, J.J.; Brass, A.L.; Ahmed, A.A.; Chi, X.; Dong, L.; et al. Distinct patterns of IFITM-mediated restriction of filoviruses, SARS coronavirus, and influenza A virus. *PLoS Pathog.* **2011**, *7*, e1001258. [CrossRef]
18. Anafu, A.A.; Bowen, C.H.; Chin, C.R.; Brass, A.L.; Holm, G.H. Interferon-inducible transmembrane protein 3 (IFITM3) restricts reovirus cell entry. *J. Biol. Chem.* **2013**, *288*, 17261–17271. [CrossRef] [PubMed]
19. Jiang, D.; Guo, H.; Xu, C.; Chang, J.; Gu, B.; Wang, L.; Block, T.M.; Guo, J.T. Identification of three interferon-inducible cellular enzymes that inhibit the replication of hepatitis C virus. *J. Virol.* **2008**, *82*, 1665–1678. [CrossRef]
20. Wang, A.; Sun, L.; Wang, M.; Jia, R.; Zhu, D.; Liu, M.; Sun, K.; Yang, Q.; Wu, Y.; Chen, X.; et al. Identification of IFITM1 and IFITM3 in Goose: Gene Structure, Expression Patterns, and Immune Reponses against Tembusu Virus Infection. *Biomed. Res. Int.* **2017**, *2017*, 5149062. [CrossRef]
21. Feeley, E.M.; Sims, J.S.; John, S.P.; Chin, C.R.; Pertel, T.; Chen, L.M.; Gaiha, G.D.; Ryan, B.J.; Donis, R.O.; Elledge, S.J.; et al. IFITM3 inhibits influenza A virus infection by preventing cytosolic entry. *PLoS Pathog.* **2011**, *7*, e1002337. [CrossRef] [PubMed]
22. Brass, A.L.; Huang, I.; Benita, Y.; John, S.P.; Manoj, N.; Feeley, E.M.; Ryan, B.; Weyer, J.L.; Weyden, L.V.D.; Fikrig, E. IFITM Proteins Mediate the Innate Immune Response to Influenza A H1N1 Virus, West Nile Virus and Dengue Virus. *Cell* **2009**, *139*, 1243. [CrossRef]
23. Pang, Z.; Hao, P.; Qu, Q.; Li, L.; Jiang, Y.; Xiao, S.; Jin, N.; Li, C. Interferon-Inducible Transmembrane Protein 3 (IFITM3) Restricts Rotavirus Infection. *Viruses* **2022**, *14*, 2407. [CrossRef] [PubMed]
24. Perreira, J.M.; Chin, C.R.; Feeley, E.M.; Brass, A.L. IFITMs restrict the replication of multiple pathogenic viruses. *J. Mol. Biol.* **2013**, *425*, 4937–4955. [CrossRef]
25. Diamond, M.S.; Farzan, M. The broad-spectrum antiviral functions of IFIT and IFITM proteins. *Nat. Rev. Immunol.* **2013**, *13*, 46–57. [CrossRef] [PubMed]
26. Xu, J.; Qian, P.; Wu, Q.; Liu, S.; Fan, W.; Zhang, K.; Wang, R.; Zhang, H.; Chen, H.; Li, X. Swine interferon-induced transmembrane protein, sIFITM3, inhibits foot-and-mouth disease virus infection in vitro and in vivo. *Antivir. Res.* **2014**, *109*, 22–29. [CrossRef]

27. Xing, H.; Ye, L.; Fan, J.; Fu, T.; Li, C.; Zhang, S.; Ren, L.; Bai, J. IFITMs of African Green Monkey Can Inhibit Replication of SFTSV but Not MNV In Vitro. *Viral Immunol.* **2020**, *33*, 634–641. [CrossRef]
28. He, Y.; Xie, Z.; Dai, J.; Cao, Y.; Hou, J.; Zheng, Y.; Wei, T.; Mo, M.; Wei, P. Responses of the Toll-like receptor and melanoma differentiation-associated protein 5 signaling pathways to avian infectious bronchitis virus infection in chicks. *Virol. Sin.* **2016**, *31*, 57–68. [CrossRef]
29. John, S.P.; Chin, C.R.; Perreira, J.M.; Feeley, E.M.; Aker, A.M.; Savidis, G.; Smith, S.E.; Elia, A.E.; Everitt, A.R.; Vora, M.; et al. The CD225 domain of IFITM3 is required for both IFITM protein association and inhibition of influenza A virus and dengue virus replication. *J. Virol.* **2013**, *87*, 7837–7852. [CrossRef]
30. Coomer, C.A.; Rahman, K.; Compton, A.A. CD225 Proteins: A Family Portrait of Fusion Regulators. *Trends Genet.* **2021**, *37*, 406–410. [CrossRef]
31. Kim, Y.C.; Jeong, M.J.; Jeong, B.H. Genetic characteristics and polymorphisms in the chicken interferon-induced transmembrane protein (IFITM3) gene. *Vet. Res. Commun.* **2019**, *43*, 203–214. [CrossRef] [PubMed]
32. Rahman, K.; Coomer, C.A.; Majdoul, S.; Ding, S.Y.; Padilla-Parra, S.; Compton, A.A. Homology-guided identification of a conserved motif linking the antiviral functions of IFITM3 to its oligomeric state. *eLife* **2020**, *9*, e58537. [CrossRef] [PubMed]
33. Smith, S.E.; Gibson, M.S.; Wash, R.S.; Ferrara, F.; Wright, E.; Temperton, N.; Kellam, P.; Fife, M. Chicken interferon-inducible transmembrane protein 3 restricts influenza viruses and lyssaviruses in vitro. *J. Virol.* **2013**, *87*, 12957–12966. [CrossRef]
34. Seo, G.S.; Lee, J.K.; Yu, J.I.; Yun, K.J.; Chae, S.C.; Choi, S.C. Identification of the polymorphisms in IFITM3 gene and their association in a Korean population with ulcerative colitis. *Exp. Mol. Med.* **2010**, *42*, 99–104. [CrossRef]
35. Andersson, M.; Ahlberg, V.; Jensen-Waern, M.; Fossum, C. Intestinal gene expression in pigs experimentally co-infected with PCV2 and PPV. *Vet. Immunol. Immunopathol.* **2011**, *142*, 72–80. [CrossRef] [PubMed]
36. Kibenge, F.S.; Gwaze, G.E.; Jones, R.C.; Chapman, A.F.; Savage, C.E. Experimental reovirus infection in chickens: Observations on early viraemia and virus distribution in bone marrow, liver and enteric tissues. *Avian Pathol.* **1985**, *14*, 87–98. [CrossRef]
37. Wan, L.; Wang, S.; Xie, Z.; Ren, H.; Xie, L.; Luo, S.; Li, M.; Xie, Z.; Fan, Q.; Zeng, T.; et al. Chicken IFI6 inhibits avian reovirus replication and affects related innate immune signaling pathways. *Front. Microbiol.* **2023**, *14*, 1237438. [CrossRef]
38. Blyth, G.A.; Chan, W.F.; Webster, R.G.; Magor, K.E. Duck Interferon-Inducible Transmembrane Protein 3 Mediates Restriction of Influenza Viruses. *J. Virol.* **2016**, *90*, 103–116. [CrossRef]
39. Chen, S.; Wang, L.; Chen, J.; Zhang, L.; Wang, S.; Goraya, M.U.; Chi, X.; Na, Y.; Shao, W.; Yang, Z.; et al. Avian Interferon-Inducible Transmembrane Protein Family Effectively Restricts Avian Tembusu Virus Infection. *Front. Microbiol.* **2017**, *8*, 672. [CrossRef]
40. Jiang, L.Q.; Xia, T.; Hu, Y.H.; Sun, M.S.; Yan, S.; Lei, C.Q.; Shu, H.B.; Guo, J.H.; Liu, Y. IFITM3 inhibits virus-triggered induction of type I interferon by mediating autophagosome-dependent degradation of IRF3. *Cell. Mol. Immunol.* **2018**, *15*, 858–867. [CrossRef]
41. Chau, T.L.; Gioia, R.; Gatot, J.S.; Patrascu, F.; Carpentier, I.; Chapelle, J.P.; O'Neill, L.; Beyaert, R.; Piette, J.; Chariot, A. Are the IKKs and IKK-related kinases TBK1 and IKK-epsilon similarly activated? *Trends Biochem. Sci.* **2008**, *33*, 171–180. [CrossRef]
42. Koop, A.; Lepenies, I.; Braum, O.; Davarnia, P.; Scherer, G.; Fickenscher, H.; Kabelitz, D.; Adam-Klages, S. Novel splice variants of human IKKepsilon negatively regulate IKKepsilon-induced IRF3 and NF-kB activation. *Eur. J. Immunol.* **2011**, *41*, 224–234. [CrossRef] [PubMed]
43. Nakajima, A.; Ibi, D.; Nagai, T.; Yamada, S.; Nabeshima, T.; Yamada, K. Induction of interferon-induced transmembrane protein 3 gene expression by lipopolysaccharide in astrocytes. *Eur. J. Pharmacol.* **2014**, *745*, 166–175. [CrossRef] [PubMed]
44. Masuda, Y.; Matsuda, A.; Usui, T.; Sugai, T.; Asano, A.; Yamano, Y. Biological effects of chicken type III interferon on expression of interferon-stimulated genes in chickens: Comparison with type I and type II interferons. *J. Vet. Med. Sci.* **2012**, *74*, 1381–1386. [CrossRef] [PubMed]
45. Kim, E.J.; Lee, J.M.; Namkoong, S.E.; Um, S.J.; Park, J.S. Interferon regulatory factor-1 mediates interferon-gamma-induced apoptosis in ovarian carcinoma cells. *J. Cell. Biochem.* **2002**, *85*, 369–380. [CrossRef] [PubMed]
46. Kano, A.; Haruyama, T.; Akaike, T.; Watanabe, Y. IRF-1 is an essential mediator in IFN-gamma-induced cell cycle arrest and apoptosis of primary cultured hepatocytes. *Biochem. Biophys. Res. Commun.* **1999**, *257*, 672–677. [CrossRef]
47. Schroder, K.; Hertzog, P.J.; Ravasi, T.; Hume, D.A. Interferon-gamma: An overview of signals, mechanisms and functions. *J. Leukoc. Biol.* **2004**, *75*, 163–189. [CrossRef]

viruses

MDPI

Article

First Detection and Molecular Characterization of Novel Variant Infectious Bursal Disease Virus (Genotype A2dB1b) in Egypt

Matteo Legnardi [1,*], Francesca Poletto [1], Shaimaa Talaat [2], Karim Selim [3], Mahmoud K. Moawad [3], Giovanni Franzo [1], Claudia Maria Tucciarone [1], Mattia Cecchinato [1] and Hesham Sultan [2,*]

[1] Department of Animal Medicine, Production and Health (MAPS), University of Padova, 35020 Legnaro, Italy; francesca.poletto@unipd.it (F.P.); giovanni.franzo@unipd.it (G.F.); claudiamaria.tucciarone@unipd.it (C.M.T.); mattia.cecchinato@unipd.it (M.C.)

[2] Department of Birds and Rabbits Medicine, Faculty of Veterinary Medicine, University of Sadat City, Menoufia 32958, Egypt; shimaa.talaat@vet.usc.edu.eg

[3] Reference Laboratory for Quality Control on Poultry Production, Animal Health Research Institute, Agriculture Research Center, Giza 12618, Egypt; dr.kareemseleem_87@yahoo.com (K.S.); mah.kamel@hotmail.com (M.K.M.)

* Correspondence: matteo.legnardi@unipd.it (M.L.); hesham.sultan@vet.usc.edu.eg (H.S.)

Abstract: Infectious bursal disease (IBD) is an immunosuppressive disease causing significant damage to the poultry industry worldwide. Its etiological agent is infectious bursal disease virus (IBDV), a highly resistant RNA virus whose genetic variability considerably affects disease manifestation, diagnosis and control, primarily pursued by vaccination. In Egypt, very virulent strains (genotype A3B2), responsible for typical IBD signs and lesions and high mortality, have historically prevailed. The present molecular survey, however, suggests that a major epidemiological shift might be occurring in the country. Out of twenty-four samples collected in twelve governorates in 2022–2023, seven tested positive for IBDV. Two of them were A3B2 strains related to other very virulent Egyptian isolates, whereas the remaining five were novel variant IBDVs (A2dB1b), reported for the first time outside of Eastern and Southern Asia. This emerging genotype spawned a large-scale epidemic in China during the 2010s, characterized by subclinical IBD with severe bursal atrophy and immunosuppression. Its spread to Egypt is even more alarming considering that, contrary to circulating IBDVs, the protection conferred by available commercial vaccines appears suboptimal. These findings are therefore crucial for guiding monitoring and control efforts and helping to track the spread of novel variant IBDVs, possibly limiting their impact.

Keywords: infectious bursal disease virus; Gumboro disease; Egypt; China; very virulent; novel variant; molecular epidemiology

Citation: Legnardi, M.; Poletto, F.; Talaat, S.; Selim, K.; Moawad, M.K.; Franzo, G.; Tucciarone, C.M.; Cecchinato, M.; Sultan, H. First Detection and Molecular Characterization of Novel Variant Infectious Bursal Disease Virus (Genotype A2dB1b) in Egypt. *Viruses* **2023**, *15*, 2388. https://doi.org/10.3390/v15122388

Academic Editor: Chi-Young Wang

Received: 20 November 2023
Revised: 2 December 2023
Accepted: 5 December 2023
Published: 7 December 2023

1. Introduction

Infectious bursal disease (IBD), also known as Gumboro disease, is an immunosuppressive infectious disease of chickens with severe implications for the global poultry industry. IBD is characterized by high morbidity and mostly occurs in chickens aged 2–6 weeks, when the bursa of Fabricius, its main target organ, reaches its full development. After a short incubation period, the disease typically manifests with non-specific signs, such as depression and dehydration, along with hemorrhagic lesions in the thigh and breast muscles. The bursa appears enlarged at first due to edema and hyperemia but rapidly undergoes atrophy, while lymphocyte depletion is observed at the microscopical level. Alternatively, IBD may follow a subclinical course with lesions limited to the bursa, which may be harder to diagnose whilst still causing immunosuppression [1]. The disease burden may be significant both in case of overt clinical outbreaks and due to the impairment of immune status, which may lead to poor productive performance, vaccine failures, secondary infections, etc. Rigorous control of the disease, primarily pursued by routine vaccination, is therefore of utmost importance [2].

The etiological agent of IBD is known as infectious bursal disease virus (IBDV) and belongs to the species *Avibirnavirus gumboroense*, genus *Avibirnavirus*, family *Birnaviridae*. IBDV features a non-enveloped virion and a double-stranded RNA genome made of two segments, named A and B. Segment A (3.2 kb) codes for a capsid protein (VP2), a scaffold protein (VP3), a protease (VP4) and a non-structural protein with regulatory and anti-apoptotic functions (VP5), whereas segment B (2.9 kb) encodes the RNA-dependent RNA polymerase [3]. Two IBDV serotypes (1 and 2) are known, but only serotype 1 is pathogenic. However, further distinctions are possible, as many different IBDV types have emerged over time, mainly through mutation and reassortment events [4].

As a matter of fact, although IBDV is globally endemic, different countries and regions are affected by a range of viral strains, whose diverse features may have profound consequences in terms of disease manifestation and impact. Historically, the first IBDVs, known as "classical" strains, have been reported in the USA since the late 1950s [5]. Two other IBDV types were then described throughout the 1980s, one grouping highly pathogenic strains (classified as "very virulent") circulating all over Europe, Africa and Asia, and another comprising the so-called "variant" strains, which were antigenically different from other IBDVs and circulated mainly in North America [6], although they eventually spread to Eastern Asia during the 2010s [7].

In recent years, it has become more and more evident that this traditional tripartite classification, albeit still valuable, is inadequate to fully capture the heterogeneity among IBDV types. Several atypical IBDVs which hardly fit in any of the three major IBDV types have been described in different continents [8–12], and reassortant strains are also being reported with increasing frequency [13–16], further complicating the evolutionary landscape.

The recent proposal of multiple classification systems relying on phylogeny, either based on a portion of the VP2 [17] or both VP2 and VP1 genes [18,19], has certainly been instrumental for characterizing such strains while retaining the information provided by the traditional classification, offering easily applicable guidelines to perform molecular surveys and generate informative and standardized results. The focus on VP2 and VP1 is motivated by their functional relevance, which makes their genes the most studied genome portions. The VP2 has a well-established role in determining antigenicity, containing the main epitopes that elicit neutralizing antibodies [20], whereas both VP2 and VP1 are known to contribute to pathogenicity determination [21]. Since they are located in different segments, considering both genes also allows to detect reassortment events, which may represent another major source of pathogenic variation [15,22].

The usefulness of this approach is obviously not limited to underinvestigated contexts for which few or no data on circulating IBDVs are available, since it is also helpful to revise the existing evidence and improve monitoring activities even in countries where more information is available. Egypt is certainly an example of the latter case, as the burden posed by IBD to the national poultry production is well-established. Since their first identification in 1989 [23], very virulent strains have consistently posed the greatest threat in the country, as confirmed by several epidemiological studies conducted over the years [24–26]. Nonetheless, steady surveillance efforts remain crucial to keep the IBD situation monitored, to assess whether existing control measures are effective and to rapidly identify new epidemiological threats. Consistent with this rationale, the present study reports the results of molecular diagnostic activities performed on samples collected in different Egyptian governorates and contextualizes them within the national and international epidemiological context according to the current classification systems.

2. Materials and Methods

2.1. Sampling Activities

This study was based on molecular diagnostic activities conducted on samples collected in Egypt for IBD investigation. Samples consisted of bursal imprints on FTA™

cards (GE Healthcare UK Limited, Amersham, UK) and were collected from broiler farms between February 2022 and August 2023 when IBD was suspected based on clinical signs (i.e., anorexia, depression, etc.), lesions (i.e., hemorrhages in the thigh and breast muscles, dehydration, enlarged or atrophic bursa, etc.) and a high mortality rate. Anamnestic information such as farm location, age at sampling, administered IBD vaccines and cumulative mortality up to the sampling date were recorded for all the investigated flocks.

2.2. Samples Processing and Nucleic Acid Extraction

Samples were processed by cutting 5 mm^2 fragments from FTA™ card circles, eluting them into 1.5 mL of 1× PBS and vortexing for 30 s. Nucleic acids were extracted from the eluates by using the High Pure Nucleic Acids kit (Roche™, Basel, Switzerland) following the manufacturer's instructions. Samples were stored at −80 °C for the entire duration of the molecular analyses and subsequently for archival purposes.

2.3. Molecular Investigation

All samples were first subjected to a one-step RT-PCR performed with the primers 743-1 and 743-2 designed by Jackwood and Sommer-Wagner [27] to amplify a portion of the VP2 gene. Additional RT-PCRs were then conducted on positive samples using multiple primer pairs partially derived from those listed by Lachheb et al. [28]. In detail, primers VP5/1+ and VP2/1263- were used to amplify the rest of the VP2 [29], whereas primers 66 and 67 [30], B-Univ-F and B-Univ-R [31], X3 [32] and VP1/1997- [33] and B3-IPP2 and B3′-P2 [34] allowed to cover the entire VP1 gene (Table 1).

The SuperScript™ III One-Step RT-PCR System with Platinum™ *Taq* DNA Polymerase kit (Invitrogen™, Waltham, MA, USA) was used to carry out all molecular assays. Whenever a positive result was evidenced by gel electrophoresis, amplicons were sent to Macrogen Europe Milan Genome Center (Milan, Italy), where Sanger sequencing was performed using the respective primer pair. The resulting chromatograms were visually inspected and appropriately trimmed using 4Peaks (Nucleobytes B.V., Aalsmer, The Netherlands), and then used to generate consensus sequences in ChromasPro (Technelysium Pty Ltd., Helensvale, QLD, Australia).

2.4. Phylogenetic Analyses

Sequencing results were used to characterize the detected strains based on the classification system proposed by Wang et al. [19], considering a portion of the hypervariable region (HVR) of the VP2 gene (nt 737–1210) and the B marker located in the VP1 gene (nt 328–756) as defined by Alfonso-Morales et al. [35]. For both genomic segments, along with the reference sequences used by Wang et al. [36], additional strains related to those detected in the present survey, retrieved through dedicated BLAST queries [37], were also considered. After aligning the reference datasets with the MUSCLE method in Mega X [38], phylogenetic trees were inferred using the same software, adopting the Maximum-Likelihood method with 1000 bootstraps and the substitution model having the lowest Bayesian information criterion (BIC) value. The resulting trees were then visualized using the Interactive Tree Of Life online tool [39]. The obtained amino acid sequences were also compared with those of reference isolates when deemed appropriate to identify relevant substitutions.

Table 1. List of primer pairs used for the amplification and sequencing of the VP2 and VP1 genes.

Genome Segment	Primer	Sequence (5′-3′)	Amplicon Length	Designed by
VP5 and VP2 (1–1263)	VP5/1+ VP2/1263-	GGATACGATCGGTCTGAC TCAGGATTTGGGATCAGC	1263 bp	Hernández et al. [29]
VP2 (736–1478)	743-1 743-2	GCCCAGAGTCTACACCAT CCCGGATTATGTCTTTGA	743 bp	Jackwood and Sommer-Wagner [27]
VP1 (1–695)	66 67	GGATACGATGGGTCTGAC ATCCTTGACGGCACCCTT	695 bp	Ruud et al. [30]
VP1 (319–1369)	B-Univ-F B-Univ-R	AATGAGGAGTATGAGACCGA CCTTCTCTAGGTCAATTGAGTACC	1051 bp	Islam et al. [31]
VP1 (756–1997)	X3 VP1/1997-	CGGTGAGGATGACAAGCCC GAACCCCTTTGCCTCCAAG	1241 bp	He et al. [32] Tiwari et al. [33]
VP1 (1839–2827)	B3-IPP2 B3′-P2	ATACAGCAAAGATCTCGGG CGATCTGCTGCAGGGGGCCCCCGCAGGCGAAGG	988 bp	Mundt and Vakharia [34]

3. Results

A total of 24 samples were collected from broiler farms located in 12 different governorates. The age at sampling was between 18 and 30 days (23.2 days on average). All flocks were reportedly immunized against IBD with a range of vaccination protocols relying on immune complex, vector or live vaccines (sometimes administered twice or after vector vaccines). Seven samples (H792, H793, H798, H800, H801, H805 and H812) tested positive for IBDV (29%). Detailed information on the sampled flocks is provided in Table 2.

Table 2. Anamnestic details recorded for each of the sampled flocks.

Sample ID	Collection Date	Farm Location	Age at Sampling	Vaccination Protocol	Mortality *	IBDV Result
H792	February 2023	Cairo	19 d	1 d: vector vaccine	11.2	A2dB1b
H793	March 2023	Giza	21 d	1 d: vector vaccine; 14 d: live vaccine	9.7	A2dB1b
H794	April 2023	Alexandria	23 d	1 d: vector vaccine	13	Negative
H795	August 2022	Damietta	21 d	1d: vector vaccine; 12 d: live vaccine	13	Negative
H796	June 2022	Beheira	25 d	1 d: vector vaccine; 14 d: live vaccine	10.5	Negative
H797	January 2023	Cairo	28 d	14 d: live vaccine; 18 d: live vaccine	12.7	Negative
H798	July 2023	Sharqia	22 d	1 d: vector vaccine; 14 d: live vaccine	9.6	A2dB1b
H799	December 2022	Giza	30 d	12 d: live vaccine; 18 d: live vaccine	22.7	Negative
H800	April 2022	Beheira	24 d	1 d: vector vaccine; 12 d: live vaccine	17	A3B2
H801	August 2023	Asyut	18 d	12 d: live vaccine	9.8	A2dB1b
H802	February 2023	Dakahlia	22 d	1 d: vector vaccine	11.6	Negative
H803	March 2023	Sharqia	25 d	1 d: immune complex vaccine	8	Negative
H804	March 2023	Sharqia	22 d	1 d: immune complex vaccine	12.4	Negative
H805	February 2022	Monufia	26 d	12 d: live vaccine; 18 d: live vaccine	13.8	A3B2
H806	February 2022	Dakahlia	26 d	1 d: vector vaccine	13.9	Negative
H807	September 2023	Minya	21 d	1 d: vector vaccine; 14 d: live vaccine	9	Negative
H809	July 2022	Alexandria	20 d	12 d: live vaccine; 20 d: live vaccine	8	Negative
H810	June 2023	Giza	27 d	1 d: immune complex vaccine	16	Negative
H811	April 2022	Giza	24 d	1 d: immune complex vaccine	11.5	Negative
H812	August 2023	Beheira	19 d	1 d: vector vaccine; 12 d: live vaccine	8.7	A2dB1b
H813	February 2022	Ismailia	24 d	1 d: vector vaccine; 12 d: live vaccine	14	Negative
H814	April 2023	Ismailia	20 d	1 d: vector vaccine; 12 d: live vaccine	10.7	Negative
H815	June 2022	Port Said	23 d	1 d: vector vaccine	11	Negative

* Cumulative mortality observed from the start of the productive cycle to the sampling date.

Five of the obtained VP2 sequences showed a reciprocal genetic identity ranging from 99.5 to 100% and belonged to genogroup A2 lineage d (novel variant). The remaining two VP2 sequences were identical to each other and fell within genogroup A3 (very virulent) (Figure 1).

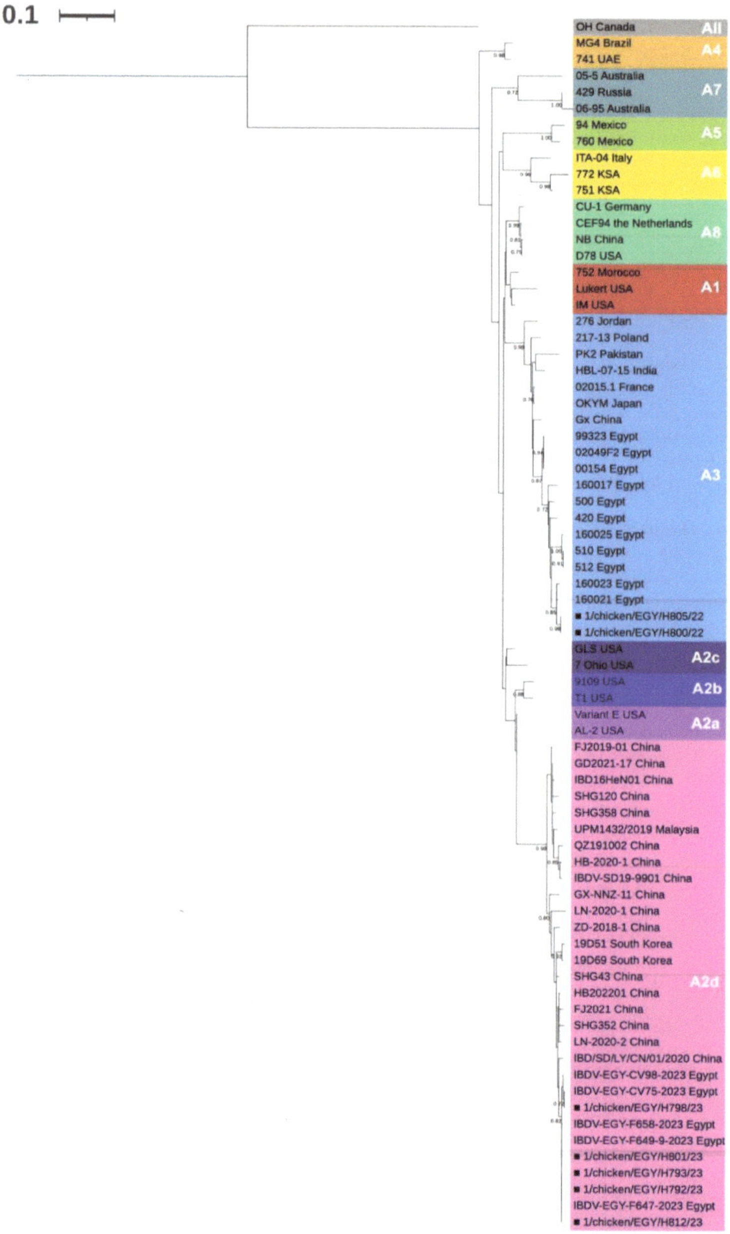

Figure 1. Classification of the detected field strains (marked with solid squares, ■) at VP2 level according to Wang et al. [19]. The evolutionary history was inferred with the Maximum Likelihood Method (1000 bootstraps) applying the K2 + G substitution model [40], based on 74 sequences and considering a 473 nt long portion. Node support values are shown only when higher than 70.

The detection of two separate strain clusters was confirmed also at the VP1 level. The five A2d strains had a 99.6–100% reciprocal genetic identity and belonged to VP1 genogroup B1 lineage b (novel variant), whereas the two A3 ones showed a 99.9% identity and were part of genogroup B2 (very virulent) (Figure 2). The two identified genotypes, both having a field origin, were thus A2dB1b and A3B2. In both cases, the most closely related sequences retrieved from GenBank belonged to recent Egyptian isolates. VP1 and VP2 sequences were submitted to GenBank under the accession numbers OR791866-OR791872 and OR79183-OR791879, respectively.

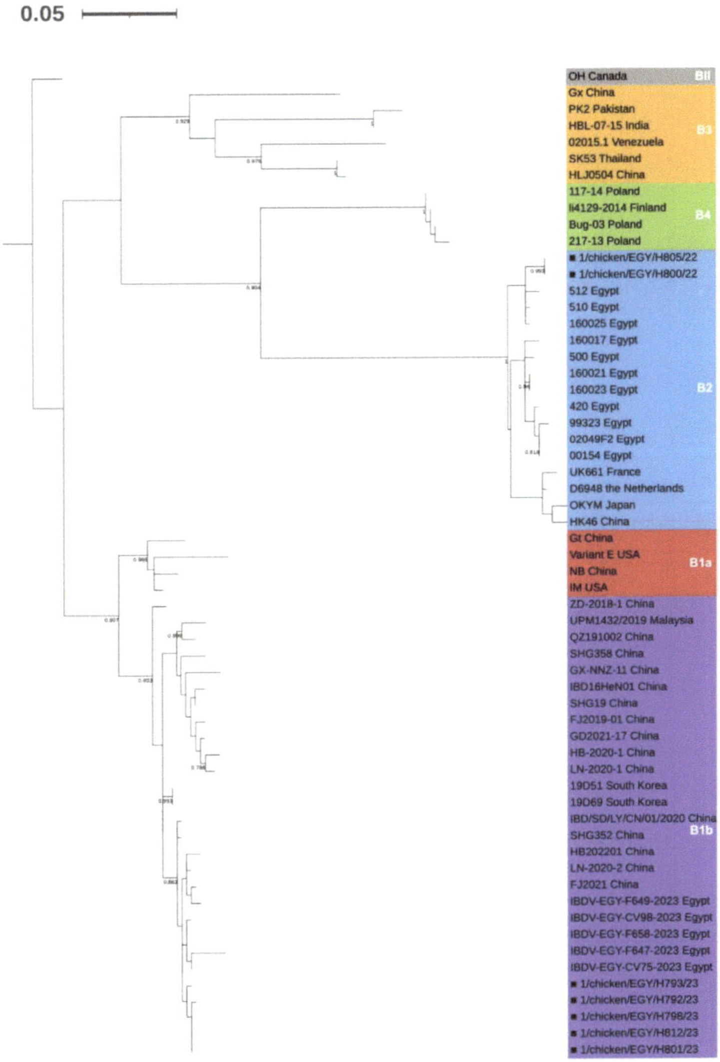

Figure 2. Classification of the detected field strains (marked with solid squares, ■) at VP1 level according to Wang et al. [19]. The evolutionary history was inferred with the Maximum Likelihood Method (1000 bootstraps) applying the K2 + G + I substitution model [40], based on 60 sequences and considering a 428 nt long portion. Node support values are shown only when higher than 70.

Positive samples were collected from farms located in six different governorates, namely Asyut, Beheira, Cairo, Giza, Monufia and Sharqia. No IBDV was detected in the remaining six governorates (Alexandria, Dakahlia, Damietta, Ismailia, Minya and Port Said). The distribution of the two detected genotypes is shown in Figure 3.

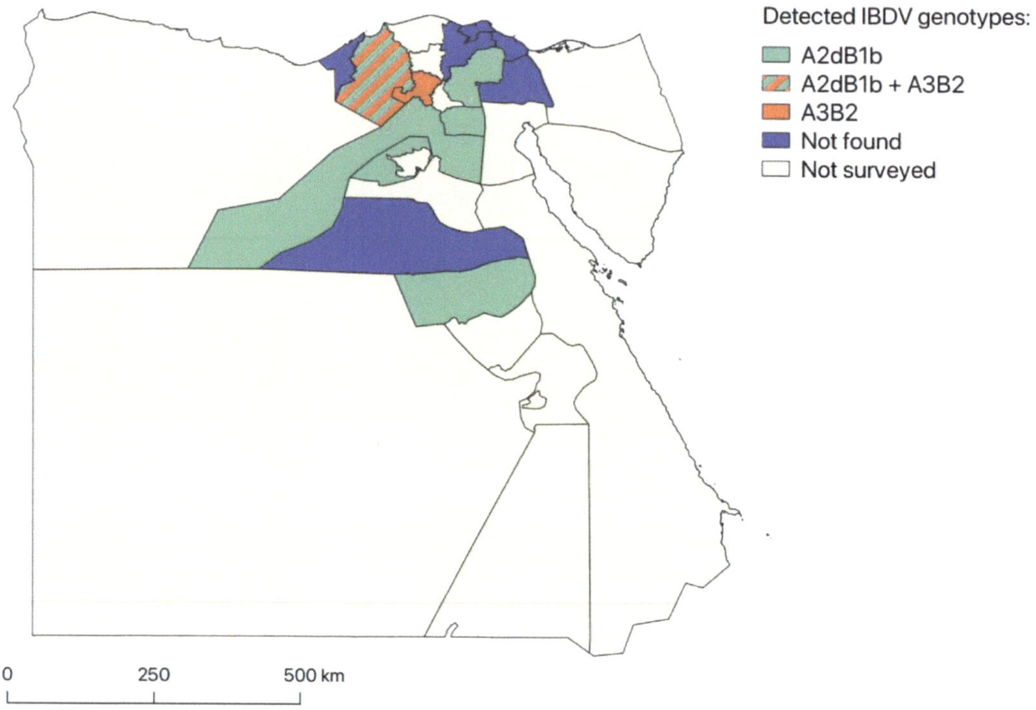

Figure 3. Distribution of IBDV field genotypes at governorate level according to the present molecular survey. The map was prepared using QGIS ver. 3.34 [41] based on a shapefile retrieved from the Dataset of Global Administrative Areas ver. 4.1 (GADM) [42].

The amino acid sequences of the detected A2dB1b strains were compared to those of other novel variant isolates to establish whether any difference was acquired at relevant sites. No consistent amino acid substitutions were unique to Egyptian strains compared to viruses of Asian origin. Nonetheless, multiple changes found in all Egyptian strains, such as A321V at the VP2 level and R511K, S687P and T859I within VP1, had previously only been encountered in a handful of Chinese novel variant IBDVs. Moreover, several substitutions were present only in some of the sequenced strains, both at the VP2 (I15M, S76N, N97K, A277V, G409A) and VP1 level (E393D, T576S, S596F, G630S, Q832R, Q879P) (Supplementary Tables S1 and S2).

4. Discussion

Despite the small scale of the study, the present results offer meaningful insights into the circulation of IBDV in Egypt, which, albeit partly in agreement with the established epidemiological scenario, also suggest that a change of great concern may be occurring.

Two of the seven field IBDVs detected were characterized as A3B2 strains, commonly referred to as very virulent strains. The enduring circulation of very virulent IBDVs in Egypt is well documented [23–25] and is further corroborated by detections in turkeys [43] and in cattle egret (*Bubulcus ibis*) [44], which suggest that interspecies transmission may play a role in their spread and maintenance. The herein described A3B2 viruses clustered with other Egyptian sequences both at the VP2 and VP1 level, thus confirming the persistence of very virulent strains with consistent features at national level. According to Samy et al. [26], very virulent Egyptian IBDVs can further be divided into antigenically typical and atypical strains based on residue 321 within VP2, with the former group featuring an alanine and the latter a threonine. The two detected strains presented an alanine in that position and can be therefore considered as typical very virulent IBDVs. Although this single mutation was shown to induce drastic changes in reactivity towards neutralizing monoclonal antibodies directed against VP2, it seems to have neither positive nor negative effects on viral fitness, as supported by the long-lasting cocirculation of these two very virulent subtypes in the country [26].

The detection of five novel variant strains, on the other hand, represents an unexpected and alarming finding. These strains have been reported since 2015 in China, where they caused a large-scale epidemic of subclinical IBD [45]. According to phylogenetic analyses, novel variants are related to North American variant IBDVs (genotype A2B1), but also sufficiently divergent to be considered as part of segregated lineage A2d [19]. Similarly, novel variant IBDVs cluster separately from other exponents of genogroup B1, leading to the definition of lineage B1b [35]. Their emergence seems to have been caused by a spread of variant IBDVs from North America to China during the 1990s, followed by a period of latent circulation until A2dB1b broke out in the 2010s [36]. A2dB1b strains were also involved in a reassortment event with an A3B3 IBDV of Chinese origin, originating a novel genotype (A2dB3) showing enhanced pathogenicity [46].

Despite their recent identification, novel variant IBDVs rapidly became one of the dominant IBDV types in Eastern and Southern Asia. Outside of China, they were also found in Malaysia [47], South Korea [48,49] and likely in Japan [50], although the unavailability of Japanese VP1 sequences does not allow to confirm this claim. The spread of novel variant IBDVs to these countries seems to have been favored by strong trade flows of live chickens and poultry products [36], but their entry into Egypt appears more difficult to explain. Interestingly, when the diagnostic activities on which this study is based were originally conducted, all the available A2dB1b sequences with a high genetic identity to the herein described strains were of Chinese origin. However, when the same BLAST query was later repeated, a group of highly homologous Egyptian sequences, which were also collected in 2022 and 2023 based on their metadata, were also retrieved. This information clearly substantiates the present results, suggesting that novel variant strains might be affirming themselves as a significant epidemiological threat in Egypt despite an apparently recent entry in the country.

The comparison of amino acid sequences did not highlight any unique substitution in the Egyptian strains. Nonetheless, some of the observed changes were only present in a minority of Asian novel variant IBDVs. Like in the case of Egyptian A3B2 strains, the most notable mutation involved residue 321 of the VP2, located in the P^{HI} loop and supposedly involved in antigenicity determination [20,26]. The A321V substitution observed in most Egyptian novel variant IBDVs was found only in Chinese strain IBD/SD/LY/CN/01/2020, whereas other novel variant viruses showed an A321T change, corroborating previous reports that this site may be prone to mutations [17]. At the VP1 level, Egyptian novel variant IBDVs showed three consistent substitutions compared to most A2dB1b strains, namely R511K, S687P and T859I. Among these, residue 687 has been proposed to play a role in the increased pathogenicity of very virulent IBDVs, which feature a proline, compared to less virulent strains, mostly featuring a serine [51]. In future studies, it will be important to monitor the evolution of Egyptian novel variant IBDVs to determine if these changes will become a permanent feature and if others will emerge as a possible consequence to the adaptation to a new epidemiological context.

Currently, novel variant strains do not seem to be circulating in countries neighboring Egypt. A recent epidemiological survey conducted in the Near and Middle East highlighted the circulation of A3B1, A3B2, A4B1 and A6B1 IBDVs [52], whereas the most recent studies conducted in Northeast Africa suggest that very virulent IBDVs still represent the main threat in the area [53,54]. Nonetheless, further monitoring activities, to be conducted not only in Egypt but also in countries where A2dB1b strains may be circulating undetected, are required to shed light on their diffusion and to track their potential spread to new territories.

Both A3B2 and A2dB1b were found in multiple governorates in the northern and central part of Egypt. The limited number of samples collected in different governorates meant that usually only one of the two genotypes was detected in each of them, with Beheira being the only exception. However, considering that very virulent IBDVs are widespread in the country and that the investigated governorates were in proximity to each other, it might be assumed that very virulent and variant strains are cocirculating in the same areas. It is also worth noting that field IBDVs have already been detected in all the governorates from which no positive samples were retrieved [24,26,55–58], suggesting that this finding was due to the small sample size rather than the actual absence of field strains in these settings.

Aside from characterizing field strains from a molecular perspective, it is essential to understand their pathogenic features and ensure that the currently enacted control measures are effective. A wealth of data has been produced in the Egyptian context on the pathogenicity of locally circulating very virulent IBDVs, which consistently cause typical IBD signs and lesions with high mortality rates [59–61], and on the protection induced by different live [61], vector [62,63] and immune complex [64] vaccines, which appears adequate. Novel variant IBDVs, on the other hand, are associated with subclinical infections with severe bursal atrophy and lymphocyte depletion [16,46,65,66]. Infections sustained by these strains may therefore be easily overlooked, favoring their spread and circulation. Another factor that likely played a role in their evolutionary success is their divergent antigenic features, which may thwart control measures. As a matter of fact, the effectiveness of currently marketed vaccines against them has been put into question [67,68]. This prompted the development of multiple vaccine candidates based on different technologies, including reassortment [67] and virus-like particle vaccines [69–71], which yielded promising results in terms of efficacy and safety but are not yet commercially available.

In partial contrast with the literature, the anamnestic information retrieved during sampling activities suggests that both very virulent and novel variant IBDVs were responsible for severe mortality. This finding might be explained by the immunosuppressive potential of A2dB1b strains, which may have favored secondary infections and reduced the efficacy of vaccination against relevant diseases affecting the Egyptian poultry sector, including avian influenza and Newcastle disease [72]. Nonetheless, it should be noted that equally high or even higher mortality rates were also encountered in IBDV-negative flocks, and that no other possible cause (neither primary nor secondary) was investigated, limiting such conclusions. Since the present research was not originally designed with this aim, additional studies, which should include viral isolation and standardized experimental infections, are therefore required to properly evaluate the pathogenic features of Egyptian novel variant strains.

The complete absence of IBDV vaccine detections represents another noteworthy finding. Detecting the administered vaccine strains is commonly considered a useful proxy for vaccine take and coverage, particularly in the case of vaccines relying on bursal colonization (i.e., live and immune complex vaccines) and to a lesser extent for vector vaccines expressing VP2 inserts, which can still be found in the bursa, although it is not their primary replication site [73]. Even if the early sampling age likely hampered vaccine detection in some cases, especially when live vaccines were used, the absence of vaccine-positive flocks suggests that the conferred protection might have been subpar, and that administration errors at hatchery or farm level cannot be excluded. On this note, many of the sampled farms were anecdotally reported to have a multi-age organization and to suffer from managerial and hygiene deficiencies, thus complicating vaccine administration and increasing the risk of exposure to field IBDVs. Regardless of the circulating field genotypes and used vaccine types, the optimization of vaccination quality and its continuous assessment should represent a priority not only to protect the immunized flock against clinical signs, but also to reduce the circulation and persistence of field viruses in the long term, eventually favoring the entire epidemiological scenario rather than just the single immunized flock.

5. Conclusions

The present study provides a crucial update on the IBDV epidemiological situation in Egypt, capturing the entry of novel variant strains in the country in a timely manner. Compared to the historically circulating very virulent IBDVs, which were still detected, such viruses, reported for the first time outside of Asia, pose an entirely different challenge both in terms of clinical manifestation, as they are mostly subclinical and thus easily overlooked despite still causing relevant losses, and required control measures, as the protection conferred by the currently marketed vaccines is likely limited by their antigenic divergence. Albeit relevant, the identification and molecular characterization of genotype A2dB1b should be intended as just the first step of a larger-scoped investigation. Its spread to Egypt could lead to its establishment as a substantial epidemiological threat in the country and neighboring regions, requiring appropriate studies to track its propagation and evolution, establish its pathogenicity and ultimately assess its impact in a different epidemiological context from the one where it originated.

Supplementary Materials: The following supporting information can be downloaded at: https://www.mdpi.com/article/10.3390/v15122388/s1, Table S1: Comparison of VP2 amino acid sequences of A2dB1b strains; Table S2: Comparison of VP1 amino acid sequences of A2dB1b strains.

Author Contributions: Conceptualization, M.L., K.S. and H.S.; formal analysis, M.L. and G.F.; investigation, M.L., F.P., S.T., M.K.M. and C.M.T.; resources, G.F.; data curation, M.L. and K.S.; writing—original draft preparation, M.L.; writing—review and editing, M.L., K.S., C.M.T., G.F., M.C. and H.S.; supervision, M.C. and H.S.; funding acquisition, M.C. All authors have read and agreed to the published version of the manuscript.

Funding: This research was supported by EU funding within the NextGeneration EU-MUR PNRR Extended Partnership initiative on Emerging Infectious Diseases (Project no. PE00000007, INF-ACT); and by the University of Padova under Grant BIRD239038/2023.

Institutional Review Board Statement: Ethical review and approval were waived for this study as the considered samples were collected within the context of routine diagnostic activities and not for experimental purposes.

Informed Consent Statement: Not applicable.

Data Availability Statement: Data are contained within the article and Supplementary Materials.

Conflicts of Interest: The authors declare no conflict of interest.

References

1. Eterradossi, N.; Saif, Y.M. Infectious bursal disease. In *Diseases of Poultry*, 14th ed.; Swayne, D.E., Boulianne, M., Logue, C.M., McDougald, L.R., Nair, V., Suarez, D.L., Eds.; Wiley-Blackwell: Hoboken, NJ, USA, 2020; Volume 1, pp. 257–283.
2. Alkie, T.N.; Rautenschlein, S. Infectious bursal disease virus in poultry: Current status and future prospects. *Vet. Med.* **2016**, *19*, 9–18.
3. Maraver, A.; Ona, A.; Abaitua, F.; Gonzalez, D.; Clemente, R.; Ruiz-Diaz, J.A.; Caston, J.R.; Pazos, F.; Rodriguez, J.F. The oligomerization domain of VP3, the scaffolding protein of infectious bursal disease virus, plays a critical role in capsid assembly. *J. Virol.* **2003**, *77*, 6438–6449. [CrossRef] [PubMed]
4. Pikuła, A.; Lisowska, A.; Jasik, A.; Perez, L.J. The Novel Genetic Background of Infectious Bursal Disease Virus Strains Emerging from the Action of Positive Selection. *Viruses* **2021**, *13*, 396. [CrossRef] [PubMed]
5. Cosgrove, A.S. An apparently new disease of chickens: Avian nephrosis. *Avian Dis.* **1962**, *6*, 385–389. [CrossRef]
6. Lasher, H.; Davis, V. History of infectious bursal disease in the U.S.A.: The first two decades. *Avian Dis.* **1997**, *41*, 11–19. [CrossRef] [PubMed]
7. Zhang, W.; Wang, X.; Gao, Y.; Qi, X. The Over-40-years-epidemic of infectious bursal disease virus in China. *Viruses* **2022**, *14*, 2253. [CrossRef] [PubMed]
8. Sapats, S.I.; Ignjatovic, J. Antigenic and sequence heterogeneity of infectious bursal disease virus strains isolated in Australia. *Arch. Virol.* **2000**, *145*, 773–785. [CrossRef] [PubMed]
9. Jackwood, D.J. Molecular epidemiologic evidence of homologous recombination in infectious bursal disease viruses. *Avian Dis.* **2012**, *56*, 574–577. [CrossRef]

10. Hernández, M.; Tomás, G.; Marandino, A.; Iraola, G.; Maya, L.; Mattion, N.; Hernández, D.; Villegas, P.; Banda, A.; Panzera, Y.; et al. Genetic characterization of South American infectious bursal disease virus reveals the existence of a distinct worldwide-spread genetic lineage. *Avian Pathol.* **2015**, *44*, 212–221. [CrossRef]
11. Lupini, C.; Giovanardi, D.; Pesente, P.; Bonci, M.; Felice, V.; Rossi, G.; Morandini, E.; Cecchinato, M.; Catelli, E. A molecular epidemiology study based on VP2 gene sequences reveals that a new genotype of infectious bursal disease virus is dominantly prevalent in Italy. *Avian Pathol.* **2016**, *45*, 458–464. [CrossRef]
12. Legnardi, M.; Franzo, G.; Tucciarone, C.M.; Koutoulis, K.; Duarte, I.; Silva, M.; Le Tallec, B.; Cecchinato, M. Detection and molecular characterization of a new genotype of infectious bursal disease virus in Portugal. *Avian Pathol.* **2022**, *51*, 97–105. [CrossRef] [PubMed]
13. Abed, M.; Soubies, S.; Courtillon, C.; Briand, F.X.; Allée, C.; Amelot, M.; De Boisseson, C.; Lucas, P.; Blanchard, Y.; Belahouel, A.; et al. Infectious bursal disease virus in Algeria: Detection of highly pathogenic reassortant viruses. *Infect. Genet. Evol.* **2018**, *60*, 48–57. [CrossRef] [PubMed]
14. Pikuła, A.; Lisowska, A.; Jasik, A.; Śmietanka, K. Identification and assessment of virulence of a natural reassortant of infectious bursal disease virus. *Vet. Res.* **2018**, *49*, 89. [CrossRef] [PubMed]
15. Mató, T.; Tatár-Kis, T.; Felföldi, B.; Jansson, D.S.; Homonnay, Z.; Bányai, K.; Palya, V. Occurrence and spread of a reassortant very virulent genotype of infectious bursal disease virus with altered VP2 amino acid profile and pathogenicity in some European countries. *Vet. Microbiol.* **2020**, *245*, 108663. [CrossRef] [PubMed]
16. Wang, Y.; Jiang, N.; Fan, L.; Niu, X.; Zhang, W.; Huang, M.; Gao, L.; Li, K.; Gao, Y.; Liu, C.; et al. Identification and Pathogenicity Evaluation of a Novel Reassortant Infectious Bursal Disease Virus (Genotype A2dB3). *Viruses* **2021**, *13*, 1682. [CrossRef]
17. Michel, L.O.; Jackwood, D.J. Classification of infectious bursal disease virus into genogroups. *Arch. Virol.* **2017**, *162*, 3661–3670. [CrossRef] [PubMed]
18. Islam, M.R.; Nooruzzaman, M.; Rahman, T.; Mumu, T.T.; Rahman, M.M.; Chowdhury, E.H.; Eterradossi, N.; Müller, H. A unified genotypic classification of infectious bursal disease virus based on both genome segments. *Avian Pathol.* **2021**, *50*, 190–206. [CrossRef]
19. Wang, Y.L.; Fan, L.J.; Jiang, N.; Li, G.A.O.; Kai, L.I.; Gao, Y.L.; Liu, C.J.; Cui, H.Y.; Pan, Q.; Zhang, Y.P.; et al. An improved scheme for infectious bursal disease virus genotype classification based on both genome-segments A and B. *J. Integr. Agric.* **2021**, *20*, 1372–1381. [CrossRef]
20. Letzel, T.; Coulibaly, F.; Rey, F.A.; Delmas, B.; Jagt, E.; Van Loon, A.A.; Mundt, E. Molecular and structural bases for the antigenicity of VP2 of infectious bursal disease virus. *J. Virol.* **2007**, *81*, 12827–12835. [CrossRef]
21. Escaffre, O.; Le Nouën, C.; Amelot, M.; Ambroggio, X.; Ogden, K.M.; Guionie, O.; Toquin, D.; Müller, H.; Islam, M.R.; Eterradossi, N. Both genome segments contribute to the pathogenicity of very virulent infectious bursal disease virus. *J. Virol.* **2013**, *87*, 2767–2780. [CrossRef]
22. He, X.; Chen, G.; Yang, L.; Xuan, J.; Long, H.; Wei, P. Role of naturally occurring genome segment reassortment in the pathogenicity of IBDV field isolates in Three-Yellow chickens. *Avian Pathol.* **2016**, *45*, 178–186. [CrossRef] [PubMed]
23. El-Batrawy, A. Studies on Severe Outbreaks of Infectious Bursal Disease. In Proceedings of the 2nd Scientific Conference of the Egyptian Veterinary Poultry Association, Cairo, Egypt, 12–14 March 1990.
24. Mawgod, S.A.; Arafa, A.S.; Hussein, H.A. Molecular genotyping of the infectious bursal disease virus (IBDV) isolated from broiler flocks in Egypt. *Int. J. Vet. Sci. Med.* **2014**, *2*, 46–52. [CrossRef]
25. Shehata, A.A.; Sultan, H.; Halami, M.Y.; Talaat, S.; Vahlenkamp, T.W. Molecular characterization of very virulent infectious bursal disease virus strains circulating in Egypt from 2003 to 2014. *Arch. Virol.* **2017**, *162*, 3803–3815. [CrossRef] [PubMed]
26. Samy, A.; Courtillon, C.; Briand, F.X.; Khalifa, M.; Selim, A.; Hegazy, A.; Eterradossi, N.; Soubies, S.M. Continuous circulation of an antigenically modified very virulent infectious bursal disease virus for fifteen years in Egypt. *Infect. Genet. Evol.* **2020**, *78*, 104099. [CrossRef]
27. Jackwood, D.J.; Sommer-Wagner, S.E. Molecular Epidemiology of Infectious Bursal Disease Viruses: Distribution and Genetic Analysis of Newly Emerging Viruses in the United States. *Avian Dis.* **2005**, *49*, 220–226. [CrossRef] [PubMed]
28. Lachheb, J.; Jbenyeni, A.; Nsiri, J.; Larbi, I.; Ammouna, F.; Ghram, A. Full-length genome sequencing of a very virulent infectious bursal disease virus isolated in Tunisia. *Poult. Sci.* **2021**, *100*, 496–506. [CrossRef]
29. Hernández, M.; Villegas, P.; Hernández, D.; Banda, A.; Maya, L.; Romero, V.; Tomás, G.; Pérez, R. Sequence variability and evolution of the terminal overlapping VP5 gene of the infectious bursal disease virus. *Virus Genes* **2010**, *41*, 59–66. [CrossRef]
30. Rudd, M.F.; Heine, H.G.; Sapats, S.I.; Parede, L.; Ignjatovic, J. Characterisation of an Indonesian very virulent strain of infectious bursal disease virus. *Arch. Virol.* **2002**, *147*, 1303–1322. [CrossRef]
31. Islam, M.R.; Rahman, S.; Noor, M.; Chowdhury, E.H.; Müller, H. Differentiation of infectious bursal disease virus (IBDV) genome segment B of very virulent and classical lineage by RT-PCR amplification and restriction enzyme analysis. *Arch. Virol.* **2011**, *157*, 333–336. [CrossRef]
32. He, X.; Xiong, Z.; Yang, L.; Guan, D.; Yang, X.; Wei, P. Molecular epidemiology studies on partial sequences of both genome segments reveal that reassortant infectious bursal disease viruses were dominantly prevalent in southern China during 2000–2012. *Arch. Virol.* **2014**, *159*, 3279–3292. [CrossRef]
33. Tiwari, A.K.; Kataria, R.S.; Prasad, N.; Gupta, R. Differentiation of infectious bursal disease viruses by restriction enzyme analysis of RT-PCR amplified VP1 gene sequence. *Comp. Immunol. Microbiol. Infect. Dis.* **2003**, *26*, 47–53. [CrossRef] [PubMed]

34. Mundt, E.; Vakharia, V.N. Synthetic transcripts of double-stranded Birnavirus genome are infectious. *Proc. Natl. Acad. Sci. USA* **1996**, *93*, 11131–11136. [CrossRef] [PubMed]
35. Alfonso-Morales, A.; Rios, L.; Martínez-Pérez, O.; Dolz, R.; Valle, R.; Perera, C.L.; Bertran, K.; Frias, M.T.; Ganges, L.; Diaz de Arce, H.; et al. Evaluation of a phylogenetic marker based on genomic segment B of infectious bursal disease virus: Facilitating a feasible incorporation of this segment to the molecular epidemiology studies for this viral agent. *PLoS ONE* **2015**, *10*, e0125853. [CrossRef] [PubMed]
36. Wang, W.; He, X.; Zhang, Y.; Qiao, Y.; Shi, J.; Chen, R.; Chen, J.; Xiang, Y.; Wang, Z.; Chen, G.; et al. Analysis of the global origin, evolution and transmission dynamics of the emerging novel variant IBDV (A2dB1b): The accumulation of critical aa-residue mutations and commercial trade contributes to the emergence and transmission of novel variants. *Transbound. Emerg. Dis.* **2022**, *69*, e2832–e2851. [CrossRef] [PubMed]
37. Altschul, S.F.; Gish, W.; Miller, W.; Myers, E.W.; Lipman, D.J. Basic local alignment search tool. *J. Mol. Biol.* **1990**, *215*, 403–410. [CrossRef]
38. Kumar, S.; Stecher, G.; Li, M.; Knyaz, C.; Tamura, K. MEGA X: Molecular evolutionary genetics analysis across computing platforms. *Mol. Biol. Evol.* **2018**, *35*, 1547–1549. [CrossRef] [PubMed]
39. Letunic, I.; Bork, P. Interactive Tree Of Life (iTOL) v5: An online tool for phylogenetic tree display and annotation. *Nucleic Acids Res.* **2021**, *49*, W293–W296. [CrossRef] [PubMed]
40. Kimura, M. A simple method for estimating evolutionary rates of base substitutions through comparative studies of nucleotide sequences. *J. Mol. Evol.* **1980**, *16*, 111–120. [CrossRef]
41. QGIS. Available online: https://www.qgis.org/ (accessed on 11 November 2023).
42. Database of Global Administrative Areas (GADM). Available online: https://gadm.org/ (accessed on 11 November 2023).
43. Mosad, S.M.; Eladl, A.H.; El-Tholoth, M.; Ali, H.S.; Hamed, M.F. Molecular characterization and pathogenicity of very virulent infectious bursal disease virus isolated from naturally infected Turkey poults in Egypt. *Trop. Anim. Health Prod.* **2020**, *52*, 3819–3831. [CrossRef]
44. El Naggar, R.F.; Rohaim, M.A.; Munir, M. Potential reverse spillover of infectious bursal disease virus at the interface of commercial poultry and wild birds. *Virus Genes* **2020**, *56*, 705–711. [CrossRef]
45. Fan, L.; Wu, T.; Hussain, A.; Gao, Y.; Zeng, X.; Wang, Y.; Gao, L.; Li, K.; Wang, Y.; Liu, C.; et al. Novel variant strains of infectious bursal disease virus isolated in China. *Vet. Microbiol.* **2019**, *230*, 212–220. [CrossRef]
46. Wang, W.; Huang, Y.; Zhang, Y.; Qiao, Y.; Deng, Q.; Chen, R.; Chen, J.; Huang, T.; Wei, T.; Mo, M.; et al. The emerging naturally reassortant strain of IBDV (genotype A2dB3) having segment A from Chinese novel variant strain and segment B from HLJ 0504-like very virulent strain showed enhanced pathogenicity to three-yellow chickens. *Transbound. Emerg. Dis.* **2022**, *69*, e566–e579. [CrossRef] [PubMed]
47. Aliyu, H.B.; Hair-Bejo, M.; Omar, A.R.; Ideris, A. Genetic diversity of recent infectious bursal disease viruses isolated from vaccinated poultry flocks in Malaysia. *Front. Vet. Sci.* **2021**, *8*, 643976. [CrossRef]
48. Thai, T.N.; Jang, I.; Kim, H.A.; Kim, H.S.; Kwon, Y.K.; Kim, H.R. Characterization of antigenic variant infectious bursal disease virus strains identified in South Korea. *Avian Pathol.* **2021**, *50*, 174–181. [CrossRef] [PubMed]
49. Thai, T.N.; Yoo, D.S.; Jang, I.; Kwon, Y.K.; Kim, H.R. Dynamics of the Emerging Genogroup of Infectious Bursal Disease Virus Infection in Broiler Farms in South Korea: A Nationwide Study. *Viruses* **2022**, *14*, 1604. [CrossRef]
50. Myint, O.; Suwanruengsri, M.; Araki, K.; Izzati, U.Z.; Pornthummawat, A.; Nueangphuet, P.; Fuke, N.; Hirai, T.; Jackwood, D.J.; Yamaguchi, R. Bursa atrophy at 28 days old caused by variant infectious bursal disease virus has a negative economic impact on broiler farms in Japan. *Avian Pathol.* **2021**, *50*, 6–17. [CrossRef] [PubMed]
51. Ren, X.; Xue, C.; Zhang, Y.; Chen, F.; Cao, Y. Genomic analysis of one Chinese strain YS07 of infectious bursal disease virus reveals unique genetic diversity. *Virus Genes* **2009**, *39*, 246–248. [CrossRef] [PubMed]
52. Legnardi, M.; Poletto, F.; Alam, S.; Cherfane, A.; Le-Tallec, B.; Franzo, G.; Tucciarone, C.M.; Lupini, C.; Pasotto, D.; Cecchinato, M. Molecular epidemiology of infectious bursal disease virus in the Near East and Persian Gulf regions. *Avian Pathol.* **2023**. *just-accepted*. [CrossRef]
53. Shegu, D.; Sori, T.; Tesfaye, A.; Belay, A.; Mohammed, H.; Degefa, T.; Getachew, B.; Abayneh, T.; Gelaye, E. Sequence-based comparison of field and vaccine strains of infectious bursal disease virus in Ethiopia reveals an amino acid mismatch in the immunodominant VP2 protein. *Arch. Virol.* **2020**, *165*, 1367–1375. [CrossRef]
54. Omer, M.G.; Khalafalla, A.I. Epidemiology and laboratory diagnosis of very virulent infectious bursal disease virus in vaccinated chickens in Khartoum, Sudan. *Open Vet. J.* **2022**, *12*, 33–43. [CrossRef]
55. Ramzy, N.; Abdel-fattah, S. Prevalence and molecular characterization of Gumboro virus in chicken farms in Ismailia. *Assiut Vet. Med. J.* **2015**, *61*, 152–159.
56. Omar, S.E.; El Sayed, W.A.E.M.; Abdelhalim, A.; Yehia, N. Genetic evolution of infectious bursal disease virus isolated from chicken poultry flocks in Egypt. *J. World Poult. Res.* **2021**, *11*, 215–222. [CrossRef]
57. Awad, N.; Morsi, H.; Eid, A.A.; Al-baqir, A. Epidemiological Occurrence of the Infectious Bursal Disease Virus in Chickens' Flocks that Had Received Various Vaccination Regimens. *Zagazig Vet. J.* **2023**, *51*, 239–262. [CrossRef]
58. Shahat, D.H. Detection and isolation of a recent infectious bursal disease virus from chicken farms in Egypt during 2021. *Benha Vet. Med. J.* **2023**, *44*, 74–78. [CrossRef]

59. Suliman, R.A.; Ahmed, B.M.; El-Safty, M.M.; Hussien, H.A. Very virulent IBDV strain Egypt/iBDV/Behera/2011: Macroscopic and microscopic lesions accompanied with induced mortalities in SPF chicks. *J. Virol. Sci.* **2017**, *2*, 79–91.
60. Gaber, H.A.H.; El-Dougdoug, K.A.; El-Masry, S.S. Isolation and Pathotyping of Infectious Bursal Disease Virus (IBDV) from Field Outbreaks among Chickens in Egypt. *J. Anim. Poult. Prod.* **2021**, *12*, 95–99. [CrossRef]
61. Hassan, M.K.; Afify, M.; Aly, M.M. Susceptibility of vaccinated and unvaccinated Egyptian chickens to very virulent infectious bursal disease virus. *Avian Pathol.* **2022**, *31*, 149–156. [CrossRef]
62. Sultan, H.; Hussein, H.A.; Abd El-Razik, A.G.; El-Balall, S.; Talaat, S.M.; Shehata, A.A. Efficacy of HVT-IBDV vector vaccine against recent Egyptian vvIBDV in commercial broiler chickens. *Int. J. Poult. Sci.* **2012**, *11*, 710. [CrossRef]
63. Rade, N.; Sultan, H.; El-Razik, A. Efficacy of The Turkey Herpes virus-IBDV Vector Vaccine Against Recent Egyptian Very Virulent IBDV in Commercial Layers. *J. Curr. Vet. Res.* **2020**, *2*, 47–56. [CrossRef]
64. Eliwa, M.G.E.D.; Talaat, S.; Tantawy, L.; El-Razik, A.; Sultan, H. Protective efficacy of IBDV winterfield H-2512 and SYZA-26 immune-complex vaccines against recent Egyptian very virulent IBDV in commercial broiler chickens. *J. Curr. Vet. Res.* **2022**, *4*, 191–200. [CrossRef]
65. Xu, A.; Pei, Y.; Zhang, K.; Xue, J.; Ruan, S.; Zhang, G. Phylogenetic analyses and pathogenicity of a variant infectious bursal disease virus strain isolated in China. *Virus Res.* **2020**, *276*, 197833. [CrossRef] [PubMed]
66. Lian, J.; Wang, Z.; Xu, Z.; Pang, Y.; Leng, M.; Tang, S.; Zhang, X.; Qin, J.; Chen, F.; Lin, W. Pathogenicity and molecular characterization of infectious bursal disease virus in China. *Poult. Sci.* **2022**, *101*, 101502. [CrossRef] [PubMed]
67. Hou, B.; Wang, C.Y.; Luo, Z.B.; Shao, G.Q. Commercial vaccines used in China do not protect against a novel infectious bursal disease virus variant isolated in Fujian. *Vet. Rec.* **2022**, *191*, e1840. [CrossRef] [PubMed]
68. Fan, L.; Wu, T.; Wang, Y.; Hussain, A.; Jiang, N.; Gao, L.; Li, K.; Gao, Y.; Liu, C.; Cui, H.; et al. Novel variants of infectious bursal disease virus can severely damage the bursa of fabricius of immunized chickens. *Vet. Microbiol.* **2020**, *240*, 108507. [CrossRef] [PubMed]
69. Fan, L.; Wang, Y.; Jiang, N.; Gao, L.; Li, K.; Gao, Y.; Cui, H.; Pan, Q.; Liu, C.; Zhang, Y.; et al. A reassortment vaccine candidate of the novel variant infectious bursal disease virus. *Vet. Microbiol.* **2020**, *251*, 108905. [CrossRef] [PubMed]
70. Li, G.; Kuang, H.; Guo, H.; Cai, L.; Chu, D.; Wang, X.; Hu, J.; Rong, J. Development of a recombinant VP2 vaccine for the prevention of novel variant strains of infectious bursal disease virus. *Avian Pathol.* **2020**, *49*, 557–571. [CrossRef] [PubMed]
71. Wang, Y.; Jiang, N.; Fan, L.; Gao, L.; Li, K.; Gao, Y.; Niu, X.; Zhang, W.; Cui, H.; Liu, A.; et al. Development of a Viral-Like Particle Candidate Vaccine Against Novel Variant Infectious Bursal Disease Virus. *Vaccines* **2021**, *9*, 142. [CrossRef]
72. El-Aried, T.A.; Mansour, S.M.; El Bakrey, R.M.; Ismail, A.E.N.; Eid, A.A. Infectious bursal disease virus: Molecular epidemiologic perspectives and impact on vaccine efficacy against avian influenza and Newcastle disease viruses. *Avian Dis.* **2019**, *63*, 606–618. [CrossRef]
73. Ramon, G.; Legnardi, M.; Cecchinato, M.; Cazaban, C.; Tucciarone, C.M.; Fiorentini, L.; Gambi, L.; Mato, T.; Berto, G.; Koutoulis, K.; et al. Efficacy of live attenuated, vector and immune complex infectious bursal disease virus (IBDV) vaccines in preventing field strain bursa colonization: A European multicentric study. *Front. Vet. Sci.* **2022**, *12*, 978901. [CrossRef]

viruses MDPI

Article

Transcriptomic and Translatomic Analyses Reveal Insights into the Signaling Pathways of the Innate Immune Response in the Spleens of SPF Chickens Infected with Avian Reovirus

Sheng Wang [1,2,†], Tengda Huang [3,†], Zhixun Xie [1,2,*], Lijun Wan [1,2], Hongyu Ren [1,2], Tian Wu [4], Liji Xie [1,2], Sisi Luo [1,2], Meng Li [1,2], Zhiqin Xie [1,2], Qing Fan [1,2], Jiaoling Huang [1,2], Tingting Zeng [1,2], Yanfang Zhang [1,2], Minxiu Zhang [1,2] and You Wei [1,2]

1 Guangxi Key Laboratory of Veterinary Biotechnology, Guangxi Veterinary Research Institute, Nanning 530000, China; wangsheng1021@126.com (S.W.); wanlijun0529@163.com (L.W.); renhongyu328@126.com (H.R.); xie3120371@163.com (L.X.); 2004-luosisi@163.com (S.L.); mengli4836@163.com (M.L.); xzqman2002@sina.com (Z.X.); fanqing1224@126.com (Q.F.); huangjiaoling728@126.com (J.H.); tingtingzeng1986@163.com (T.Z.); zhangyanfang409@126.com (Y.Z.); zhminxiu2010@163.com (M.Z.); weiyou0909@163.com (Y.W.)
2 Key Laboratory of China (Guangxi)-ASEAN Cross-Border Animal Disease Prevention and Control, Ministry of Agriculture and Rural Affairs of China, Nanning 530000, China
3 Division of Liver Surgery, Department of General Surgery, Laboratory of Liver Surgery, and State Key Laboratory of Biotherapy, West China Hospital, Sichuan University, Chengdu 610041, China; 2022324065113@stu.scu.edu.cn
4 NHC Key Laboratory of Transplant Engineering and Immunology, Regenerative Medicine Research Center, Frontiers Science Center for Disease-Related Molecular Network, West China Hospital of Sichuan University, Chengdu 610041, China; wutian980518@126.com
* Correspondence: xiezhixun@126.com
† These authors contributed equally to this work.

Citation: Wang, S.; Huang, T.; Xie, Z.; Wan, L.; Ren, H.; Wu, T.; Xie, L.; Luo, S.; Li, M.; Xie, Z.; et al. Transcriptomic and Translatomic Analyses Reveal Insights into the Signaling Pathways of the Innate Immune Response in the Spleens of SPF Chickens Infected with Avian Reovirus. *Viruses* **2023**, *15*, 2346. https://doi.org/10.3390/v15122346

Academic Editor: Chi-Young Wang

Received: 9 November 2023
Revised: 23 November 2023
Accepted: 24 November 2023
Published: 29 November 2023

Abstract: Avian reovirus (ARV) infection is prevalent in farmed poultry and causes viral arthritis and severe immunosuppression. The spleen plays a very important part in protecting hosts against infectious pathogens. In this research, transcriptome and translatome sequencing technology were combined to investigate the mechanisms of transcriptional and translational regulation in the spleen after ARV infection. On a genome-wide scale, ARV infection can significantly reduce the translation efficiency (TE) of splenic genes. Differentially expressed translational efficiency genes (DTEGs) were identified, including 15 upregulated DTEGs and 396 downregulated DTEGs. These DTEGs were mainly enriched in immune regulation signaling pathways, which indicates that ARV infection reduces the innate immune response in the spleen. In addition, combined analyses revealed that the innate immune response involves the effects of transcriptional and translational regulation. Moreover, we discovered the key gene IL4I1, the most significantly upregulated gene at both the transcriptional and translational levels. Further studies in DF1 cells showed that overexpression of IL4I1 could inhibit the replication of ARV, while inhibiting the expression of endogenous IL4I1 with siRNA promoted the replication of ARV. Overexpression of IL4I1 significantly downregulated the mRNA expression of IFN-β, LGP2, TBK1 and NF-κB; however, the expression of these genes was significantly upregulated after inhibition of IL4I1, suggesting that IL4I1 may be a negative feedback effect of innate immune signaling pathways. In addition, there may be an interaction between IL4I1 and ARV σA protein, and we speculate that the IL4I1 protein plays a regulatory role by interacting with the σA protein. This study not only provides a new perspective on the regulatory mechanisms of the innate immune response after ARV infection but also enriches the knowledge of the host defense mechanisms against ARV invasion and the outcome of ARV evasion of the host's innate immune response.

Keywords: translatomics; Ribo-seq; avian reovirus; spleen; innate immunity; IL4I1

1. Introduction

Avian reovirus (ARV) is part of the genus Orthoreovirus in the Spinareoviridae family, and the main symptoms it causes include viral arthritis, chronic respiratory disease, growth retardation and malabsorption syndrome. In addition, ARV infection can cause severe immunosuppression and predispose patients to other complications or secondary infections. ARV infection is widespread in the global poultry industry; vaccination is mainly used to prevent it in the fowl industry, but it is still not well prevented or controlled. ARV infection causes major economic losses for farmers [1–3].

At present, good progress has been made in the research and development of ARV vaccines and the establishment of detection methods, but research on the pathogenic mechanism of ARV and the antiviral response of host innate immunity is still in the development stage. Furthermore, clarifying the interaction mechanism of ARV is necessary for its prevention, control and treatment.

Innate immunity is the body's first line of defense against ARV invasion. The body activates the production of inflammatory factors and interferons by recognizing pathogenic pattern-related molecules through pattern recognition receptors and activates acquired immunity to trigger a comprehensive immune response [4,5]. Many studies have been conducted on the regulation of innate immune-related pattern recognition receptors and their effector factors during ARV infection. In the early period of ARV infection, the PI3K/Akt/NF-κB and STAT3 signaling pathways can be activated to induce an inflammatory response [6,7]. Lostalé-Seijo et al. found that ARV infection of chicken embryonic fibroblasts induced the expression of interferon and interferon-stimulated genes Mx and double-stranded RNA-dependent protein kinases (PKRs) to exert antiviral effects [8].

In the early stage of ARV infection, the virus can induce the activation of MDA5 signaling pathway-related molecules in chicken peripheral blood lymphocytes, thereby inducing the production of inflammatory factors and interferons [9]. In a previous study, we detected the transcriptional expression level changes in interferon and interferon-stimulated genes (Mx, IFITM3, IFI6 and IFIT5) in several different tissues and organs of ARV-infected specific pathogen-free (SPF) chickens using real-time PCR, and the results suggested that ARV infection can cause significant changes in these effector factors, indicating that the process of ARV infection is closely linked to the recognition of host innate immune-related model receptors and the production of effector factors [10,11]. However, the limited number of genes that were tested made it impossible to fully characterize the gene regulation of innate immunity during ARV infection.

Next-generation sequencing technology has become an effective tool for studying the interaction between viruses and hosts. However, due to the poor correlations between mRNA abundance and protein abundance, traditional mRNA sequencing (RNA-seq) cannot accurately depict the whole realm of gene expression, particularly in regards to reflecting the actual expression levels of proteins [12]. Ribosome profiling, also known as ribosomal footprint sequencing (Ribo-seq), is a new high-throughput sequencing technology developed in recent years that sequences ribosome-protected mRNA fragments (RPFs) [13]. Ribo-seq can accurately measure translational activity and abundance genome-wide [14], making it possible to investigate the ribosome density profile of the translatome [15,16]. Association analysis combined with RNA-seq and Ribo-seq methods can be used to study post-transcriptional regulation and translational regulation mechanisms. Ribo-seq has been used to explore the mechanisms of translation regulation in different species, such as humans [17], mice [18], zebrafish [19], Drosophila [20], rice [21], Arabidopsis [22] and maize [23]. However, the translational regulation mechanisms in chickens remain poorly studied.

The spleen is the largest and most important peripheral immune organ in chickens, and it plays a major role in maintaining the balance of immune function and evading the invasion of pathogenic microorganisms. Previous studies have found that ARV infection can cause harm to the spleen, which leads to immunosuppression [24,25]. The results of our previous study showed that the viral load in the spleen after ARV infection was noticeably above those in the thymus and bursa of Fabricius, suggesting that the spleen is the main immune organ attacked by ARV. In addition, the mRNA expression of various interferon-stimulated genes in the spleen after ARV infection was rapidly upregulated in the early stage of infection, indicating that ARV infection can induce a strong innate immune response in the spleen. Analysis of the pathological changes in the spleen after ARV infection showed that there were no obvious lesions on days 1 to 2, while generalized necrotic degeneration of the lymphocytes and homogeneous red staining of the splenic body were observed on day 3. This pathological injury continued until day 7 and was gradually relieved. Interestingly, the ARV viral load in the spleen remained high for 1 to 3 days after infection and then decreased sharply on day 4 [11]. Therefore, it is speculated that the early stage of ARV infection, especially day 3, is a critical period for ARV invasion of the spleen. Transcriptional and translational regulation play major roles in host innate immunity against viral infection. In this research, SPF chickens artificially infected with the ARV S1133 strain were used as subjects. Their splenic tissues were dissected on the third day after infection, and RNA-seq and Ribo-seq analyses were performed to study chicken spleen gene regulation after ARV infection at the transcriptional and translational levels. Finally, functional genes that play an important part in the innate immune response were identified, and their functions were further analyzed. Our results provide a comprehensive understanding of the immune evasion of ARVs in the spleen and of the host immune defense against ARVs.

2. Results

2.1. Overview of High-Throughput Sequencing Data between the Spleens of Control Group and ARV SPF Chickens

To explore genome-wide innate immune response regulation from a translational perspective, we compared the ribosomal maps of the spleens of control group (CON) and ARV SPF chickens using ribosomal footprint sequencing and mRNA sequencing. The Ribo-seq and RNA-seq libraries of the CON and ARV groups were prepared and sequenced on HiSeq-2000 platforms, resulting in 13.1–14.8 million and 16–16.2 million ribosome profiling clean reads for the CON and ARV groups, as well as 17.3–17.8 million and 14.5–16.5 million RNA-seq clean reads for the CON and ARV groups, respectively (Supplemental Table S1). RNA-seq identified and quantified 17,721 genes and 17,693 genes in the CON and ARV groups, respectively (Supplemental Figure S1A,B). Ribo-seq identified and quantified 15,760 genes and 14,776 genes in the CON and ARV groups, respectively (Supplemental Figure S1C,D), and their expression abundance levels all had a similar normal distribution. Supplemental Tables S2 and S3 display the gene expression abundance information of the transcriptome and translatome. The Pearson correlation analysis of RNA-seq and Ribo-seq exhibited similarities and differences between the CON and ARV groups ($R^2 > 0.92$, Supplemental Figure S1E,F). These results indicate that subsequent analyses are performed on the basis of reliable data.

2.2. Global Translatome Characteristics

To investigate whether the characteristics of the ribosome-protected fragments change with innate immune response regulation in the spleen, the basic ribosome profiles of RPFs were compared between the CON and ARV groups. The length distribution of RPF peaks at 28 nt for both the CON and ARV groups (Figure 1A). Figure 1B shows that the distribution patterns of RPFs for the CON and ARV groups were similar, with the vast majority of ribosome footprints located at the CDS of both CON and ARV mRNAs. These results are similar to those in most eukaryotes, suggesting that the translation process is highly conserved [26]. However, compared to the CON group, the RPFs of the ARV group in the CDSs and 5′ UTRs decreased to 3.87% and 3.31%, respectively. The ARV RPFs in 3′ UTRs increased from 8.02% to 15.19%. These results suggest that the apparent activation of RPFs in 3′ UTRs may be caused by ARV infection in chickens. In addition, three-nucleotide periodicity was clearly observed around the start and stop codon regions of RPFs at different read lengths of 28 nt. A vast number of RPFs were enriched in the region approximately from position −12 nt to the annotated start codon (Figure 1C and Supplemental Figure S1G), indicating that the initiation stage is the principal rate-limiting stage of translation.

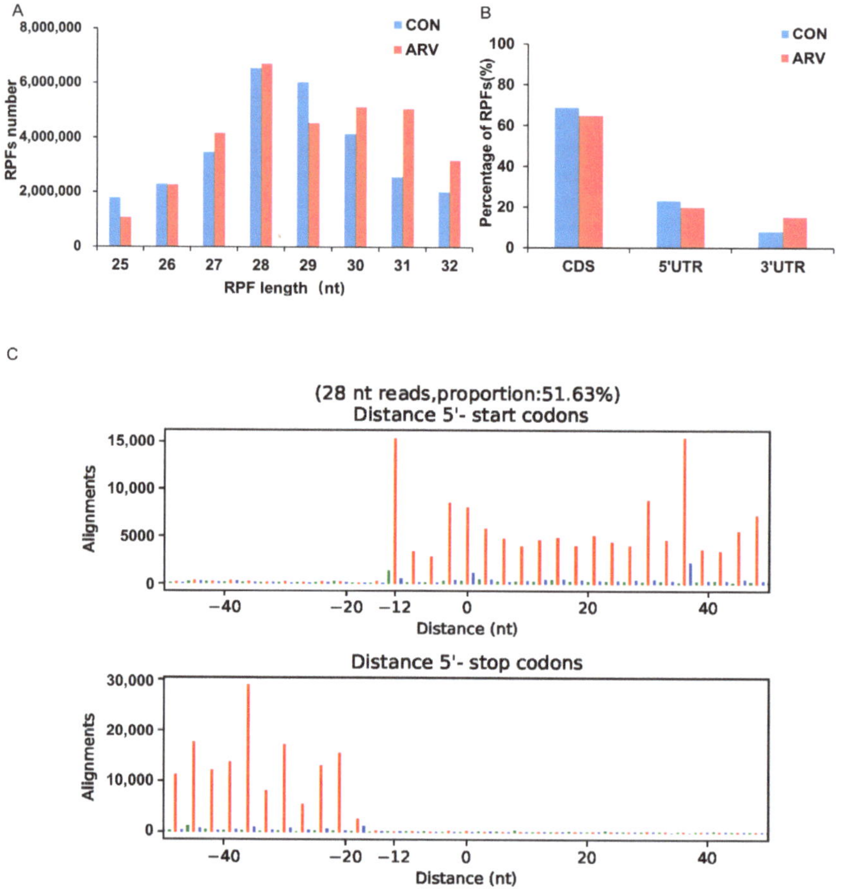

Figure 1. Characteristics of ribosome profiling data in the CON and ARV groups. (**A**) Length distribution of RPFs. (**B**) The percentage of RPFs located in CDS, 5′ UTR and 3′ UTR. (**C**) The total number of RPFs along CDS start and stop codon regions in ARV group. A codon contains three bases, which are represented by red, blue and green.

2.3. Translational Efficiency Significantly Decreased after ARV Infection

TE is an important index of translation that reflects the efficiency of mRNA utilization, and the formula is as follows: TE = (RPKM from translatome)/(FPKM from transcriptome) [14,27]. The average TE of genes across the whole genome decreased significantly after ARV infection (log2 mean TE of CON = −0.09297, log2 mean TE of ARV = −0.6425; Figure 2A). In addition, the ratio of genes with higher TE (log2TE > 1) in the ARV group was lower than that in the CON group (Figure 2B). Moreover, there were 15 upregulated, differentially expressed TE genes and 396 downregulated, differentially expressed TE genes after ARV infection compared to the CON group (Figure 2C). In regard to the functions of the differentially expressed TE genes, GO and KEGG analyses were conducted. The GO analysis displayed the top 20 terms, which mainly included cell activation, regulation of response to stimulus, regulation of immune system process, etc. (Figure 2D). The KEGG pathway enrichment analysis showed the top 20 pathways for which gene expression was enriched. Among the top 20 pathways, 7 pathways belonged to the "immune system" category, including the chemokine signaling pathway, Fc epsilon RI signaling pathway, T-cell receptor signaling pathway, intestinal immune network for IgA production, complement and coagulation cascades, B-cell receptor signaling pathway and hematopoietic cell lineage. The rheumatoid arthritis pathway was also among the top 20 pathways and belonged to the "immune diseases" category (Figure 2E). The above results indicate that after infection with ARV, gene translation efficiency is reduced at the overall level, and the translation efficiency of immune-related genes is significantly affected.

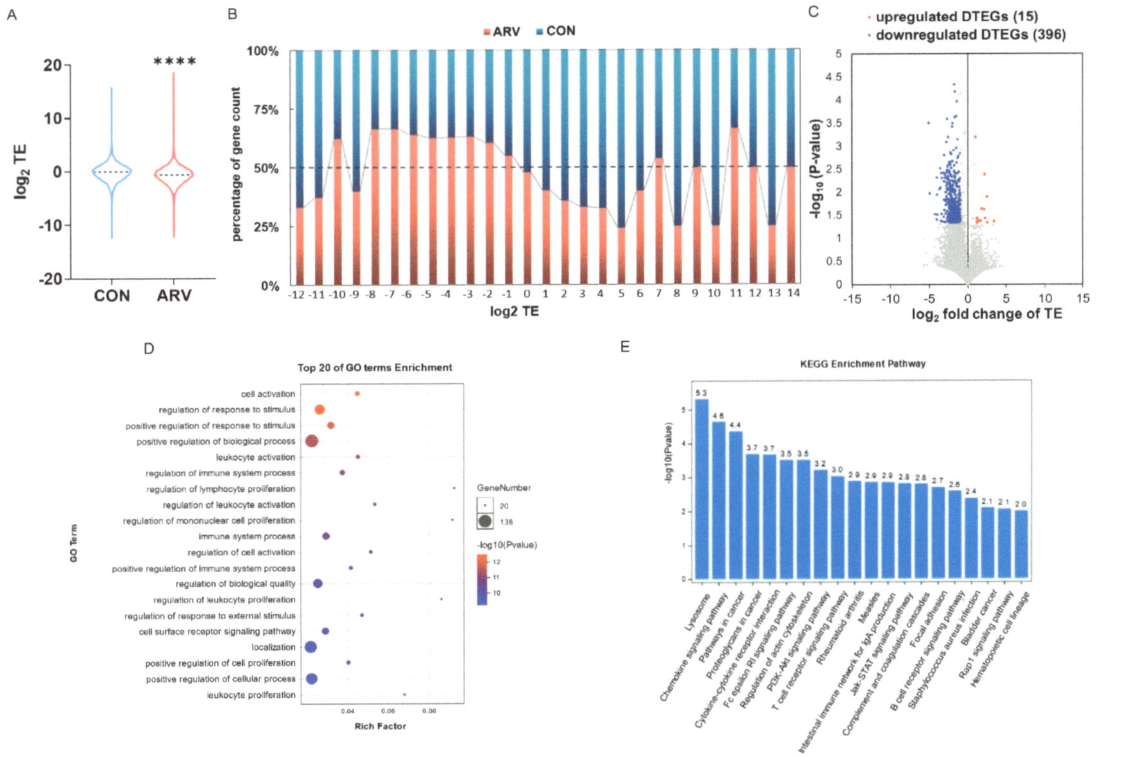

Figure 2. Translation efficiency analysis. (**A**) Violin plot of TE in the CON and ARV groups. Asterisk indicates significant difference (**** $p < 0.0001$). (**B**) Relative TE ratio. Genes were classified based on their rounded $\log_2$ TE values. (**C**) Volcano map of DTEGs. The gray dot represents the non-differentially expressed translation efficiency genes. (**D**) Gene ontology (GO) analysis of DTEGs. (**E**) Kyoto Encyclopedia of Genes and Genomes (KEGG) analysis of DTEGs.

2.4. Regulation Patterns of the Transcriptome and Translatome

Based on both ribosome profiling and RNA sequencing data, the transcriptional and translational expression differences between the CON and ARV groups were examined. The CON and ARV groups had high correlations for transcriptome and translatome ($R^2 = 0.8364$ in RNA-seq, $R^2 = 0.8531$ in Ribo-seq; Supplemental Figure S2A,B), which illustrates that transcriptome analysis and translatome analysis are reliable. The differentially expressed genes in both the RNA-seq and Ribo-seq data sets were filtered based on the criteria of $|\log2 \text{ fold change}| > 1$ and FDR < 0.01. There were 225 transcriptionally upregulated and 439 downregulated DEGs in the ARV group compared to the CON group, corresponding to 851 upregulated and 1128 downregulated DEGs at the translational level (Supplemental Figure S2C,D). The quantities of downregulated genes were much greater than those of the upregulated genes at two levels, suggesting a global decline in gene expression in the ARV group.

To explore the relationships and differences in the regulation of gene expression in the spleen at the transcriptional level and the translation level after ARV infection, we conducted a combined analysis of the transcriptome and the translatome. Figure 3A displays the scatter plot of the fold changes in transcriptional and translational expression. The scatter plot was classified into nine categories based on the criteria of | log2 fold change in RPKM | > 1 and FDR < 0.01. The gene information of the nine categories can be found in Supplemental Table S4. Our results revealed that 81.96% of genes were categorized in the unchanged class (quadrant E), and 14.7% of genes were in the discordant classes (quadrants A, B, D, F, H, I). Notably, 1.31% (154) and 2.02% (238) of genes were located in quadrants C and G, respectively, which meant that the expression of genes changed congruously at the transcriptional and translational levels (upregulation for quadrant C; downregulation for quadrant G). Furthermore, to explore the synergistic functions of transcription and translation, GO analysis of the biological processes enriched for the congruous DEGs (quadrants C and G) was conducted. The results showed that the congruous DEGs were significantly enriched for terms related to innate immunity such as cell surface receptor signaling pathway, immune response, innate immune response, immune system process and regulation of immune system process (Figure 3B). These results suggest that the innate immune response of the body to ARV infection involves co-regulation of transcription and translation.

2.5. Screening Functional Genes after ARV Infection

The above association analysis showed that genes in quadrants C and G were mainly enriched for biological processes related to immune regulation, indicating that these DEGs may be involved in the innate immune response to ARV infection. We identified 392 DEGs in quadrants C and G. We compared the top 30 DEGs at the transcriptional and translational levels (Figure 4A,B). Based on the significance of the DEGs, the most significant DEG at the transcriptional and translational levels was determined to be IL4I1 (FDR in transcriptome = 1.85×10^{-27}, FDR in translatome = 6.2×10^{-57}). According to the RNA-seq and Ribo-seq data, the expression level of IL4I1 significantly increased after ARV infection (Figure 4C). The RT-qPCR results were consistent with the RNA-seq and Ribo-seq results (Figure 4D).

2.6. IL4I1 Expression Reduced ARV Replication

To verify the effect of IL4I1 overexpression on ARV replication, we transfected the pEF1α-Myc-IL4I1 recombinant plasmid into DF1 cells, then verified IL4I1 overexpression by real-time PCR and Western blotting 24 h later. Real-time PCR showed that IL4I1 gene expression in DF1 cells was significantly upregulated after transfection with the pEF1α-Myc-IL4I1 (Figure 5A). Detection at approximately 60 kDa using Myc-tagged antibodies showed that IL4I1 was correctly expressed in DF1 cells transfected with the pEF1α-Myc-IL4I1, while IL4I1 protein expression was not detected in cells transfected with empty vectors (Figure 5B). Cells were infected with ARV after 24 h of transfection, and cell samples and supernatants were collected after another 24 h. Real-time PCR detection showed that the expression of the ARV σC gene at the mRNA level was significantly reduced (Figure 5C), and the ARV virus titer in the cell supernatant was also significantly reduced (Figure 5D). These results suggest that the overexpression of IL4I1 in DF1 cells inhibits the replication of ARV.

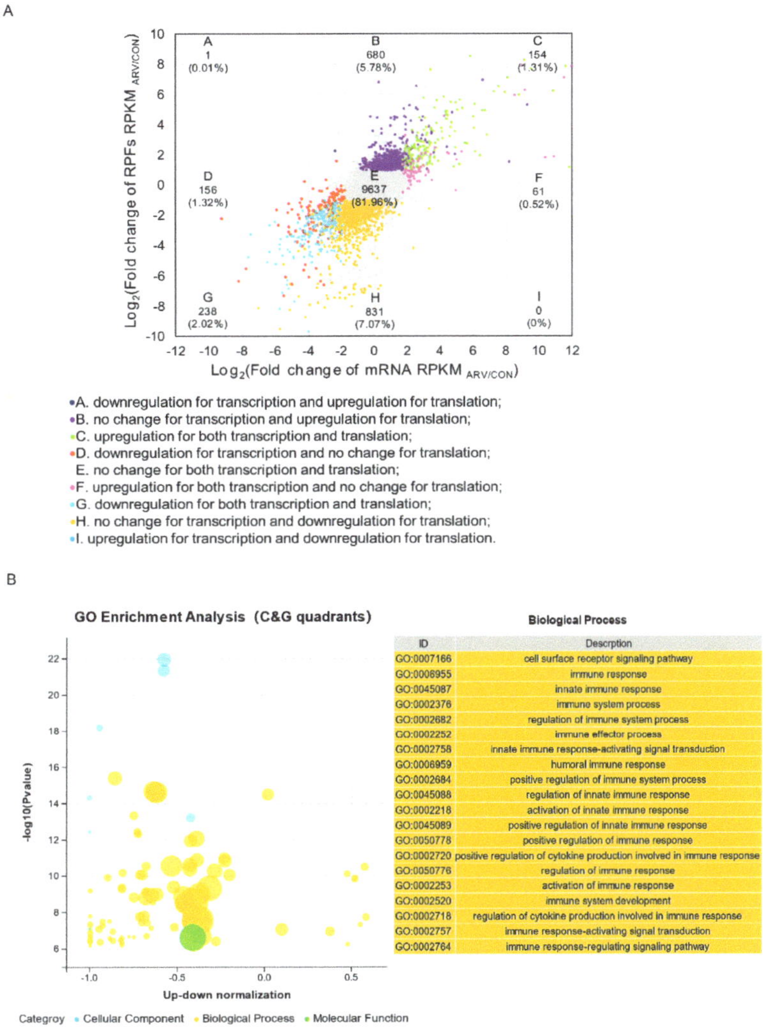

ID	Descrption
GO:0007166	cell surface receptor signaling pathway
GO:0006955	immune response
GO:0045087	innate immune response
GO:0002376	immune system process
GO:0002682	regulation of immune system process
GO:0002252	immune effector process
GO:0002758	innate immune response-activating signal transduction
GO:0006959	humoral immune response
GO:0002684	positive regulation of immune system process
GO:0045088	regulation of innate immune response
GO:0002218	activation of innate immune response
GO:0045089	positive regulation of innate immune response
GO:0050778	positive regulation of immune response
GO:0002720	positive regulation of cytokine production involved in immune response
GO:0050776	regulation of immune response
GO:0002253	activation of immune response
GO:0002520	immune system development
GO:0002718	regulation of cytokine production involved in immune response
GO:0002757	immune response-activating signal transduction
GO:0002764	immune response-regulating signaling pathway

Figure 3. Avian reovirus altered gene expression at both the transcriptional and translational levels. (**A**) Scatter plot of the fold change in the ARV/CON group at the transcriptional and translational levels. Nine squares in different colors indicate nine response groups ($|\log_2$ fold change$| \geq 1$ and FDR < 0.01). (**B**) GO enrichment analysis of genes in quadrants C and G.

Therefore, we speculated that IL4I1 can cause negative feedback in the replication of ARV and that inhibiting the expression of IL4I1 can promote the replication of ARV. We designed and synthesized three siRNAs against the IL4I1 gene to inhibit the expression of IL4I1, of which siRNA1357 was the most ideal (Figure 5E). siRNA1357 was transfected into DF1 cells, and the cells were infected with ARV virus after 24 h of transfection. Then, cell samples and supernatants were collected at 24 h postinfection to detect ARV replication at the gene expression and viral titer levels, and the results were consistent with expectations (Figure 5F,G). The above results show that inhibiting the expression of IL4I1 can promote the replication of ARV.

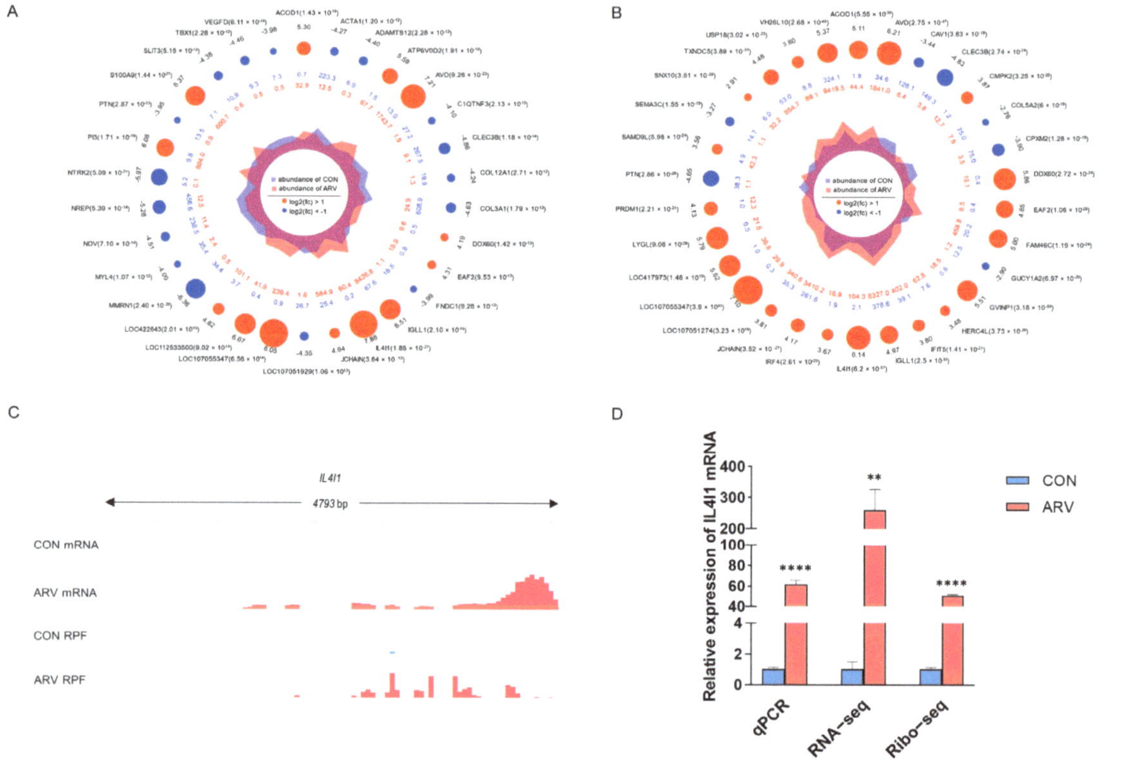

Figure 4. Functional gene screening. The circle maps of the top 30 DEGs in the transcriptome (**A**) and translatome (**B**). (**C**) The expression abundance of IL4I1 at the transcriptional and translational levels. (**D**) The relative level of IL4I1 mRNA expression. Asterisks indicate significant differences (** $p < 0.01$, **** $p < 0.0001$).

2.7. The Effect of IL4I1 Expression on the Innate Immune Response during ARV Infection

To investigate how IL4I1 regulates the innate immune response induced by ARV infection, we overexpressed or inhibited IL4I1 and detected the effect of IL4I1 expression on the expression of innate immune signaling pathway-correlated factors during ARV infection by real-time PCR. The results showed that the mRNA expression of MDA5, TRAF3 and TRAF6 was significantly upregulated after overexpression or inhibition of IL4I1. The mRNA expression of MAVS was upregulated after overexpression of IL4I1 and downregulated after inhibition of IL4I1. The mRNA expression of IKKε did not differ significantly after overexpression of IL4I1 and was significantly upregulated after inhibition of IL4I1. The mRNA expression of IRF7 was significantly upregulated after overexpression of IL4I1, but there was no significant difference after IL4I1 inhibition. There was no significant difference in the mRNA expression of IFN-α after overexpression or inhibition of IL4I1. The mRNA expression of IFN-β, LGP2, TBK1 and NF-κB was significantly downregulated after overexpression of IL4I1 and upregulated after inhibition of IL4I1 (Figure 6A,B). These results suggest that IL4I1 may be a negative feedback regulator of innate immune signaling pathways and that IL4I1 expression may reduce IFN-β production by inhibiting the expression of LGP2, TBK1 and NF-κB.

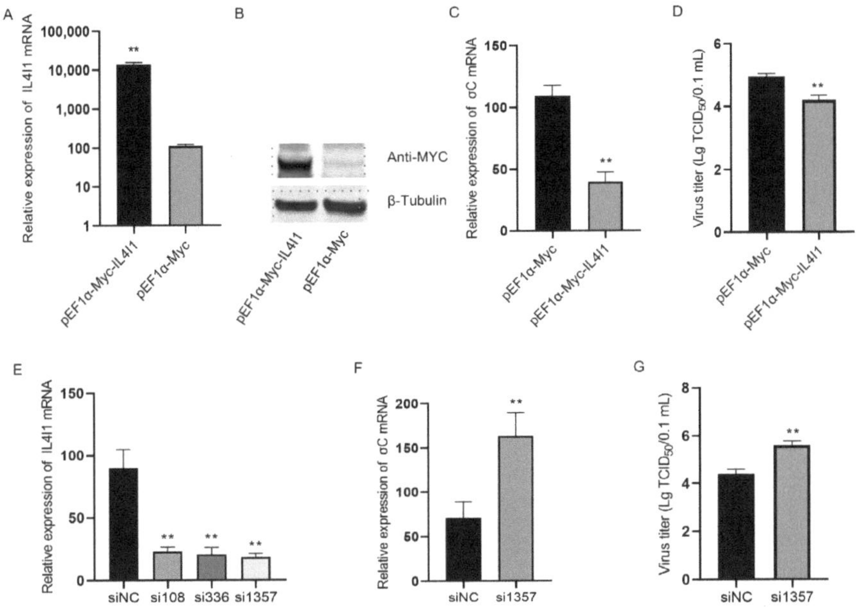

Figure 5. IL4I1 inhibits the replication of ARV in DF1 cells. DF-1 cells were transfected with pEF1α-Myc-IL4I1 or pEF1α-Myc plasmids, and both real-time PCR (**A**) and Western blot (**B**) confirmed high levels of IL4I1 expression in DF-1 cells. DF-1 cells were transfected with pEF1α-Myc-IL4I1 or pEF1α-Myc plasmids and infected with the ARV S1133 strain at an MOI of 1. Viral replication was detected by real-time PCR (**C**) and viral titer (**D**) 24 h postinfection. Comparison of the inhibition efficiency of three siRNAs of IL4I1 by real-time PCR (**E**). DF1 cells were transfected with si1357 or siNC and infected with the ARV S1133 strain of virus at an MOI of 1. Viral replication was detected by real-time PCR (**F**) and viral titer (**G**) 24 h postinfection. Data are represented as the mean ± SD of three independent experiments. Asterisks indicate significant differences (** $p < 0.01$).

2.8. Interaction between IL4I1 and ARV σA/σC Proteins

The σA and σC proteins are important structural proteins of ARV and play a significant part in the interaction between ARV and the host. Therefore, we studied the relationship between IL4I1 and ARV σA/σC. We transfected the eukaryotic expression plasmids pEF1α-HA-σA and pEF1α-HA-σC into DF1 cells and overexpressed ARV σA and σC proteins in DF1 cells. Real-time PCR detection showed that the expression of IL4I1 was significantly upregulated after the overexpression of σA and σC proteins in DF1 cells. The overexpression of σA in particular upregulated IL4I1 by a relatively high fold change (Figure 7A).

Subsequently, we used Co-IP to determine whether IL4I1 interacted with ARV σA and σC proteins in vitro. The Co-IP results of IL4I1 protein and ARV σA protein showed that when Co-IP immobilization used the anti-Myc monoclonal antibody, the σA-HA protein could be identified by Western blot. However, when Co-IP immobilization used the anti-HA monoclonal antibody, the IL4I1-Myc protein was not identified by Western blot (Figure 7B).

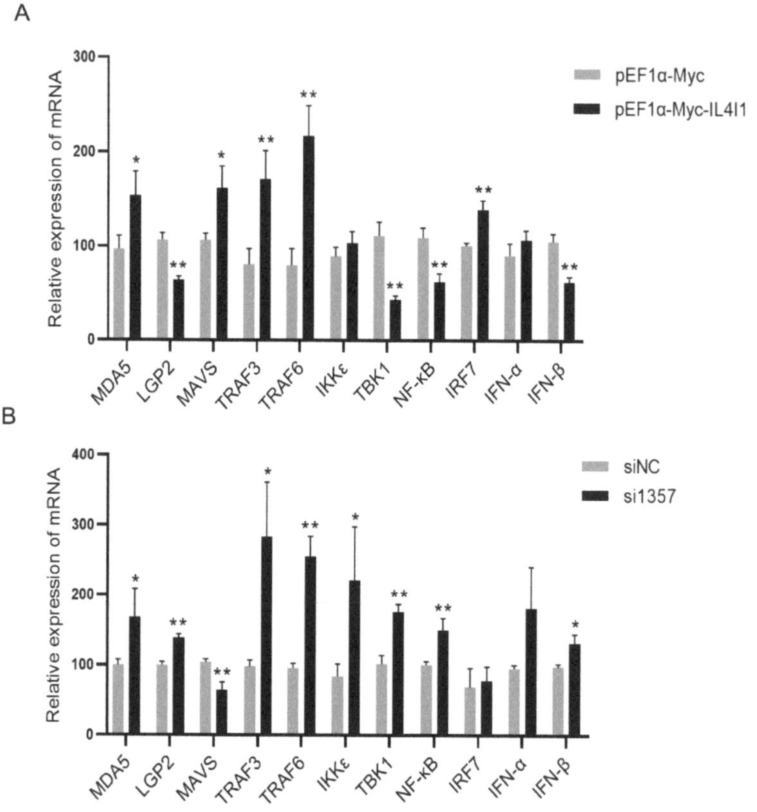

Figure 6. Effect of IL4I1 on the innate immune response during ARV infection. DF-1 cells were transfected with pEF1α-Myc-IL4I1 or pEF1α-Myc plasmids and then infected with the ARV S1133 strain at an MOI of 1. Expression changes in genes associated with the innate immune signaling pathway were detected by real-time PCR (**A**) 24 h postinfection. DF1 cells were transfected with si1357 or siNC and infected with the ARV S1133 strain of virus at an MOI of 1. Expression changes in genes associated with the innate immune signaling pathway were detected by real-time PCR (**B**) 24 h postinfection. Data are represented as the mean ± SD of three independent experiments. Asterisks indicate significant differences (* $p < 0.05$, ** $p < 0.01$).

The Co-IP results of IL4I1 protein and ARV σC protein showed that when Co-IP immobilization used the anti-Myc monoclonal antibody, no σC-HA protein was identified by Western blot. IL4I1-Myc protein was also not identified by Western blot when Co-IP immobilization used the anti-HA monoclonal antibody (Figure 7C). Therefore, there may be an interaction between the IL4I1 and ARV σA proteins.

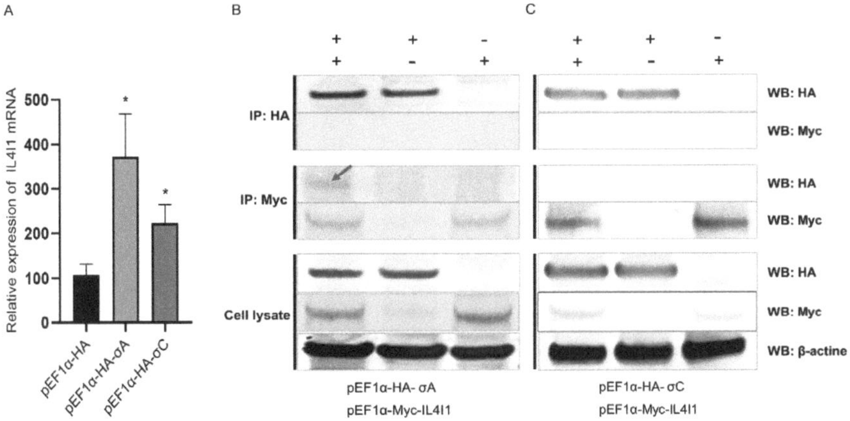

Figure 7. IL4I1 in DF1 cells interacts with ARV σA and σC proteins. PEF1α-HA-σA or pEF1α-HA-σC were transfected into DF1 cells to overexpress ARV σA or σC proteins, respectively. Determination of IL4I1 expression by real-time PCR (**A**). We cotransfected cells with pEF1α-Myc-IL4I1 and pEF1α-HA-σA/σC in the experimental group and pEF1α-Myc-IL4I1 and pEF1α-HA or pEF1α-Myc and pEF1α-HA-σA/σC in the control group. After 24 h of transfection, cells were lysed to collect protein samples, and the interaction of IL4I1 with ARV σA and σC proteins in DF-1 cells was verified by Co-IP. Verification of IL4I1 interaction with ARV σA by Co-IP (**B**). Verification of IL4I1 interaction with ARV σC by Co-IP (**C**). Asterisks indicate significant differences (* $p < 0.05$).

3. Discussion

Gene expression is closely related to the occurrence and development of various physiological and pathological activities and diseases. High-throughput sequencing technology enables the sequencing and identification of millions of nucleotide molecules simultaneously. To date, it is widely used in the screening of important functional genes and research on animal diseases [28]. Translation regulation is a key element in the regulation of gene expression. Omics studies have shown that translation regulation accounts for more than half of all regulation overseeing gene expression, and the translational differences better reflect the expression changes in the proteome than those of the transcriptome [29,30].

In this study, Ribo-seq was conducted to reveal the gene expression profile of the spleen after ARV infection. We analyzed the characteristics of RPFs in the spleen; after ARV infection, the abundance of splenic RPFs in the CDS region and the 5′ UTR was lower than that in the control group, which also indicated that ARV infection inhibited the process of protein synthesis in the spleen. After ARV infection, the abundance of splenic RPFs in the 3′ UTR was higher than that in the CON group. In the eukaryotic translational process, the 5′ UTR and the 3′ UTR play important roles in post-transcriptional regulation. The 5′ UTR mediates post-transcriptional regulation through the main elements present in this region, such as uORFs, secondary structures and RPF-binding motifs, and the 3′ UTR contains a large number of regulatory elements, such as microRNA binding sites and protein binding sites [31–33]. After ARV infection, the abundance of splenic RPFs increased significantly in the 3′ UTR, suggesting that there may be potential translational regulation of ARV infection in the 3′ UTR, which may be related to the innate immune regulation process of the host after ARV infection. These complex regulatory mechanisms still need to be further studied.

Studies have confirmed that genes with higher translation efficiency perform more important biological functions, and in addition, the specific array of genes with high translation efficiency or upregulated translation efficiency reflect the function and phenotype of a particular cell [14]. Our sequencing results showed that ARV infection significantly reduced the overall translation efficiency of splenic genes. Further analysis showed that, compared with the control group, there were 15 significantly upregulated DTEGs and

369 significantly downregulated DTEGs in the ARV infection group. These DTEGs were mainly enriched in signaling pathways related to immune regulation, which led to speculation that ARV infection would reduce the immune response ability of the spleen. Recent studies have confirmed that ARV infection causes immunosuppression [34]. However, the specific mechanism of ARV-induced immunosuppression still needs to be studied in greater depth. After ARV infection, the translation efficiency of immune regulation-related signaling pathways in the spleen is reduced, which we speculate is one of the important reasons for immunosuppression caused by ARV infection.

The transcriptome and translatome association data analysis showed that 392 genes were expressed in common with significant differences at the transcription and translation levels. GO enrichment analysis showed that the 20 most significant GO terms were all enriched in signaling pathways related to immune regulation. This suggests that these DEGs play important roles in the innate immune response to ARV infection. We further analyzed the significance of these 392 congruous DEGs and screened the 30 genes with the highest significance. The most significantly differentially expressed gene was IL4I1 in both the transcriptome and translatome. The expression of IL4I1 was highly induced after ARV infection, suggesting that IL4I1 plays an important part in the response to ARV infection. Interleukin-4-induced-1 (IL4I1) is a less-studied amino acid catabolic enzyme that belongs to the L-amino acid oxidase family. IL4I1 plays an important role in the body's defense against infection, regulation of immune homeostasis and injury response. In recent years, it has been found that IL4I1 is closely related to the regulatory process of human immune metabolism, and it is an important immunosuppressive factor and a key metabolic immune checkpoint [35]. Tumor cells produce large amounts of the IL4I1 metabolic enzyme, which promotes the spread of tumor cells and suppresses the immune system. IL4I1 breaks down tryptophan to form indole metabolites and kynurequinolinic acid, which are agonists of the aryl hydrocarbon receptor (AHR). Indole metabolites and kynurequinolinic acid bind to and activate AHR receptors, thereby mediating the toxic effects of dioxins, which reduces the utilization of essential or semi-essential amino acids. At the same time, toxic metabolites are produced, which cause damage to antitumor T lymphocytes and promote the growth of tumor cells [36].

There are few reports on the role and mechanism of IL4I1 in avian virus infection. Studies by high-throughput sequencing technology have found that a large amount of IL4I1 expression can be induced after a variety of viral infections. Hu et al. found that IL4I1 expression was significantly upregulated in chicken embryo fibroblasts infected by the J subpopulation of avian leukemia virus (ALV-J) by transcriptome sequencing [37]. Feng et al. used transcriptome sequencing analysis to find that the expression of IL4I1 in chicken primary mononuclear macrophages infected with ALV-J was significantly upregulated 3 h and 36 h after infection, and overexpression of IL4I1 at the gene level could facilitate the replication of ALV-J in chicken macrophages [38]. Dong et al. found that the IL4I1 gene was upregulated in chicken spleen tissues infected with Marek virus (MDV) by transcriptome sequencing technology [39]. Conversely, our study showed that IL4I1 inhibits the replication of the ARV virus. This suggests that there may be differences in the roles of IL4I1 in the replication of different viruses. We found that IL4I1 was able to prevent the replication of ARV in DF1 cells by overexpression or inhibition assays. Our previous studies showed that the ARV viral load in the spleen was high on days 1 to 3 after ARV infection and then decreased sharply on day 4 [11]. Therefore, we speculate that the rapid upregulation of IL4I1 expression in the spleen after ARV infection is beneficial to inhibiting the proliferation of ARV in the spleen. However, IL4I1 was able to promote the replication of ALV-J in chicken macrophages, suggesting that there may be differences in the roles of IL4I1 in the replication of different avian viruses. We also detected a regulatory role for IL4I1 on innate immune signaling pathway-correlated factors during ARV infection by real-time PCR. The mRNA expression of IFN-β, LGP2, TBK1 and NF-κB was significantly downregulated after overexpression of IL4I1, and the mRNA expression of IFN-β, LGP2, TBK1 and NF-κB was significantly upregulated after inhibiting IL4I1. This suggests that IL4I1 may be a negative feedback effect of innate immune signaling pathways during ARV infection, and IL4I1 may reduce the production of IFN-β by inhibiting the expression of LGP2, TBK1 and NF-κB. The current study has shown that IL4I1 is an important immunosuppressive molecule that plays a key role in the immune evasion of tumors [36]. Previous studies have also found that IL4I1 can inhibit the production of IFN-γ and inflammatory cytokines, limit local Th1 inflammation and inhibit the inflammatory response [40]. ARV is an important avian immunosuppressive disease, and our sequencing analysis found that ARV infection can significantly reduce the translational efficiency of immunomodulatory-related genes in chicken spleen. ARV, ALV-J and MDV infection can cause avian immunosuppressive diseases, and IL4I1 expression was upregulated after each of these three viral infections. Whether the regulation of IL4I1 expression is related to the immunosuppressive processes caused by avian immunosuppressive viruses is an interesting mechanism that deserves more in-depth study.

Virus-encoded proteins play a crucial part in virus interactions with its host. The σA protein of ARV plays a vital role in the pathogenesis of ARV infection. A study found that the ARV σA protein binds irreversibly to viral dsRNA, thereby inhibiting the dsRNA-dependent protein kinases activation and ultimately interfering with the antiviral effects of interferon [41,42]. In addition, the ARV σA protein can also activate the PI3K/Akt signal transduction pathways in cells, increase the expression of phosphorylated Akt (p-Akt) in cells and, thus, inhibit the apoptosis of infected cells to facilitate ARV infection and replication [43]. It has also been showed that the ARV σA protein affects the replication of ARV in DF1 cells by interacting with the NME2 protein of the host [44]. The ARV σC protein is related to the adsorption and proliferation of virions [45]. The ARV σC protein is able to induce apoptosis by interacting with the host protein EFF1A1 [46]. In this study, we found that overexpression of ARV σA and σC proteins in DF1 cells can cause significant upregulation of IL4I1 expression at the transcriptional level. The interaction between IL4I1 and ARV σC proteins was not found by co-immunoprecipitation experiments, while the co-immunoprecipitation analysis of IL4I1 protein and ARV σA proteins uncovered an interesting phenomenon. When we used the anti-Myc antibody to fix IL4I1 protein in the Co-IP experiment, σA protein interacted with IL4I1 protein, but when we fixed σA protein using the anti-HA antibody in the Co-IP experiment, the interaction between σA protein and IL4I1 protein could not be detected. To ensure the rigor of the experimental data, we performed multiple replicates using antibodies and Co-IP kits of different brands, all with the same results. We reviewed the literature and found that the human IL4I1 protein is a glycosylated secreted protein [47]. The structure and function of avian IL4I1 protein have not been reported, and our online software analysis shows that avian IL4I1 protein is also a secreted protein. We hypothesize that the IL4I1 protein failed to be detected by Western blot analysis when the σA protein was immobilized in the Co-IP experiment, which is related to the fact that IL4I1 is secreted extracellularly after synthesis. Therefore, we speculate that there may be an interaction between the IL4I1 protein and the ARV σA protein, and that the IL4I1 protein may actively bind to the σA protein. We speculate that the IL4I1 protein may play a regulatory role by interacting with the ARV σA protein. We further speculate that after ARV infection, IL4I1 is modulated and then transcribed and expressed in large quantities, and the IL4I1 protein competitively binds to the ARV σA protein, thereby affecting the function of the ARV σA protein and inhibiting the replication of ARV. However, due to a lack of avian-derived IL4I1 protein-specific antibodies, it is difficult to further verify the interaction between the IL4I1 and ARV σA proteins. In future studies, we will prepare monoclonal antibodies against avian IL4I1 protein and conduct in-depth research on the role and regulatory mechanism of IL4I1 in the interaction network of ARV or σA protein.

4. Materials and Methods

4.1. Ethics Statement

This study was approved by the Animal Ethics Committee of Guangxi Veterinary Research Institute. Animal experiments and sample collection were conducted in accordance with the guidance of protocol #2019C0406 issued by the Animal Ethics Committee of Guangxi Veterinary Research Institute.

4.2. Viral Inoculations and Animal Experiments

The ARV S1133 strain used in the study was purchased from the China Institute of Veterinary Drug Control. "White Leghorn" SPF chicken eggs were purchased from Beijing Boehringer Ingelheim Vital Biotechnology Co., Ltd. (Beijing, China). Incubation was performed using a fully automated incubator, after which chicks were raised in SPF chicken isolators. A total of twenty 7-day-old SPF chickens were randomized into two groups and raised aseptically in an SPF chicken isolator. Group A was the experimental group (ARV), and each chicken was inoculated with 0.1 mL 10^4 $TCID_{50}/0.1$ mL ARV S1133 virus by foot pad injection. Group B was the control group (CON), which was inoculated with the same amount of PBS via foot pad injection. Samples were collected on day 3 after infection. The chickens were taken from the ARV infection group and the control group for dissection and collection of spleens, and then the collected samples were snap-frozen in liquid nitrogen and stored in a -80 °C freezer for subsequent analysis. The standard for selecting sequencing samples in this study was to use the two samples whose viral load of spleen was closest to the mean in the group as 2 biological replicates.

4.3. RNA Extraction and Transcriptome Sequencing

Total RNA of the spleen in each group was extracted by using TRIzol® RNA extraction reagent (Invitrogen, Carlsbad, CA, USA) according to the manufacturer's instructions. The integrity of RNA was examined by agarose gel electrophoresis, and the concentration of RNA was measured by NanoDrop 2000 spectrophotometers (Thermo Fisher Scientific, Boston, MA, USA). The mRNA was purified by oligo (dT) magnetic beads and fragmented into short fragments using fragmentation buffer. First-strand cDNA was synthesized with SuperScript II Reverse Transcriptase (Invitrogen) using random primers, and second-strand cDNA was synthesized using the synthesized first strand of cDNA as a template. The obtained double-stranded cDNA was purified by a VAHTS® mRNA-seq V3 Library Prep Kit for Illumina (Vazyme, Nanjing, China), end repaired, poly(A) added and then ligated to Illumina sequencing adapters. Sequencing was performed on the Illumina HiSeq-2000 platform for 50 cycles. High-quality reads passed through the Illumina quality filter were retained in fastq.gz format for sequence analysis.

4.4. Preparation of Ribosome-Protected Fragments and Ribosome Profiling

RPF extraction and sequencing were performed by a commercial company (Chi-Biotech, Wuhan, China) according to a previous study [17]. Spleen tissue from each group was added to lysis buffer, ground at low temperature and then low concentrations of RNase I were added for digestion. The digested samples were pooled and layered on the surface of 15 mL sucrose buffer (30% sucrose in RB buffer). The ribosomes were pelleted by ultracentrifugation at 42,500 rpm for 5 h at 4 °C. RPF extraction was then performed using TRIzol, and ribosomal RNA (rRNA) was depleted using the Ribo-off® rRNA Depletion Kit (Vazyme) following the manufacturer's instructions. Sequencing libraries of RPFs were constructed following the VAHTS® Small RNA Library Prep Kit for Illumina (Vazyme). The library was resolved by a 6% polyacrylamide gel. The fraction with an insertion size of ~28 nt was excised and purified from the gel. This fraction was sequenced by an Illumina HiSeq-2000 sequencer for 50 cycles. High-quality reads that passed the Illumina quality filters were kept for sequence analysis.

4.5. Sequence Analysis

For both mRNA and RPF sequencing data sets, high-quality reads were mapped to the mRNA reference sequence (GRCg6a) through the FANSe2 algorithm [48] with the parameters -E5% --indel -S14. The expression abundance of mRNA and RPFs was normalized by RPKM (reads per kilobase per million reads) [49]. Differentially expressed genes (DEGs) in RNA-seq and Ribo-seq were identified via the edgeR package [50] with $|\log_2$ fold change$| > 1$ and false discovery rate (FDR) < 0.01. The quotient of RPFs and mRNA expression abundance is translation efficiency (TE) [51,52]. Differential TE genes (DTEGs) were calculated by a t test with $|\log_2$ fold change$| > 1$ and p value < 0.05. Bioinformatic analysis was performed using Omicsmart, a real-time, interactive online platform for data analysis (http://www.omicsmart.com, accessed on 20 November 2023).

4.6. Overexpression of IL4I1 Protein

The recombinant plasmid pEF1α-Myc-IL4I1 was constructed from the IL4I1 gene sequence (Genbank accession number NM_001099351.3) from chicken. DF1 cells were cultured in 6-well plates. When the cell confluency reached 70–80%, the recombinant IL4I1 plasmid was transfected with liposome Lipofectamine™ 3000 (Invitrogen) to overexpress IL4I1 protein. After 24 h of transfection, DF1 cells were infected with the ARV S1133 strain at a multiplicity of infection (MOI) of 1. Then, the sample of cells and medium supernatant were gathered at 24 h postinfection. RNA was extracted from the above cell samples and reverse-transcribed to synthesize cDNA using the GeneJET RNA Purification Kit and Maxima™ H minus cDNA synthesis master mix (Thermo Fisher Scientific). Real-time PCR detected the replication of ARV at the gene level and the expression changes in innate immune signaling pathway-related molecules. The primer sequences of molecules associated with the innate immune signaling pathway and ARV σC gene are shown in Table 1 [53]. In addition, the above medium supernatant was used to infect DF1 cells and the virulence was determined by the Reed–Muench method to detect the replication of ARV.

Table 1. Primers used in this study.

Gene	Genbank Accession Number	Primer Sequences (5′-3′)
ARV σC	L39002.1	F: CCACGGGAAATCTCACGGTCACT, R: TACGCACGGTCAAGGAACGAATGT
IL4I1	NM_001099351.3	F: CACGCCGTATCAGTTCACC, R: CCTCACCGCAGCCTTCAT
IFN-α	AB021154.1	F: ATGCCACCTTCTCTCACGAC, R: AGGCGCTGTAATCGTTGTCT
IFN-β	X92479.1	F: ACCAGGATGCCAACTTCT, R: TCACTGGGTGTTGAGACG
MDA5	NM_001193638	F: CAGCCAGTTGCCCTCGCCTCA, R: AACAGCTCCCTTGCACCGTCT
LGP2	MF563595.1	F: CCAGAATGAGCAGCAGGAC, R: AATGTTGCACTCAGGGATGT
MAVS	MF289560.1	F: CCTGACTCAAACAAGGGAAG, R: AATCAGAGCGATGCCAACAG
TRAF3	XM_040672281.1	F: GGACGCACTTGTCGCTGTTT, R: CGGACCCTGATCCATTAGCAT
TRAF6	XM_040673314.1	F: GATGGAGACGCAAAACACTCAC, R: GCATCACAACAGGTCTCTCTTC
IKKε	XM_428036.4	F: TGGATGGGATGGTGTCTGAAC, R: TGCGGAACTGCTTGTAGATG
TBK1	MF159109.1	F: AAGAAGGCACACATCCGAGA, R: GGTAGCGTGCAAATACAGC
IRF7	NM_205372.1	F: CAGTGCTTCTCCAGCACAAA, R: TGCATGTGGTATTGCTCGAT
NF-κB	NM_205129.1	F: CATTGCCAGCATGGCTACTAT, R: TTCCAGTTCCCGTTTCTTCAC
GAPDH	NM_204305.1	F: GCACTGTCAAGGCTGAGAACG, R: GATGATAACACGCTTAGCACCAC

4.7. RNA Interference Assay

According to the sequence of IL4I1 genes, three small interfering RNAs (siRNAs) (Table 2) were designed and synthesized (GenePharma, Shanghai, China). IL4I1 siRNA inhibitory molecules were transfected into DF1 cells using Lipofectamine® RNAiMAX Reagent (Invitrogen) to inhibit IL4I1 protein expression. After 24 h of transfection, cells were infected with the ARV S1133 strain at a MOI of 1, and after another 24 h, cell samples and medium supernatants were collected to detect replication of ARV virus.

Table 2. siRNA sequence targeting the IL4I1 gene.

siRNA	Sense	Antisense
si108	GCUGCUGAGUAUUGUGAAATT	UUUCACAAUACUCAGCAGCTT
si336	GCUGGUGCGUGAGUUUAUATT	UAUAAACUCACGCACCAGCTT
si1357	CCGUAUCAGUUCACCGAUUTT	AAUCGGUGAACUGAUACGGTT
siNC	UUCUCCGAACGUGUCACGUTT	ACGUGACACGUUCGGAGAATT

4.8. Real-Time PCR

Real-time PCR was performed using the PowerUpTM SYBRTM Green Master Mix (Thermo Scientific) via the QuantStudio 5 real-time PCR system (Thermo Lifetech ABI, Boston, MA, USA).

4.9. Co-immunoprecipitation (Co-IP) Assays

The interactions between IL4I1 and ARV σA or σC protein were detected by Co-IP. We designed three experimental groups: the test group was cotransfected with pEF1α-Myc-IL4I1 and pEF1α-HA-σA/σC and the control group was cotransfected with pEF1α-Myc-IL4I1 and pEF1α-HA or pEF1α-Myc and pEF1α-HA-σA/σC. Three biological replicates were assigned to each group. After 24 h of transfection, cells were lysed, protein samples were collected and Co-IP analysis with the Pierce Classic IP Kit (Thermo Scientific) was performed. The forward Co-IP test used rabbit-derived HA antibody (Invitrogen) for fixed adsorption samples, and Western blot analysis used murine Myc antibody and murine HA antibody (Invitrogen) as primary antibodies for detection. The reverse Co-IP used rabbit-derived Myc antibody (Invitrogen) for fixed adsorbed samples, and Western blot analysis used murine HA antibody and murine Myc antibody (Invitrogen) as primary antibodies. Goat anti-murine IgG (Beyotime, Shanghai, China) labeled with alkaline phosphatase was the secondary antibody.

4.10. Statistical Analysis

At least three valid repeat tests were performed for each treatment, and the results are expressed as the mean ± SD. Graph analysis and statistical comparisons used GraphPad Prism statistical software, version 9.5.0. The unpaired two tailed *t*-test (for two groups) and one-way ANOVA (for multiple groups) were used to identify the significance of difference. The results' difference were considered statistically significant at $p < 0.05$.

5. Conclusions

In this study, we determined that the spleen produces a strong innate immune response at both the transcriptional and translational levels after ARV infection and that the spleen is an important immune response organ in ARV infection. ARV infection reduces the translation efficiency of innate immunity-related genes, and we speculate that the decrease in translation efficiency is the key cause of immunosuppression caused by ARV infection. ARV infection can significantly upregulate the expression of IL4I1, while the upregulation of IL4I1 helps to inhibit the replication of ARV. IL4I1 may inhibit the innate immune response triggered by ARV infection. In addition, the IL4I1 protein may interact with the viral protein σA of ARV. These results provide new insights into ARV–host interactions and will facilitate the development of new vaccines or other therapeutic agents to control ARV based on the IL4I1 gene in chickens.

Supplementary Materials: The following supporting information can be downloaded at: https://www.mdpi.com/article/10.3390/v15122346/s1, Figure S1. Overview of transcriptome and translatome. (A–D) Distribution of the mRNA and RPFs abundance in CON and ARV groups. (E–F) Pearson correlation analysis of RNA-seq and Ribo-seq. (G) The total number of RPFs along CDS start and stop codon regions in CON group. Figure S2. Differential analysis. (A–B) Venn diagram showing the distinct and over-lapping genes of the transcriptome and translatome. Scatter diagram showing the correlation of gene abundance in RNA-seq and Ribo-seq. (C–D) Volcano plots of DEGs of the transcriptome and translatome. Table S1. Statistic on the ribosomal profiling data and RNA-Seq data. Table S2. The identification and quantification information of the transcriptome. Table S3. The identification and quantification information of the translatome. Table S4. The gene information in different quadrants.

Author Contributions: Z.X. (Zhixun Xie) designed and coordinated the study and helped to review the manuscript. S.W. performed the experiments, analyzed the data and wrote the manuscript. T.H. analyzed the data and wrote the manuscript. L.W. and H.R. assisted in completion of the experiment. T.W. analyzed the data. L.X., S.L., M.L., Z.X. (Zhiqin Xie), Q.F., J.H., T.Z., Y.Z., M.Z. and Y.W. assisted in the animal experiments. All authors have read and agreed to the published version of the manuscript.

Funding: This work was supported by the Natural Science Foundation of China (project 32300148), Guangxi Basic research Funds supported by the Special project (Guike special 20-1), the Guangxi BaGui Scholars Program Foundation (2019A50) and Guangxi Key Laboratory of Veterinary Biotechnology Projects (23-035-32-A-01).

Institutional Review Board Statement: The animal study was reviewed and approved by the Animal Ethics Committee of Guangxi Veterinary Research Institute (No. #2019C0406).

Informed Consent Statement: Not applicable.

Data Availability Statement: The data sets presented in this study can be found in online repositories. The names of the repository/repositories and accession number(s) can be found below: https://www.ncbi.nlm.nih.gov/geo/query/acc.cgi?acc=GSE241418, accessed on 20 November 2023.

Conflicts of Interest: The authors declare no conflict of interest.

References

1. Van der Heide, L. The history of avian reovirus. *Avian Dis.* **2000**, *44*, 638–641. [CrossRef] [PubMed]
2. Dandar, E.; Balint, A.; Kecskemeti, S.; Szentpali-Gavaller, K.; Kisfali, P.; Melegh, B.; Farkas, S.L.; Banyai, K. Detection and characterization of a divergent avian reovirus strain from a broiler chicken with central nervous system disease. *Arch. Virol.* **2013**, *158*, 2583–2588. [CrossRef] [PubMed]
3. Teng, L.; Xie, Z.; Xie, L.; Liu, J.; Pang, Y.; Deng, X.; Xie, Z.; Fan, Q.; Luo, S.; Feng, J.; et al. Sequencing and phylogenetic analysis of an avian reovirus genome. *Virus Genes* **2014**, *48*, 381–386. [CrossRef] [PubMed]
4. Green, A.M.; Beatty, P.R.; Hadjilaou, A.; Harris, E. Innate immunity to dengue virus infection and subversion of antiviral responses. *J. Mol. Biol.* **2014**, *426*, 1148–1160. [CrossRef] [PubMed]
5. Iwasaki, A.; Pillai, P.S. Innate immunity to influenza virus infection. *Nat. Rev. Immunol.* **2014**, *14*, 315–328. [CrossRef] [PubMed]
6. Lin, P.Y.; Liu, H.J.; Liao, M.H.; Chang, C.D.; Chang, C.I.; Cheng, H.L.; Lee, J.W.; Shih, W.L. Activation of PI 3-kinase/Akt/NF-kappaB and Stat3 signaling by avian reovirus S1133 in the early stages of infection results in an inflammatory response and delayed apoptosis. *Virology* **2010**, *400*, 104–114. [CrossRef] [PubMed]
7. Neelima, S.; Ram, G.C.; Kataria, J.M.; Goswami, T.K. Avian reovirus induces an inhibitory effect on lymphoproliferation in chickens. *Vet. Res. Commun.* **2003**, *27*, 73–85. [CrossRef]
8. Lostale-Seijo, I.; Martinez-Costas, J.; Benavente, J. Interferon induction by avian reovirus. *Virology* **2016**, *487*, 104–111. [CrossRef]
9. Xie, L.; Xie, Z.; Wang, S.; Huang, J.; Deng, X.; Xie, Z.; Luo, S.; Zeng, T.; Zhang, Y.; Zhang, M. Altered gene expression profiles of the MDA5 signaling pathway in peripheral blood lymphocytes of chickens infected with avian reovirus. *Arch. Virol.* **2019**, *164*, 2451–2458. [CrossRef]
10. Wang, S.; Xie, L.; Xie, Z.; Wan, L.; Huang, J.; Deng, X.; Xie, Z.Q.; Luo, S.; Zeng, T.; Zhang, Y.; et al. Dynamic Changes in the Expression of Interferon-Stimulated Genes in Joints of SPF Chickens Infected with Avian Reovirus. *Front. Vet. Sci.* **2021**, *8*, 618124. [CrossRef]
11. Wang, S.; Wan, L.; Ren, H.; Xie, Z.; Xie, L.; Huang, J.; Deng, X.; Xie, Z.; Luo, S.; Li, M.; et al. Screening of interferon-stimulated genes against avian reovirus infection and mechanistic exploration of the antiviral activity of IFIT5. *Front. Microbiol.* **2022**, *13*, 998505. [CrossRef] [PubMed]
12. Huang, T.; Yu, J.; Luo, Z.; Yu, L.; Liu, S.; Wang, P.; Jia, M.; Wu, T.; Miao, W.; Zhou, L.; et al. Translatome analysis reveals the regulatory role of betaine in high fat diet (HFD)-induced hepatic steatosis. *Biochem. Biophys. Res. Commun.* **2021**, *575*, 20–27. [CrossRef] [PubMed]
13. Huang, T.; Yu, J.; Ma, Z.; Fu, Q.; Liu, S.; Luo, Z.; Liu, K.; Yu, L.; Miao, W.; Yu, D.; et al. Translatomics Probes into the Role of Lycopene on Improving Hepatic Steatosis Induced by High-Fat Diet. *Front. Nutr.* **2021**, *8*, 727785. [CrossRef] [PubMed]
14. Ingolia, N.T.; Ghaemmaghami, S.; Newman, J.R.; Weissman, J.S. Genome-wide analysis in vivo of translation with nucleotide resolution using ribosome profiling. *Science* **2009**, *324*, 218–223. [CrossRef]

15. Ingolia, N.T.; Lareau, L.F.; Weissman, J.S. Ribosome profiling of mouse embryonic stem cells reveals the complexity and dynamics of mammalian proteomes. *Cell* **2011**, *147*, 789–802. [CrossRef] [PubMed]
16. Ingolia, N.T. Ribosome profiling: New views of translation, from single codons to genome scale. *Nat. Rev. Genet.* **2014**, *15*, 205–213. [CrossRef]
17. Lian, X.; Guo, J.; Gu, W.; Cui, Y.; Zhong, J.; Jin, J.; He, Q.; Wang, T.; Zhang, G. Genome-Wide and Experimental Resolution of Relative Translation Elongation Speed at Individual Gene Level in Human Cells. *PLoS Genet.* **2016**, *12*, e1005901. [CrossRef]
18. Huang, T.; Yu, L.; Pan, H.; Ma, Z.; Wu, T.; Zhang, L.; Liu, K.; Qi, Q.; Miao, W.; Song, Z.; et al. Integrated Transcriptomic and Translatomic Inquiry of the Role of Betaine on Lipid Metabolic Dysregulation Induced by a High-Fat Diet. *Front. Nutr.* **2021**, *8*, 751436. [CrossRef]
19. Bazzini, A.A.; Lee, M.T.; Giraldez, A.J. Ribosome profiling shows that miR-430 reduces translation before causing mRNA decay in zebrafish. *Science* **2012**, *336*, 233–237. [CrossRef]
20. Zhang, H.; Dou, S.; He, F.; Luo, J.; Wei, L.; Lu, J. Genome-wide maps of ribosomal occupancy provide insights into adaptive evolution and regulatory roles of uORFs during Drosophila development. *PLoS Biol.* **2018**, *16*, e2003903. [CrossRef]
21. Xiong, Q.; Zhong, L.; Du, J.; Zhu, C.; Peng, X.; He, X.; Fu, J.; Ouyang, L.; Bian, J.; Hu, L.; et al. Ribosome profiling reveals the effects of nitrogen application translational regulation of yield recovery after abrupt drought-flood alternation in rice. *Plant Physiol. Bioch.* **2020**, *155*, 42–58. [CrossRef] [PubMed]
22. Juntawong, P.; Girke, T.; Bazin, J.; Bailey-Serres, J. Translational dynamics revealed by genome-wide profiling of ribosome footprints in Arabidopsis. *Proc. Natl. Acad. Sci. USA* **2014**, *111*, E203–E212. [CrossRef]
23. Lei, L.; Shi, J.; Chen, J.; Zhang, M.; Sun, S.; Xie, S.; Li, X.; Zeng, B.; Peng, L.; Hauck, A.; et al. Ribosome profiling reveals dynamic translational landscape in maize seedlings under drought stress. *Plant J.* **2015**, *84*, 1206–1218. [CrossRef] [PubMed]
24. Rosenberger, J.K.; Sterner, F.J.; Botts, S.; Lee, K.P.; Margolin, A. In vitro and in vivo characterization of avian reoviruses. I. Pathogenicity and antigenic relatedness of several avian reovirus isolates. *Avian Dis.* **1989**, *33*, 535–544. [CrossRef] [PubMed]
25. Roessler, D.E.; Rosenberger, J.K. In vitro and in vivo characterization of avian reoviruses. III. Host factors affecting virulence and persistence. *Avian Dis.* **1989**, *33*, 555–565. [CrossRef] [PubMed]
26. Fujita, T.; Kurihara, Y.; Iwasaki, S. The Plant Translatome Surveyed by Ribosome Profiling. *Plant Cell Physiol.* **2019**, *60*, 1917–1926. [CrossRef]
27. Dunn, J.G.; Foo, C.K.; Belletier, N.G.; Gavis, E.R.; Weissman, J.S. Ribosome profiling reveals pervasive and regulated stop codon readthrough in Drosophila melanogaster. *eLife* **2013**, *2*, e1179. [CrossRef]
28. Maier, T.; Guell, M.; Serrano, L. Correlation of mRNA and protein in complex biological samples. *FEBS Lett.* **2009**, *583*, 3966–3973. [CrossRef]
29. Ingolia, N.T.; Brar, G.A.; Rouskin, S.; McGeachy, A.M.; Weissman, J.S. The ribosome profiling strategy for monitoring translation in vivo by deep sequencing of ribosome-protected mRNA fragments. *Nat. Protoc.* **2012**, *7*, 1534–1550. [CrossRef]
30. Schafer, S.; Adami, E.; Heinig, M.; Rodrigues, K.; Kreuchwig, F.; Silhavy, J.; van Heesch, S.; Simaite, D.; Rajewsky, N.; Cuppen, E.; et al. Translational regulation shapes the molecular landscape of complex disease phenotypes. *Nat. Commun.* **2015**, *6*, 7200. [CrossRef]
31. Cabrera-Quio, L.E.; Herberg, S.; Pauli, A. Decoding sORF translation—From small proteins to gene regulation. *RNA Biol.* **2016**, *13*, 1051–1059. [CrossRef] [PubMed]
32. Araujo, P.R.; Yoon, K.; Ko, D.; Smith, A.D.; Qiao, M.; Suresh, U.; Burns, S.C.; Penalva, L.O. Before It Gets Started: Regulating Translation at the 5′ UTR. *Comp. Funct. Genom.* **2012**, *2012*, 475731. [CrossRef] [PubMed]
33. Chaudhury, A.; Hussey, G.S.; Howe, P.H. 3′-UTR-mediated post-transcriptional regulation of cancer metastasis: Beginning at the end. *RNA Biol.* **2011**, *8*, 595–599. [CrossRef] [PubMed]
34. Lin, H.Y.; Chuang, S.T.; Chen, Y.T.; Shih, W.L.; Chang, C.D.; Liu, H.J. Avian reovirus-induced apoptosis related to tissue injury. *Avian Pathol.* **2007**, *36*, 155–159. [CrossRef]
35. Mason, J.M.; Naidu, M.D.; Barcia, M.; Porti, D.; Chavan, S.S.; Chu, C.C. IL-4-induced gene-1 is a leukocyte L-amino acid oxidase with an unusual acidic pH preference and lysosomal localization. *J. Immunol.* **2004**, *173*, 4561–4567. [CrossRef] [PubMed]
36. Sadik, A.; Somarribas, P.L.; Ozturk, S.; Mohapatra, S.R.; Panitz, V.; Secker, P.F.; Pfander, P.; Loth, S.; Salem, H.; Prentzell, M.T.; et al. IL4I1 Is a Metabolic Immune Checkpoint that Activates the AHR and Promotes Tumor Progression. *Cell* **2020**, *182*, 1252–1270. [CrossRef] [PubMed]
37. Hu, X.; Chen, S.; Jia, C.; Xue, S.; Dou, C.; Dai, Z.; Xu, H.; Sun, Z.; Geng, T.; Cui, H. Gene expression profile and long non-coding RNA analysis, using RNA-Seq, in chicken embryonic fibroblast cells infected by avian leukosis virus J. *Arch. Virol.* **2018**, *163*, 639–647. [CrossRef]
38. Feng, M.; Xie, T.; Li, Y.; Zhang, N.; Lu, Q.; Zhou, Y.; Shi, M.; Sun, J.; Zhang, X. A balanced game: Chicken macrophage response to ALV-J infection. *Vet. Res.* **2019**, *50*, 20. [CrossRef]
39. Dong, K.; Chang, S.; Xie, Q.; Zhao, P.; Zhang, H. RNA Sequencing revealed differentially expressed genes functionally associated with immunity and tumor suppression during latent phase infection of a vv + MDV in chickens. *Sci. Rep.* **2019**, *9*, 14182. [CrossRef]
40. Marquet, J.; Lasoudris, F.; Cousin, C.; Puiffe, M.L.; Martin-Garcia, N.; Baud, V.; Chereau, F.; Farcet, J.P.; Molinier-Frenkel, V.; Castellano, F. Dichotomy between factors inducing the immunosuppressive enzyme IL-4-induced gene 1 (IL4I1) in B lymphocytes and mononuclear phagocytes. *Eur. J. Immunol.* **2010**, *40*, 2557–2568. [CrossRef]

41. Vazquez-Iglesias, L.; Lostale-Seijo, I.; Martinez-Costas, J.; Benavente, J. Avian reovirus σA localizes to the nucleolus and enters the nucleus by a nonclassical energy- and carrier-independent pathway. *J. Virol.* **2009**, *83*, 10163–10175. [CrossRef] [PubMed]
42. Gonzalez-Lopez, C.; Martinez-Costas, J.; Esteban, M.; Benavente, J. Evidence that avian reovirus σA protein is an inhibitor of the double-stranded RNA-dependent protein kinase. *J. Gen. Virol.* **2003**, *84*, 1629–1639. [CrossRef] [PubMed]
43. Xie, L.; Xie, Z.; Huang, L.; Fan, Q.; Luo, S.; Huang, J.; Deng, X.; Xie, Z.; Zeng, T.; Zhang, Y.; et al. Avian reovirus σA and σNS proteins activate the phosphatidylinositol 3-kinase-dependent Akt signalling pathway. *Arch. Virol.* **2016**, *161*, 2243–2248. [CrossRef] [PubMed]
44. Xie, L.; Wang, S.; Xie, Z.; Wang, X.; Wan, L.; Deng, X.; Xie, Z.; Luo, S.; Zeng, T.; Zhang, M.; et al. Gallus NME/NM23 nucleoside diphosphate kinase 2 interacts with viral σA and affects the replication of avian reovirus. *Vet. Microbiol.* **2021**, *252*, 108926. [CrossRef]
45. Shmulevitz, M.; Yameen, Z.; Dawe, S.; Shou, J.; O'Hara, D.; Holmes, I.; Duncan, R. Sequential partially overlapping gene arrangement in the tricistronic S1 genome segments of avian reovirus and Nelson Bay reovirus: Implications for translation initiation. *J. Virol.* **2002**, *76*, 609–618. [CrossRef]
46. Zhang, Z.; Lin, W.; Li, X.; Cao, H.; Wang, Y.; Zheng, S.J. Critical role of eukaryotic elongation factor 1 alpha 1 (EEF1A1) in avian reovirus sigma-C-induced apoptosis and inhibition of viral growth. *Arch. Virol.* **2015**, *160*, 1449–1461. [CrossRef]
47. Castellano, F.; Molinier-Frenkel, V. An Overview of l-Amino Acid Oxidase Functions from Bacteria to Mammals: Focus on the Immunoregulatory Phenylalanine Oxidase IL4I1. *Molecules* **2017**, *22*, 2151. [CrossRef]
48. Xiao, C.L.; Mai, Z.B.; Lian, X.L.; Zhong, J.Y.; Jin, J.J.; He, Q.Y.; Zhang, G. FANSe2: A robust and cost-efficient alignment tool for quantitative next-generation sequencing applications. *PLoS ONE* **2014**, *9*, e94250. [CrossRef]
49. Mortazavi, A.; Williams, B.A.; McCue, K.; Schaeffer, L.; Wold, B. Mapping and quantifying mammalian transcriptomes by RNA-Seq. *Nat. Methods* **2008**, *5*, 621–628. [CrossRef]
50. Robinson, M.D.; McCarthy, D.J.; Smyth, G.K. edgeR: A Bioconductor package for differential expression analysis of digital gene expression data. *Bioinformatics* **2010**, *26*, 139–140. [CrossRef]
51. Wang, T.; Cui, Y.; Jin, J.; Guo, J.; Wang, G.; Yin, X.; He, Q.; Zhang, G. Translating mRNAs strongly correlate to proteins in a multivariate manner and their translation ratios are phenotype specific. *Nucleic Acids Res.* **2013**, *41*, 4743–4754. [CrossRef] [PubMed]
52. Li, G.W.; Burkhardt, D.; Gross, C.; Weissman, J.S. Quantifying absolute protein synthesis rates reveals principles underlying allocation of cellular resources. *Cell* **2014**, *157*, 624–635. [CrossRef] [PubMed]
53. He, Y.; Xie, Z.; Dai, J.; Cao, Y.; Hou, J.; Zheng, Y.; Wei, T.; Mo, M.; Wei, P. Responses of the Toll-like receptor and melanoma differentiation-associated protein 5 signaling pathways to avian infectious bronchitis virus infection in chicks. *Virol. Sin.* **2016**, *31*, 57–68. [CrossRef] [PubMed]

viruses

MDPI

Article

Comparison of Infectious Bronchitis Virus (IBV) Pathogenesis and Host Responses in Young Male and Female Chickens

Ishara M. Isham [1], Reham M. Abd-Elsalam [1,2], Motamed E. Mahmoud [1,3], Shahnas M. Najimudeen [1], Hiruni A. Ranaweera [1], Ahmed Ali [1,4], Mohamed S. H. Hassan [1,5], Susan C. Cork [1], Ashish Gupta [1] and Mohamed Faizal Abdul-Careem [1,*]

1. Health Research Innovation Center 2C53, Faculty of Veterinary Medicine, University of Calgary, 3330 Hospital Drive NW, Calgary, AB T2N 4N1, Canada; fathimaishara.muhamm@ucalgary.ca (I.M.I.); reham.abdelsalam1@ucalgary.ca (R.M.A.-E.); motamed.ali@ucalgary.ca (M.E.M.); fathimashahnas.moham@ucalgary.ca (S.M.N.); hiruni.ranaweera@ucalgary.ca (H.A.R.); ahmed.ali@ucalgary.ca (A.A.); msh.hassan@ucalgary.ca (M.S.H.H.); sccork@ucalgary.ca (S.C.C.); ashish.gupta1@ucalgary.ca (A.G.)
2. Faculty of Veterinary Medicine, Cairo University, Giza 12211, Egypt
3. Department of Animal Husbandry, Faculty of Veterinary Medicine, Sohag University, Sohag 82524, Egypt
4. Department of Pathology, Beni-Suef University, Beni Suef 62521, Egypt
5. Department of Avian and Rabbit Medicine, Faculty of Veterinary Medicine, Assiut University, Assiut 71515, Egypt

* Correspondence: faizal.abdulcareem@ucalgary.ca; Tel.: +1-403-220-4462

Abstract: Infectious bronchitis virus (IBV) is an avian coronavirus that causes a disease in chickens known as infectious bronchitis (IB). The pathogenesis of IBV and the host immune responses against it depend on multiple factors such as the IBV variant, breed and age of the chicken, and the environment provided by the management. Since there is limited knowledge about the influence of the sex of chickens in the pathogenesis of IBV, in this study we aim to compare IBV pathogenesis and host immune responses in young male and female chickens. One-week-old specific pathogen-free (SPF) White Leghorn male and female chickens were infected with Canadian Delmarva (DMV)/1639 IBV variant at a dose of 1×10^6 embryo infectious dose $(EID)_{50}$ by the oculo-nasal route while maintaining uninfected controls, and these chickens were euthanized and sampled 4- and 11-days post-infection (dpi). No significant difference was observed between the infected male and female chickens in IBV shedding, IBV genome load in the trachea, lung, kidney, bursa of Fabricius (BF), thymus, spleen, and cecal tonsils (CT), and IBV-induced lesion in all the examined tissues at both 4 and 11 dpi. In addition, there was no significant difference in the percentage of IBV immune-positive area observed between the infected male and female chickens in all tissues except for the kidney, which expressed an increased level of IBV antigen in infected males compared with females at both 4 and 11 dpi. The percentage of B lymphocytes was not significantly different between infected male and female chickens in all the examined tissues. The percentage of CD8+ T cells was not significantly different between infected male and female chickens in all the examined tissues except in the trachea at 11 dpi, where female chickens had higher recruitment when compared with male chickens. Overall, although most of the findings of this study suggest that the sex of chickens does not play a significant role in the pathogenesis of IBV and the host immune response in young chickens, marginal differences in viral replication and host responses could be observed to indicate that IBV-induced infection in male chickens is more severe.

Keywords: infectious bronchitis virus (IBV); male chicken; female chicken; pathogenesis; immune response

check for updates

Citation: Isham, I.M.; Abd-Elsalam, R.M.; Mahmoud, M.E.; Najimudeen, S.M.; Ranaweera, H.A.; Ali, A.; Hassan, M.S.H.; Cork, S.C.; Gupta, A.; Abdul-Careem, M.F. Comparison of Infectious Bronchitis Virus (IBV) Pathogenesis and Host Responses in Young Male and Female Chickens. *Viruses* **2023**, *15*, 2285. https://doi.org/10.3390/v15122285

Academic Editor: Chi-Young Wang

Received: 27 October 2023
Revised: 17 November 2023
Accepted: 20 November 2023
Published: 22 November 2023

1. Introduction

Infectious bronchitis virus (IBV) is an avian gamma coronavirus that belongs to the order Nidovirales, family Coronoviridae, and subfamily Orthocoronavirinae, and it causes infectious bronchitis (IB) [1]. IBV was first reported in North Dakota, United States of America (USA), in young chickens [2]. Although both the chicken (*Gallus gallus*) and pheasant (*Phasianus* spp.) are reported to be natural hosts of IBV, clinical IBV infections are predominantly reported in chickens [3]. IB is common and has a high morbidity; hence, it is one of the most frequently reported diseases in chickens. Furthermore, reports state that IB is second only to highly pathogenic avian influenza (HPAI) virus infection in terms of poultry diseases causing a significant impact on the global economy [4]. HPAI may be more frequently reported as it is a regulated and reportable disease. In addition, the emergence of new strains of IB and the failure of current vaccines to provide efficient and effective cross-protection to these new strains has led to an increase in the occurrence of IB in poultry farms. Hence, IB is one of the major challenges faced by the poultry industry, and major steps are used to control the spread of IB in order to prevent any significant economic losses [5]. Therefore, a better understanding of the pathogenesis of IBV and the immune responses generated against IBV is essential to combat IB. The pathogenesis of IBV and the host's immune responses against it depend on multiple factors such as the characteristics of the pathogen (IBV), host (chicken), and environment.

The pathogenesis of IBV in chickens depends on the different variants of the virus, as different variants can lead to different tropisms of IBV and differing levels of severity of the disease. The gene coding for the spike (S)1 glycoprotein, which is the IBV receptor-binding domain (RBD), is a highly variable region in the IBV genome [6,7]. Hence, variations in the S1 protein can determine the virulence and tissue tropism of IBV as tissue tropism is determined by the avidity of the S1 protein to the α 2,3-linked sialic acid receptors in the host tissues [6,7]. The previous literature demonstrates that IBV is a multisystem disease that affects respiratory, reproductive, and renal tract tissues [8,9]. Some studies have also reported that IBV could infect the lymphoid organs of chickens [5,10,11]. In addition to the tropism of the virus, several comparative studies have demonstrated that the virulence of the virus differs between different variants within the respiratory [12,13], reproductive [14,15], and renal [16,17] systems. Studies have also described that the nutrition provided to chickens and their environmental conditions such as temperature, air quality, and light could also play some roles in the susceptibility of chickens to IBV infection [18,19].

Previously, it was shown that the age and breed of a chicken could play a role in the pathogenesis of IBV. Chickens of all ages are susceptible to IBV infection, but the severity of the disease is higher in younger chickens [20]. Studies report that with an increase in the age of chickens, the immune response and, thereby, the resistance to IBV infection and pathogenesis increases, hence resulting in lower IBV-induced nephropathic effects [16,20] and oviduct lesions [15]. However, another study by Macdonald and colleagues reported that younger chickens had a higher resistance to IBV than older chickens [21]. Another major factor of the host that could determine the pathogenesis of IBV is the breed of the chicken. Several experimental studies have demonstrated that the breed of the chicken could play a decisive role in susceptibility to IBV infection [18,22,23]. One such study reported that line 151 chickens are more susceptible to IBV M41 infection in comparison with line C White Leghorn chickens [23]. Another study reported that higher mortality was observed in IBV-infected broilers compared with layers [9].

A few studies have reported that the sex of a chicken could play a role in susceptibility to Arkansas (Ark), Australian T, and Australian N1/88 strains of IBV infection. A report by Cumming in 1969 stated that the susceptibility of male chickens is two-fold higher than that of female chickens [18]. In addition, a study in broiler chickens disclosed that female chickens developed immune responses faster than males by measuring the production of antibodies using a hemagglutination-inhibition assay and by evaluating antigen-specific T-lymphocyte proliferation experiments. Hence, the authors predicted that this difference in the rate of immune response development could be the leading cause of higher susceptibility to IBV infection in males [24]. Their study further stated that the mortality rate in male chickens was significantly higher than that of female chickens [24]. In another study on broiler chickens, female chickens had a higher phagocytic activity compared with male chickens, indicating that the innate immune response in females is more efficient than that observed in males [25]. However, a study on 18-day-old White Leghorn chickens hatched from specific-pathogen-free (SPF) fertile eggs reported that there was no significant difference in Ark-type IBV pathogenesis between sexes by assessing the viral load in the trachea and cecal tonsil (CT) and by assessing tracheal histomorphometry [26].

The existence of a relationship between steroid sex hormones and host immune response in humans, mice, and birds has been proclaimed [27–29]. It is widely suggested that sex hormones such as testosterone have an immunosuppressive effect, while estrogen has an immunoenhancing effect in hosts. A recent meta-analysis by Foo and colleagues in 2016 supported the past literature indicating that steroid sex hormones in males and females may affect immune responses in opposite directions, where testosterone in males resulted in an immunosuppressive effect while estrogen in females had an immunoenhancing effect [30]. Another review further reported that sex hormones could impact the strength of immune responses in males and females, where females demonstrated a stronger immune response than males [31]. In addition, a report on humans, rodents, and birds stated that estrogen stimulates humoral and cell-mediated immune responses in females, while testosterone has an opposite function in males [29]. Moreover, a study on broiler chicken demonstrated that the administration of estradiol 3-benzoate resulted in enhanced immune responses against *Escherichia coli* (*E. coli*) and sheep erythrocytes [24].

In recent years, a high incidence of the Delmarva (DMV)/1639 variant of IBV has been reported in layer flocks of Eastern Canada [32,33]. The DMV/1639 IBV causes cystic oviducts and false layer syndrome outbreaks in layers [34]. It is also responsible for a 30% drop in egg production in adult hens during the peak of lay [35]. Hence, it is imperative to study the factors that influence the pathogenesis of DMV/1639 in chickens. There is a scarcity of knowledge regarding the role of the sex of chickens in the pathogenesis of IBV infection and host immune response. Moreover, there are no studies comparing the pathogenicity of DMV/1639 IBV variants in young male and female chickens. Hence, in this study, we aimed to compare the IBV pathogenesis and host immune responses in young male and female chickens.

2. Materials and Methods

2.1. Virus

The Canadian IBV DMV/1639 strain (IBV/Ck/Can/17-036989) isolated from the kidney tissues of 22-week-old-infected chickens in a commercial layer flock in Eastern Canada was used as the challenge virus in this study [33]. The propagation of this viral strain was conducted by inoculating the allantoic cavities of 9-day-old SPF embryonated chicken eggs and harvesting the allantoic fluid 48 h post-inoculation after incubation (37.6 °C at 60% relative humidity from day 1 to 18 and 37.2 °C at 70% relative humidity from day 19 to 21). Following this, the virus was titrated, as previously described [34,35], where the 50% chicken embryo infectious dose (EID_{50}) of the virus was calculated using the Reed and Muench method [36].

2.2. Experimental Animals

White Leghorn SPF one-day-old chickens were purchased from the Canadian Food Inspection Agency (CFIA), in Ottawa, Ontario, Canada, and they were sexed as described in Section 2.3. The male (number of chicken/n = 20) and female (n = 20) chickens were housed in two separate isolators at the Veterinary Science Research Station (VSRS) facility at the Spy Hill campus, University of Calgary. The chickens were allowed to adapt to the new environment for 6 days by providing feed and lighting according to the recommended management guidelines. The Veterinary Science Animal Care Committee (VSACC) of the University of Calgary provided ethical approval for this work (Protocol number: AC19-0011).

2.3. Sex Determination in Chickens

The sex of the chickens was determined using a conventional polymerase chain reaction (PCR) assay, as previously described by He and colleagues, with some modifications [37]. Briefly, deoxyribonucleic acid (DNA) was extracted from the feather follicles of the chickens using a commercial DNA extraction kit (Qiagen, Hilden, North Rhine-Westphalia, Germany). The extracted DNA was amplified in a CFX 96-c1000 Thermocycler (Bio- Rad Laboratories, Mississauga, ON, Canada), where each reaction volume consisted of 2.5 µL 10X PCR buffer, 0.75 µL 50 mM $MgCl_2$, 0.5 µL 10 mM dNTP, 0.5 µL 10 mM forward primer, 0.5 µL 10 mM reverse primer, and 0.1 µL of Taq DNA polymerase (ThermoFisher Scientific, Wilmington, DE, USA). The thermal profile for the amplification was, initial denaturation at 94 °C for 2 min; and 35 cycles of amplification with 30 s of denaturation at 94 °C, and 30 s of annealing at 55 °C and 30 s of elongation at 72 °C, followed by a final extension at 72 °C for 5 min. The forward and reverse primers used targeted the SWIM gene located on the W sexual chromosome, hence serving as a specific marker for females. The sequences of the forward and reverse primers were 5′GAGATCACGAACTCAACCAG-3′ and 5′CCAGACCTAATACGGTTTTACAG-3′, respectively [37]. Following the amplification of DNA, the PCR products were analyzed using agarose gel electrophoresis as described by He and colleagues [37].

2.4. Experimental Design

One-week-old male and female chickens were each randomly divided into two groups and housed in four separate isolators. One group of male and female chickens ($n = 10$ per each group) were challenged with 100 µL of the IBV DMV/1639 strain at a dose of 1×10^6 EID_{50} by the oculo-nasal route, while the other group of male and female chickens were mock challenged with 100 µL of phosphate-buffered saline (PBS, Invitrogen Canada Inc., Burlington, ON, Canada) and maintained as uninfected controls. At 4 and 11 days post-infection (dpi), 1 mL of blood was collected from a randomly selected subset of chicken ($n = 5$) from the four experimental groups for the separation of serum. In addition, oropharyngeal (OP) and cloacal (CL) swabs were procured from the chicken from all the groups and were stored in 1 mL aliquots of cold PBS. Isoflurane anesthesia was performed on the chickens before euthanizing them by cervical dislocation. Subsequently, trachea, lung, kidney, bursa of Fabricius (BF), thymus, CTs, and spleen tissue samples were collected in ribonucleic acid (RNA) Save® (Invitrogen Canada Inc., Burlington, ON, Canada) for extraction of RNA and in 10% neutral buffered formalin (VWR International, Edmonton, AB, Canada) for histopathology. The separated serum samples were stored at −20 °C, while the swab and tissue samples collected for RNA extraction were stored at −80 °C until further processing. The tissue samples fixed in 10% neutral buffered formalin were stored at room temperature.

2.5. Techniques

2.5.1. Enzyme-Linked Immunosorbent Assay (ELISA)

The ELISA performed to quantify the serum anti-IBV antibody titer in chicken was performed with a commercial ELISA kit (IDEXX Laboratories, Inc., Westbrook, ME, USA). The ELISA was carried out according to the manufacturer's instructions, and the antibody titers were calculated using the formula provided by the manufacturer. Accordingly, the titers above 396 (cut-off) were considered positive.

2.5.2. RNA Extraction and cDNA Synthesis

The Trizol LS® reagent (Invitrogen Canada Inc., Burlington, ON, Canada) and the Trizol reagent (Invitrogen Canada Inc., Burlington, ON, Canada) were used in accordance with the manufacturer's instructions to extract RNA from swab and tissue samples, respectively. Then, the amount of extracted RNA was quantified at 260 nm wavelength with a Nanodrop 1000 spectrophotometer (ThermoFisher Scientific, Wilmington, DE, USA). Complementary DNA (cDNA) was synthesized using 1000 ng of RNA from swab samples and 2000 ng of RNA from tissue samples with the RT random primers high-capacity cDNA reverse transcriptase kit (Invitrogen Life Technologies, Carlsbad, CA, USA) following the manufacturer's guidelines.

2.5.3. IBV Genome Load Quantification

The quantification of IBV genome load in swab and tissue cDNA samples was performed with quantitative PCR (qPCR) assay using Fast SYBR® Green Master Mix (Quntabio®, Beverly, MA, USA). Each reaction volume incorporated 10 μL of SYBR Green master mix, 100 ng of interested cDNA sample, 0.5 μL 10 μM of forward primer, 0.5 μL 10 μM of reverse primer, and molecular biology-grade water to reach a final reaction volume of 20 μL. The qPCR assays were performed in a CFX 96-c1000 Thermocycler (Bio-Rad Laboratories, Mississauga, ON, Canada) with a thermal profile of 20 s of initial denaturation at 95 °C, 40 cycles of amplification with 3 s of denaturation at 95 °C, and 30 s of annealing at 60 °C. The forward and reverse primers used in this qPCR assay were 5′GACGGAGGACCTGATGGTAA-3′ and 5′CCCTTCTTCTGCTGATCCTG-3′, respectively, and they were targeted against the conserved IBV N gene [38].

2.5.4. Immunohistochemistry (IHC)

IHC was performed on the paraffin sections of the tissue samples to quantify IBV nucleoprotein, CD8+ cells, and B cells. IHC was performed as previously described [10]. Briefly, the paraffin tissue sections on positively charged slides (VWR International, Radnor, PA, USA) were deparaffinized with xylene and then rehydrated in a descending serial concentration of alcohol. Subsequently, the endogenous peroxidase activity of the tissue specimens was blocked by incubating them in a 3% H_2O_2 solution in methanol for 10 min at room temperature. Following this, the viral epitopes in the tissue sections were unmasked by microwaving the sections at 850 W for 10–15 min with a 10 mM citrate buffer at pH 6.0. Then, the tissue sections were incubated overnight at 4 °C in a humidified chamber with the respective primary antibody. The mouse primary anti-IBV nucleoprotein antibody (Novus Biological, Bio-Techne, Toronto, ON, Canada) targeting the IBV antigen in cells, mouse anti-chicken CD8a antibody (SouthernBiotech, Birmingham, AL, USA) targeting the CD8 positive cells in tissues, and mouse anti-chicken Bu-1 antibody (SouthernBiotech, Birmingham, AL, USA) targeting the Bu-1 positive cells in tissues at dilutions of 1:400, 1:100, and 1:200 in PBS, respectively, were used for IHC staining. Succeeding this the tissue sections were incubated with goat anti-mouse IgG (H + L) secondary antibody (Vector Laboratories Inc., Newark, CA, USA) for 1 h at room temperature. Then, an ABC peroxidase kit and a 3,3′-Diaminobenzidine (DAB) substrate solution (Vector Laboratories, Newark, CA, USA) were used according to the manufacturer's instructions to detect antibody binding. Washing of the tissue sections with Tris-buffered saline (TBS) for 5 min was performed following all the incubation steps described above. Then, the slides were counterstained with hematoxylin (Vector Laboratories, Newark, CA, USA) for 8 min, and bluing was accomplished by running the tissue sections under tap water for 30 min. Then, the tissue sections were dehydrated and cleaned with an ascending series of alcohol and xylene, respectively. The tissue sections were mounted in a toluene mounting solution (Vector Laboratories, Newark, CA, USA) and cover-slipped.

2.5.5. Histopathology

The formalin-fixed tissue samples were sent to the Diagnostic Services Unit (DSU) at the University of Calgary, Faculty of Veterinary Medicine (UCVM), to prepare paraffin-embedded tissue blocks and hematoxylin–eosin (H&E)-stained tissue sections. The H&E stained tissue sections were examined under the light microscope (Olympus BX51, Center Valley, PA, USA) for histopathological lesions and scored as previously described with some modifications [39]. Each organ was scored based on several criteria, and the scoring system was performed as follows: normal (0), mild (1), moderate (2), and severe (3) for each criterion. Then, the total score was calculated for each organ per group.

2.6. Statistical Analyses

The IBV genome load in swabs and tissues, percentage of IBV antigen, and histopathological lesion scores between the four groups were compared using the Kruskal–Wallis test followed by Dunn's multiple comparisons test. The percentage of B (Bu-1+) and T (CD8+) lymphocytes in the tissues were compared with ordinary one-way ANOVA followed by Tukey's multiple comparisons test. All the statistical analyses were performed with GraphPad Prism 9.2.0 Software (GraphPad Software, San Diego, CA, USA), and this software was also used to generate graphs. All the IHC images at 20× magnification stained for the IBV antigen were analyzed with Image J analyzer software version 1.46a (National Institute of Health, Bethesda, MD, USA). The immunostained B (Bu-1+) and T (CD8+) lymphocytes were counted at 20× magnification, and the percentage of positive cells was calculated relative to the total nuclei in each field using Fiji software as per the prior description [40]. For the analysis of all IHC images, five different fields from each tissue section were photographed and then analyzed.

3. Results

3.1. Clinical Manifestations

Only the DMV/1639-infected males showed clinical signs such as a mild increase in respiration at 4 dpi. Furthermore, the DMV1639-infected male or female birds did not reach the endpoints in the DMV/1639-infected male and female chickens during the period of this experiment.

3.2. Anti-IBV Antibody Titer

In all four experimental groups, the anti-IBV antibody titers in the serum were observed to be within the negative range (<396) at both 4 and 11 dpi.

3.3. Viral Shedding

The IBV genome was not detected in OP and CL swabs from uninfected male and female chickens at 4 and 11 dpi, while it was detected in the IBV-challenged chickens (Figure 1). A statistically significant difference in IBV genome load was not observed between the infected male and female chickens in the viral shedding via OP and CL swabs at 4 and 11 dpi (Figure 1, $p > 0.05$).

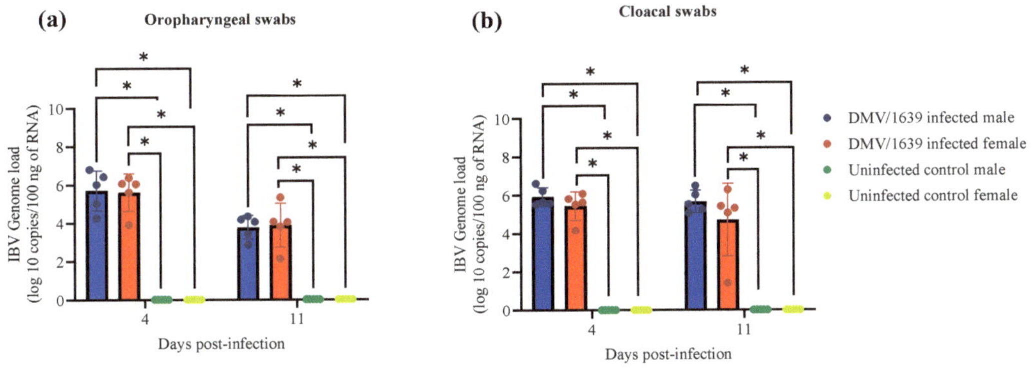

Figure 1. IBV genome load in (**a**) OP and (**b**) CL swabs at 4 and 11 dpi following infection with the Canadian DMV/1639 strain (IBV/Ck/Can/17–036989) of IBV. The average starting IBV genome load was quantified per 100 ng of the extracted RNA, and a comparison between groups was performed using the Kruskal–Wallis test followed by Dunn's multiple comparisons test. The error bars represent the standard deviation (SD). Statistical significance: * $p < 0.05$.

3.4. IBV Genome Loads in Tissues

The IBV genome was not detected with qPCR assays in all target organs of the uninfected male and female control chickens at both 4 and 11 dpi, thus stipulating no other source of IBV challenge (Figure 2). In addition, a significant difference in quantified IBV genome load was not demonstrated in all the targeted organs of the DMV/1639-infected male and female chickens at 4 and 11 dpi (Figure 2, $p > 0.05$).

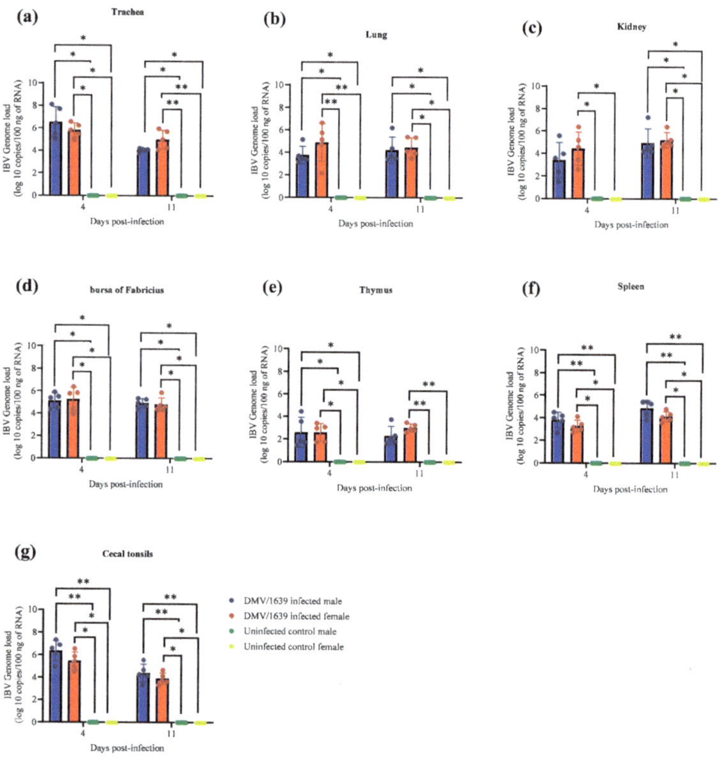

Figure 2. IBV genome loads in (**a**) trachea, (**b**) lung, (**c**) kidney, (**d**) bursa of Fabricius, (**e**) thymus, (**f**) spleen, and (**g**) cecal tonsils at 4 and 11 dpi following challenge with the Canadian DMV/1639 strain of IBV. The average starting IBV genome load was quantified per 100 ng of the extracted RNA, and a comparison between groups was performed using the Kruskal–Wallis test followed by Dunn's multiple comparisons test. The error bars represent the SD. Statistical significance: * $p < 0.05$, ** $p < 0.01$.

3.5. IBV Antigen in Tissues

IBV immune-positive staining was not observed in all the target organs of the uninfected male and female control chickens at both 4 and 11 dpi (Figures 3–6). On the contrary, immune-positive staining of IBV nucleoprotein was observed in the trachea, lung, kidney, BF, and CTs of DMV/1639-infected male and female chickens at 4 and 11 dpi (Figures 3–6). The cells exhibiting IBV nucleoprotein revealed intra-cytoplasmic, brown fine to coarse crumbs, and IBV immune-positive cells were mostly distributed in the epithelial lining of the mucosa, renal tubular epithelium, and macrophages. The percentage of IBV immune-positive areas in the kidney of infected male chickens was significantly higher than that in infected female chickens at 4 and 11 dpi (Figure 3, $p < 0.05$). However, no significant difference was detected in the percentage of IBV immune-positive areas of the trachea, lung, BF, and CTs between DMV/1639-infected male and female chickens at 4 and 11 dpi (Figure 3, $p > 0.05$). Moreover, immune-positive staining of IBV nucleoprotein was not observed in the spleen or thymus of DMV/1639-infected male and female chickens at 4 and 11 dpi.

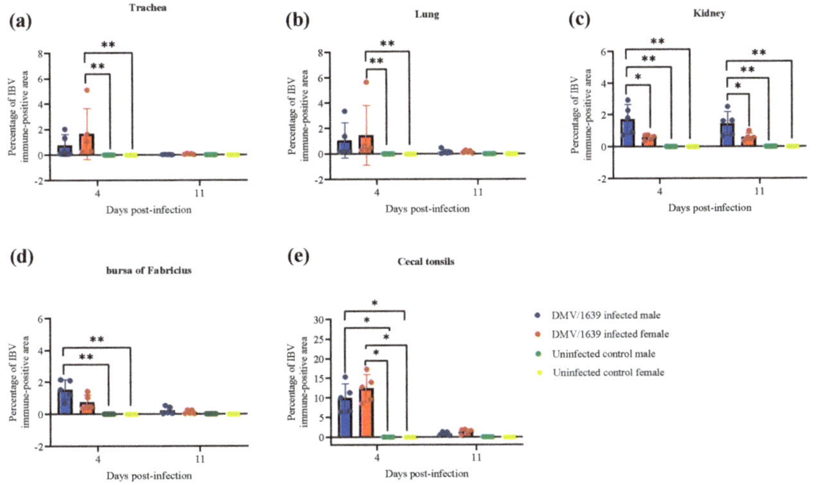

Figure 3. Percentage of IBV immune-positive area for IBV nucleoprotein in the (**a**) trachea, (**b**) lung, (**c**) kidney, (**d**) bursa of Fabricius, and (**e**) cecal tonsils at 4 and 11 dpi following challenge with the Canadian DMV/1639 strain of IBV. The comparison between groups was performed using the Kruskal–Wallis test followed by the Dunn's multiple comparisons test, and the error bars represent the SD. Statistical significance: * $p < 0.05$ and ** $p < 0.01$.

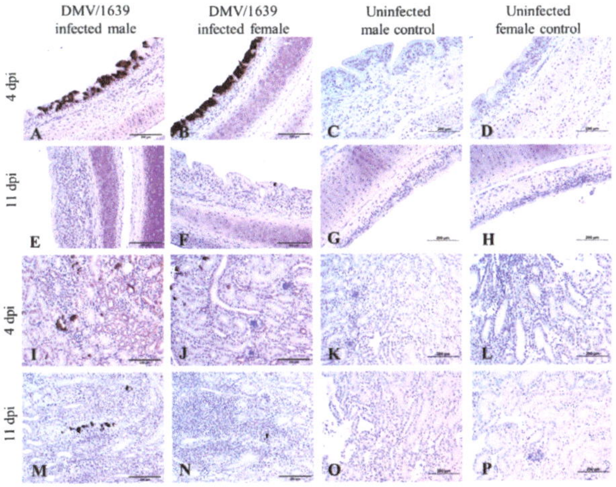

Figure 4. Photomicrograph of IBV nucleoprotein in the trachea and kidney. (**A–D**) Trachea of IBV DMV/1639-infected male, IBV DMV/1639-infected female, uninfected control male, and uninfected control female chickens at 4 dpi, respectively. (**E–H**) Trachea of IBV DMV/1639-infected male, IBV DMV/1639-infected female, uninfected control male, and uninfected control female chickens at 11 dpi, respectively. (**I–L**) Kidney of IBV DMV/1639-infected male, IBV DMV/1639-infected female, uninfected control male, and uninfected control female chickens at 4 dpi, respectively. (**M–P**) Kidney of IBV DMV/1639-infected male, IBV DMV/1639-infected female, uninfected control male, and uninfected control female chickens at 11 dpi, respectively.

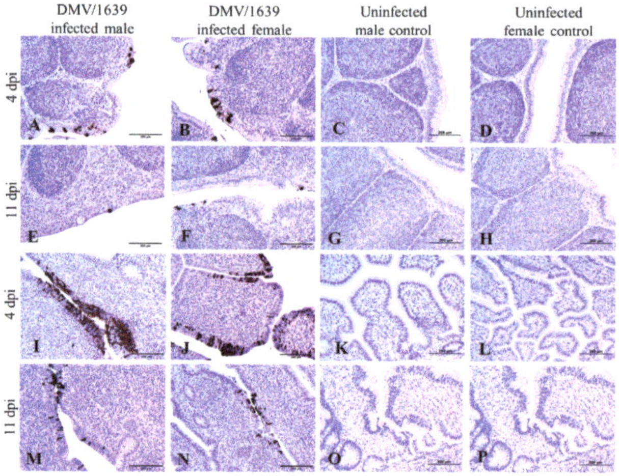

Figure 5. Photomicrograph of IBV nucleoprotein in the bursa of Fabricius and cecal tonsils. (**A–D**) bursa of Fabricius of IBV DMV/1639-infected male, IBV DMV/1639-infected female, uninfected control male, and uninfected control female chickens at 4 dpi, respectively. (**E–H**) bursa of Fabricius of IBV DMV/1639-infected male, IBV DMV/1639-infected female, uninfected control male, and uninfected control female chickens at 11 dpi, respectively. (**I–L**) Cecal tonsils of IBV DMV/1639-infected male, IBV DMV/1639-infected female, uninfected control male, and uninfected control female chickens at 4 dpi, respectively. (**M–P**) Cecal tonsils of IBV DMV/1639-infected male, IBV DMV/1639-infected female, uninfected control male, and uninfected control female chickens at 11 dpi, respectively.

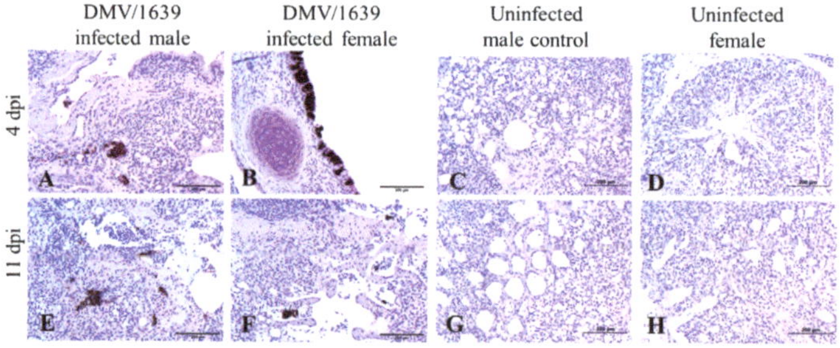

Figure 6. Photomicrograph of IBV nucleoprotein in the lung. (**A–D**) The lungs of IBV DMV/1639-infected male, IBV DMV/1639-infected female, uninfected control male, and uninfected control female chickens at 4 dpi, respectively. (**E–H**) The lungs of IBV DMV/1639-infected male, IBV DMV/1639-infected female, uninfected control male, and uninfected control female chickens at 11 dpi, respectively. The 4 dpi lung section of a female DMV1639-infected chicken shows a primary bronchus within lung tissue.

3.6. Histopathology

The control uninfected male and female chickens at 4 and 11 dpi revealed normal histological architecture of the trachea, lung, kidney, thymus, spleen, BF, and CTs (Figure 7). IBV-induced lesions were observed in the trachea, lung, kidney, BF, and CTs of IBV-challenged male and female chickens, and there was no significant difference recorded in lesion scores between male and female IBV DMV/1639-infected chickens at 4 and 11 dpi (Figure 7, $p > 0.05$). IBV-induced lesions were not observed in the thymus or spleen of both IBV DMV/1639-infected male and female chickens at 4 and 11 dpi.

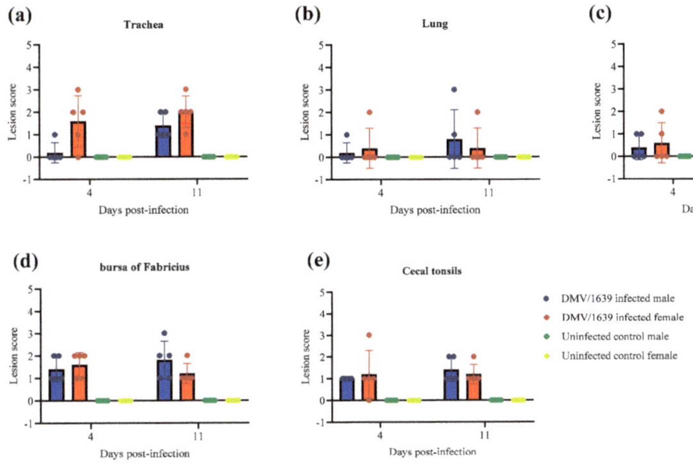

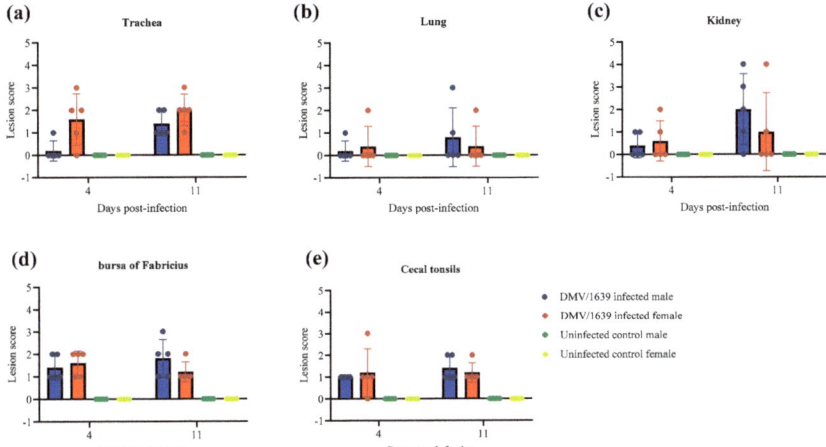

Figure 7. Lesion scores in the (**a**) trachea, (**b**) lung, (**c**) kidney, (**d**) bursa of Fabricius, and (**e**) cecal tonsils at 4 and 11 dpi following challenge with the Canadian IBV DMV/1639 strain. The comparison between groups was performed using the Kruskal–Wallis test followed by Dunn's multiple comparisons test, and the error bars represent the SD.

The male and female IBV DMV/1639-infected chickens showed mild to moderate tracheal lesions at 4 dpi in the form of loss of cilia, degeneration and necrosis of columnar epithelium, mucus cell gland depletion, and lymphocytic infiltration in the mucosa and submucosa (Figure 8A,B). While at 11 dpi, the trachea showed focal areas of epithelium loss with alternated areas of epithelium and mucus cell gland hyperplasia and mononuclear cell infiltration in the mucosa and submucosa, leading to an increase in tracheal thickness (Figure 8E,F).

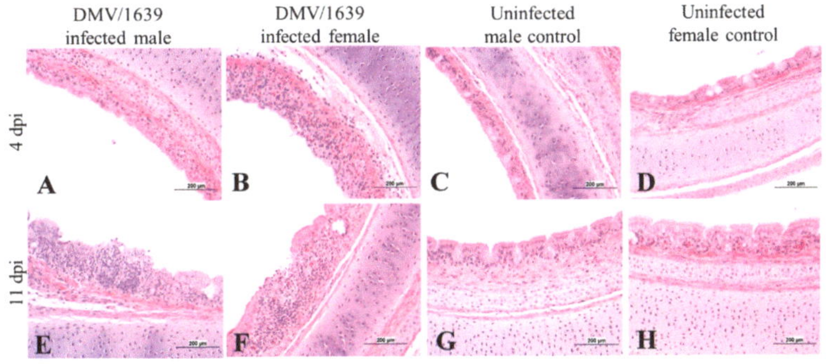

Figure 8. Photomicrographs of the trachea of (**A**) an IBV DMV/1639-infected male chicken at 4 dpi, (**B**) an IBV DMV/1639-infected female chicken at 4 dpi showing loss of cilia, degeneration, and necrosis of the epithelial lining, and mucosal and submucosal inflammatory cell infiltration, (**C**) an uninfected control male chicken at 4 dpi, and (**D**) an uninfected control female chicken at 4 dpi showing a normal histological picture, (**E**) an IBV DMV/1639-infected male at 11 dpi showing hyperplasia of the epithelial lining and focal area of epithelial necrosis with mucosal mononuclear cell aggregation, (**F**) an IBV DMV/1639-infected female chicken at 11 dpi showing focal epithelial loss with mucosal mononuclear inflammatory cell infiltration, (**G**) an uninfected control male chicken at 11 dpi, and (**H**) an uninfected control female chicken at 11 dpi.

The histopathological changes in the lungs of both male and female infected chickens were minimal at 4 dpi with more severe lesions at 11 dpi (Figure 9A,B,E,F). Moderate bronchitis was detected in two male chickens and one female chicken in the IBV DMV/1639-infected groups at 11 dpi (Figure 9E,F).

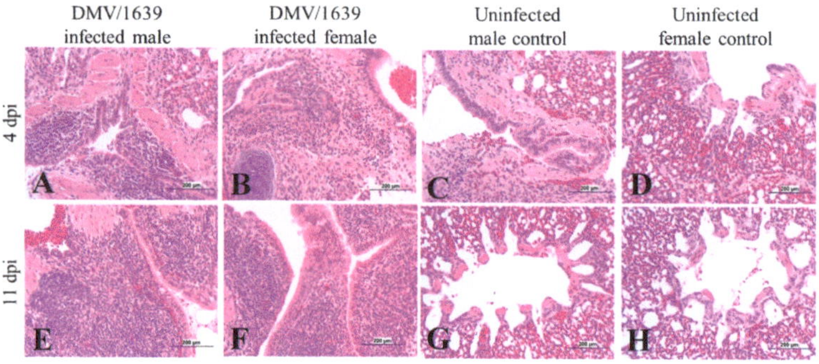

Figure 9. Photomicrographs of the lung of (**A**) IBV DMV/1639-infected male chicken at 4 dpi, (**B**) IBV DMV/1639-infected female chicken at 4 dpi showing mild bronchitis, (**C**) an uninfected control male chicken at 4 dpi, (**D**) an uninfected control female chicken at 4 dpi showing a normal histological picture, (**E**) an IBV DMV/1639-infected male chicken at 11 dpi, (**F**) an IBV DMV/1639-infected female chicken at 11 dpi showing moderate bronchitis, (**G**) an uninfected control male chicken at 11 dpi, and (**H**) an uninfected control female chicken at 11 dpi.

The male and female infected chickens exhibited mild renal tubular degeneration with focal aggregation of lymphoplasmocytes in the interstitial tissue of the kidney at 4 dpi (Figure 10A,B). However, moderate to severe lymphoplasmocytic interstitial nephritis was observed in both male and female infected chickens at 11 dpi (Figure 10E,F).

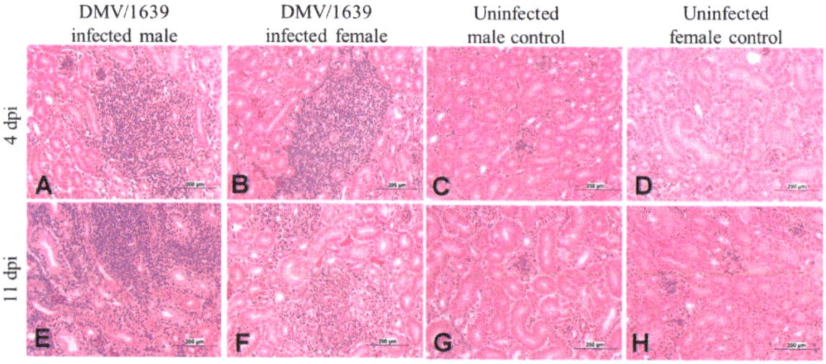

Figure 10. Photomicrographs of the kidney of (**A**) an IBV DMV/1639-infected male chicken at 4 dpi, (**B**) an IBV DMV/1639-infected female chicken at 4 dpi showing focal interstitial nephritis, (**C**) an uninfected control male chicken at 4 dpi, (**D**) an uninfected control female chicken at 4 dpi showing a normal histological architecture, (**E**) an IBV DMV/1639-infected male chicken at 11 dpi, (**F**) an IBV DMV/1639-infected female chicken at 11 dpi showing diffuse lymphoplasmocytic interstitial nephritis, (**G**) an uninfected control male chicken at 11 dpi, and (**H**) uninfected control female chicken at 11 dpi.

The BF of male and female IBV DMV/1639-infected chickens exhibited mild to moderate histopathological changes at 4 and 11 dpi (Figure 11A,B,E,F). Mild to moderate lining epithelial cells hyperplasia, with degeneration and necrosis of some cells, epithelial and subepithelial infiltration with heterophils, lymphocytes, and macrophages were recorded at 4 dpi (Figure 11A,B). Moreover, the expansion of interfollicular and subepithelial tissues with edema and mononuclear cells and mild lymphoid depletion were also recorded. The nature of the BF lesions at 11 dpi was less severe (Figure 11E,F).

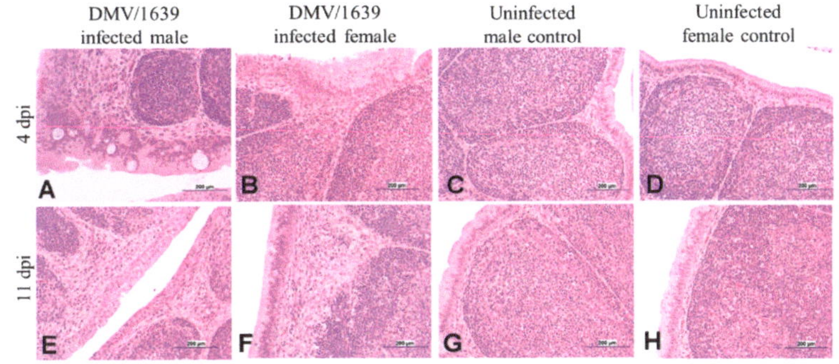

Figure 11. Photomicrographs of the bursa of Fabricius of (**A**) an IBV DMV/1639-infected male chicken at 4 dpi showing severe hyperplasia of lining epithelium with squamous cell metaplasia with ballooning and degeneration of some cells, (**B**) an IBV DMV/1639-infected female chicken at 4 dpi showing hyperplasia and squamous cell metaplasia of the plical lining epithelium, (**C**) an uninfected control male chicken at 4 dpi, (**D**) an uninfected control female chicken at 4 dpi showing normal epithelial lining and lymphoid follicles, (**E**) an IBV DMV/1639 infected male chicken at 11 dpi, (**F**) an IBV DMV/1639 infected female chicken at 11 dpi showing marked expansion of sub-epithelial and interfollicular tissue with mononuclear inflammatory cells, (**G**) uninfected control male chicken at 11 dpi, and (**H**) an uninfected control female chicken at 11 dpi.

The histopathological examination of the CTs of IBV DMV/1639-infected chickens revealed mild to moderate lymphoepithelial necrosis with sub-epithelial mononuclear cell aggregation, lymphoidal apoptosis, and lymphoidal depletion in interfollicular area at 4 and 11 dpi (Figure 12A,B,E,F).

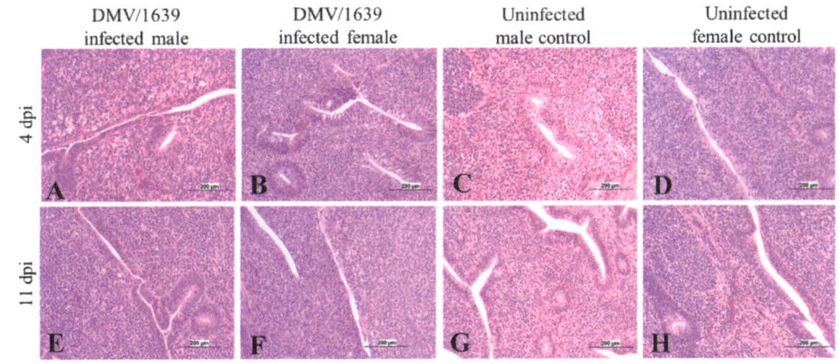

Figure 12. Photomicrograph of the cecal tonsils of (**A**) an IBV DMV/1639-infected male chicken at 4 dpi showing degeneration and necrosis of lining epithelium with vacuolation of sub-epithelial mononuclear cells, (**B**) an IBV DMV/1639-infected female chicken at 4 dpi showing mild degeneration of the epithelium, (**C**) an uninfected control male at 4 dpi, (**D**) an uninfected control female chicken at 4 dpi showing normal epithelial lining and lymphoid follicles, (**E**) an IBV DMV/1639-infected male chicken at 11 dpi, (**F**) an IBV DMV/1639 infected female chicken at 11 dpi show mild epithelial degeneration and necrosis, (**G**) an uninfected control male chicken at 11 dpi, and (**H**) an uninfected control female at 11 dpi.

3.7. Immunohistochemical Staining of B (BU-1+) and T (CD+8) Cells

Figure 13 illustrates the percentage of B lymphocytes in the trachea, lung, kidney, CT, spleen, BF, and thymus of IBV-infected groups. No significant difference in B lymphocyte percentage was observed between the uninfected control male and female groups and the IBV-infected male and female groups in the trachea and lung at 4 dpi and in the kidney at both 4 and 11 dpi (Figure 13, $p > 0.05$). The percentage of B lymphocytes in the trachea and lung at 11 dpi was significantly higher in the IBV-infected male and female groups compared with the uninfected control male and female groups (Figure 13, $p < 0.05$). In addition, no significant difference was observed in the percentage of B lymphocytes in the trachea, lung, and kidney of IBV-infected male and female chickens (Figure 13, $p > 0.05$). In the BF, IBV-infected male and female chickens showed a significant reduction in the percentage of B lymphocytes compared with uninfected control male and female chickens (Figure 13, $p < 0.01$) at 11 dpi. However, a significant difference was not observed in the percentage of B lymphocytes in the BF of IBV-infected male and female chicken at 4 and 11 dpi (Figure 13, $p > 0.05$). Similarly, there was no significant difference in the percentage of B lymphocytes in the CT, spleen, and thymus between IBV-infected male and female chicken at both 4 and 11 dpi (Figure 13, $p > 0.05$). Figure S1 illustrates the distribution of B lymphocytes in all the examined tissues, and these B lymphocytes are stained brown and are indicated by arrows in the figures.

The percentages of T (CD8+) lymphocytes in the trachea, lung, kidney, BF, CTs, spleen, and thymus of the IBV-infected groups are demonstrated in Figure 14. A significant difference in the CD8+ T cell percentage was not discerned between the IBV-infected male and female groups and the uninfected control male and female groups in the lung and BF at both 4 and 11 dpi (Figure 14, $p > 0.05$). In addition, there was no statistically significant difference in the CD8+ T cell percentage in the IBV-infected male and female groups in comparison with the uninfected control male and female groups at 11 dpi in the kidney, CTs, spleen, and thymus (Figure 14, $p > 0.05$). Furthermore, a significantly higher percentage of CD8+ T cells were recorded in IBV-infected male and female chickens in comparison with uninfected control male and female chickens at 4 dpi in the trachea, CTs, and thymus (Figure 14, $p < 0.05$). The percentage of CD8+ T cells in IBV-infected female chickens was significantly higher in comparison with uninfected control male and female chickens at 4 dpi in the spleen, whilst the CD8+ T cell percentage in IBV-infected male was significantly higher than in the uninfected control female chickens at 4 dpi in the kidney (Figure 14, $p < 0.05$). However, there was no significant difference in the percentage of CD8+ T cells recorded between IBV-infected male and female chickens in all the tissues of interest at both 4 and 11 dpi except for the trachea (Figure 14, $p > 0.05$). The recruitment of CD8+ T cells in the IBV-infected female chickens was significantly higher than that in the IBV-infected male chickens in the trachea at 11 dpi (Figure 14, $p < 0.05$), whilst there was no significant difference in the levels of CD8+ T cells between IBV-infected male and female chickens in the trachea at 4 dpi (Figure 14, $p > 0.05$). Figure S2 shows the distribution of CD8+ T lymphocytes in all the examined tissues, and these CD8+ T lymphocytes are stained brown and are indicated by arrows in the figures.

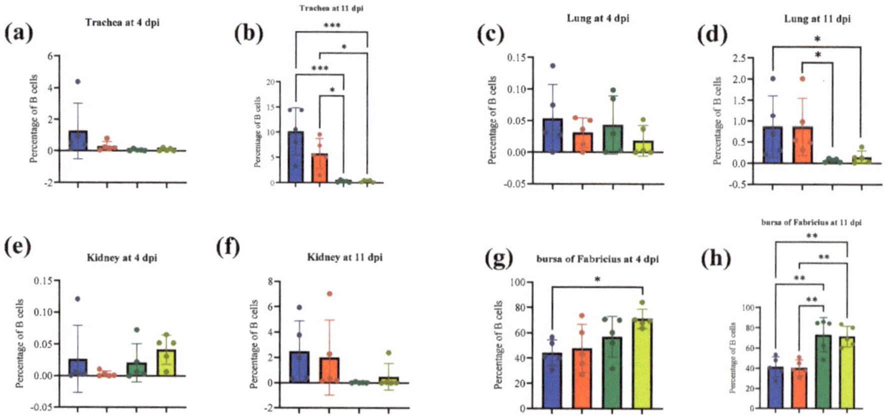

Figure 13. *Cont.*

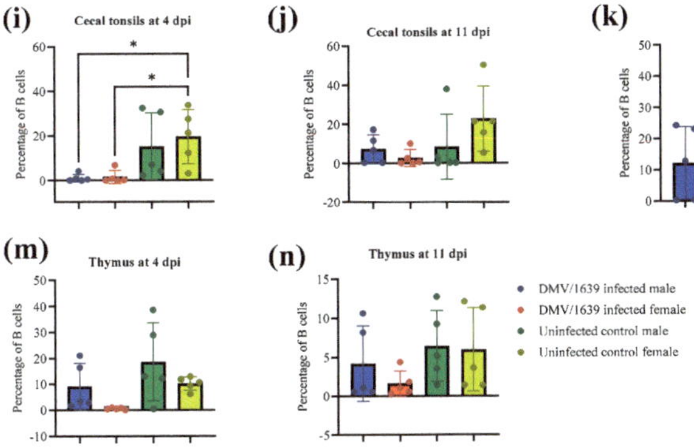

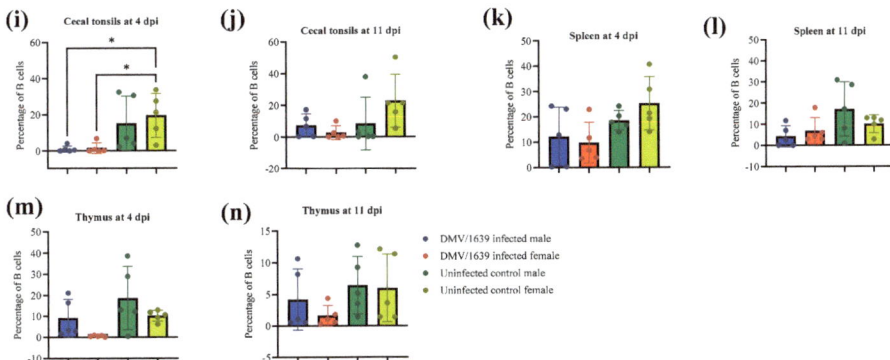

Figure 13. Percentage of B (BU-1+) cells in tissues infected with Canadian IBV DMV/1639 strain in male and female chickens and uninfected control male and female chickens at 4 and 11 dpi. (**a**,**b**) trachea, (**c**,**d**) lung, (**e**,**f**) kidney, (**g**,**h**) bursa of Fabricius, (**i**,**j**) cecal tonsils, (**k**,**l**) spleen and (**m**,**n**) thymus. The comparison between groups was performed using one-way ANOVA followed by Turkey's multiple comparisons test, and the error bars represent the SD. Statistical significance: * $p < 0.05$, ** $p < 0.01$ and *** $p < 0.001$.

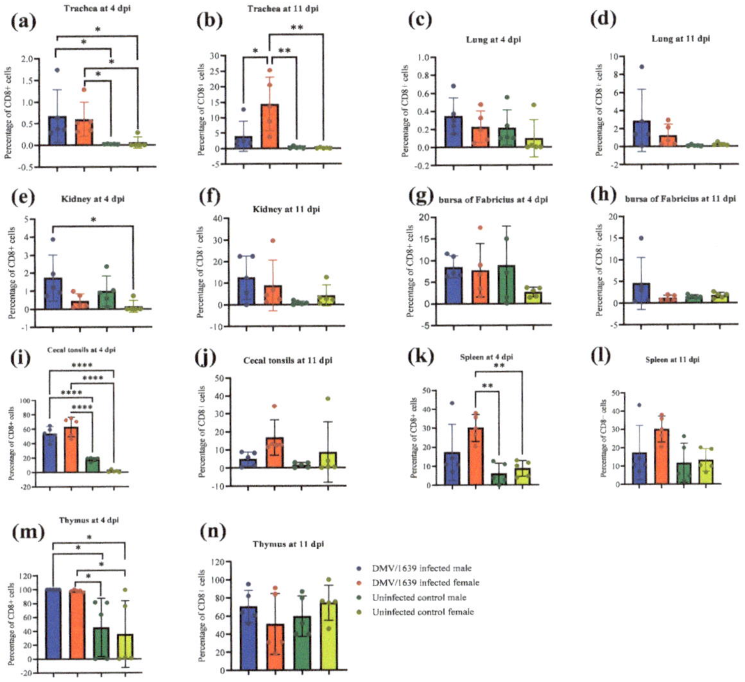

Figure 14. Percentage of T (CD8+) cells in tissues infected with the Canadian IBV DMV/1639 strain in male and female chickens and uninfected control male and female chickens at 4 and 11 dpi: (**a**,**b**) trachea, (**c**,**d**) lung, (**e**,**f**) kidney, (**g**,**h**) bursa of Fabricius, (**i**,**j**) cecal tonsils, (**k**,**l**) spleen, and (**m**,**n**) thymus. The comparison between groups was performed using one-way ANOVA followed by Turkey's multiple comparisons test, and the error bars represent the SD. Statistical significance: * $p < 0.05$, ** $p < 0.01$, and **** $p < 0.0001$.

4. Discussion

Due to its high rate of morbidity and challenges with disease control, IBV poses a significant economic threat to the poultry industry [4]. In addition, the prevalence of the DMV/1639 IBV strain in poultry farms in Eastern Canada has become alarmingly high [32,33]. Hence it is essential to understand the factors that govern the pathogenesis of the DMV/1639 IBV strain in chickens. Therefore, in this study, we aimed to determine if the sex of a chicken plays a role in the pathogenesis of DMV/1639 IBV and host immune responses in young male and female chickens. The results of this study were multifold. There was no significant difference in IBV genome load detected between DMV/1639 infected male and female chickens in viral shedding via OP and CL swabs and in tissue samples from all the targeted organs at both 4 and 11 dpi. Although no significant difference was detected in the percentage of IBV immune-positive areas of the trachea, lung, BF, and CTs between DMV/1639-infected male and female chickens at 4 and 11 dpi, the percentage of IBV immune-positive areas in the kidney tissues of infected male chickens was significantly higher than that of infected female chickens. In addition, no significant difference in IBV-induced lesion scores was detected between DMV/1639-infected male and female chicken at 4 and 11 dpi for all the targeted tissues. Furthermore, there was no significant difference in host response in terms of recruitment of B lymphocytes in all the tissues of interest at both 4 and 11 dpi. Moreover, the percentage of CD8+ T cells was not significantly different between infected male and female chickens in all the examined tissues except in the trachea at 11 dpi, where female chickens had higher recruitment of CD8+ T cells when compared with male chickens.

Although there are several previous studies determining the impact that the IBV variant [12–17], age of chicken [16,20,21], and breed of chicken [9,18,22,23] have on the pathogenesis of IBV, there are very limited studies examining the role that the sex of a chicken plays in the pathogenesis of IBV and host immune response. In order to determine the role that the sex of a chicken plays in the pathogenesis of IBV and the subsequent immune response against the virus, we maintained all the other influencing factors at constant values. Hence, the breed and age of the chickens, the time of challenge, and the dose of IBV were kept the same between the infected male and female chickens. In addition, the condition of the isolators that housed these chickens and the feed and water were also maintained as uniformly as possible throughout the duration of the experiment for both male and female chickens. Furthermore, in order to minimize the variation in susceptibility to IBV, purebred White Leghorn chickens were used in this experiment instead of a crossbred chicken line, similar to a previous study aiming to investigate if sex influences the pathogenesis of IBV [26].

The anti-IBV antibody titers in the serum of all the experimental groups were within the negative range at both 4 and 11 dpi. The negative results in the IBV-infected male and female chickens at 4 dpi could be because the antibody-mediated immune response in chickens only starts at 4–5 dpi and the level of anti-IBV antibody in serum at this time will be very low [41,42]. In addition, the anti-IBV antibody titers in the serum of infected male and female chickens at 11 dpi were also negative. This could be because the birds in this study are very young, and hence, the amount of antibody produced by these birds will be low. ELISA has a comparatively lower assay sensitivity, and this could be a reason for obtaining negative results for infected chickens at 11 dpi [43]. In future studies, different commercial ELISA kits other than the kit used in this study could be used to quantify the anti-IBV antibody titers in the serum of young chickens.

In terms of viral shedding, there was no statistically significant difference in the IBV genome load between the infected male and female chickens in both OP and CL swabs at 4 and 11 dpi. Although a few studies have reported a significant difference in IBV pathogenesis in the trachea of male and female chickens, these studies did not analyze viral shedding from the infected chickens [26,44]. Hence, this study provides some preliminary data comparing the IBV genome load in male and female chickens during the shedding of the virus. In addition, a significant difference was not observed in the IBV genome load between infected male and female chickens in the trachea, lung, kidney, BF, thymus, spleen, and CTs at both 4 and 11 dpi. In agreement, a previous study performed on 18-day-old White Leghorn chickens infected with the Ark type IBV variant also reported that there was no significant difference in the IBV genome load in the CTs between infected male and female chickens at 5 dpi [26]. However, in contrast to our finding, that study further reported that male chickens exhibited significantly higher viral loads in the trachea than that in females at 5 dpi [26]. This difference in the findings of the IBV genome load data in the two studies could be due to the difference in the IBV challenge strain (IBV DMV1639 vs. IBV Ark) and the dose used in the two studies.

To further determine the replication of IBV in the examined tissues, we stained the tissues for IBV nucleoprotein and analyzed the percentage of immune-positive areas with Image J software. In general, IBV antigen staining in the trachea was more intense than in the kidney tissues (Figure 4). In the trachea, lung, BF and CTs, a significant difference was not detected in the percentage of IBV immune-positive areas in DMV/1639-infected male and female chickens at 4 and 11 dpi. However, the percentage of IBV immune-positive areas in the kidney of infected male chickens was significantly higher than that in infected female chickens at 4 and 11 dpi. This lower percentage of IBV antigen in females could be due to the ability of females to prevent initial IBV infection. However, further studies are necessary to conclude if males are more susceptible to IBV DMV/1639 infection in kidney tissues compared with females. Since there are no past studies comparing and quantifying the distribution of IBV antigen in tissues of infected male and female chickens, this study provides some important preliminary data to design future studies. In this study, we observed a discrepancy in the detection of the IBV genome load and IBV antigen in the examined tissues. There was no significant difference in the IBV genome load between infected male and female chickens in all the examined tissues at both 4 and 11 dpi, while a higher expression of IBV antigen was observed in infected male chickens compared with the infected females in the kidney at 4 and 11 dpi. Furthermore, although the IBV genome was detected in all the examined tissues, the IBV antigen was not detected in the spleen or thymus of infected chickens. This discrepancy is not alarming since the qPCR technique detects both replicating and non-replicating IBV in tissues, while the immunohistochemistry technique detects only the IBV antigen expressed by the replicating IBV [45,46]. In addition, since the qPCR technique has a higher sensitivity compared with the immunohistochemistry technique, some tissues positive for the IBV viral genome could be negative for the IBV antigen [47,48].

Furthermore, histopathology was performed to compare IBV-induced lesions in the trachea, lung, kidney, BF, and CTs, and we observed no significant difference in the lesion scores between IBV DMV/1639-infected male and female chickens at 4 and 11 dpi. In agreement with these results, a previous study observing and comparing the tracheal histomorphometry in terms of mucosal thickness and lymphocyte infiltration in the trachea of IBV-infected male and female chickens reported that there was no significant difference in both the thickness of the tracheal mucosa and lymphocytic infiltration in trachea between the two sexes [26]. However, another study on 65-week-old hens and cockerels, challenged with T and N1/88 Australian IBV strains, reported that the cockerels had more severe tracheal lesions in terms of edema in mucosa and alveolar mucous gland hypertrophy compared with the hens [44]. That study further stated that there was no significant difference in lymphocytic infiltration in the trachea of the challenged hens and cockerels [44]. The contradiction between the results of that study and our study could be due to the difference in the age of chickens during the IBV challenge and the difference in the IBV strains used for the challenge (IBV DMV1639 vs IBV Australian T and N1/88). Moreover, similar to the observations of our study, that study also reported that no significant difference was observed in the histopathological lesions between male and female chickens in the kidneys [44].

The host immune response in chickens during an IBV infection is mediated by innate and adaptive immune responses. The adaptive immune response is essential to reduce and control an IBV infection in tissues, clearance of IBV, and the reduction in the shedding of

IBV [49]. Several previous studies have reported the recruitment of lymphocytes in the target organs following IBV infection [13,35,50]. In this study, the recruitment of B and T lymphocytes in the target organs was examined and compared between IBV DMV/1639-infected male and female chickens. Recruitment of B lymphocytes in the trachea and lung was illustrated with the significant increase in the percentage of B cells at 11 dpi in IBV-infected male and female chickens compared with uninfected control male and female chickens. This could be indicative of the initiation of an adaptive immune response in chickens and the lymphocyte infiltration in infected tissues [51]. On the contrary, a significant decline was noted in the percentage of B cells in BF of IBV DMV/1639 infected male and female chickens compared with the uninfected controls at both 4 and 11 dpi. A prior study reported similar observations of depleted B cells in the BF of IBV-infected birds due to indirect follicular destruction in the BF [52]. However, no significant difference was discovered in the percentage of B cells at 4 and 11 dpi between IBV DMV/1639-infected male and female chickens in all the tissues of interest at both 4 and 11 dpi. These findings could indicate that there is no difference in the B cell response mounted by the chicken based on sex. Since there are no past studies comparing the recruitment of B cells in male and female chickens, the results of this study could be used as basic data to design future studies to investigate the difference in host immune response in male and female chickens.

Cytotoxic T cells (CD8+ T-cells) are essential in eliminating IBV-infected cells during an infection [53]. The influx of CD8+ T cells at the site of IBV infection to control the replication and spread of the virus has been documented in the past literature [35,49,54]. A significantly higher percentage of CD8+ T cells were recorded in IBV-infected male and female chickens in comparison with uninfected control male and female chickens at 4 dpi in the trachea, CTs, and thymus in this study. These observations are in agreement with the findings reported in previous studies, which showed increased levels of recruitment of CD8+ T cells in the kidney of infected birds from 3 dpi onward [49,55]. Moreover, no significant difference was revealed in the percentage of CD8+ T cells between IBV-infected male and female chickens at both 4 and 11 dpi in all the examined tissues except for the trachea. This could suggest that no significant difference exists in the host immune response against IBV infection in most organs. Although there are no prior studies examining and comparing the recruitment of CD8+ T cells in IBV-infected male and female chickens, a study by Leitner and colleagues described that there was no significant difference in the T cells in peripheral blood lymphocytes in infected male and female chickens [24]. However, in our study, in the trachea of IBV-infected female chickens, the recruitment of CD8+ T cells was significantly higher than that in IBV-infected male chickens at 11 dpi. This observation is in support of some previous studies that reported that males are more susceptible to viral infection than females [18,24].

This study presented some evidence to indicate a difference in the pathogenesis of IBV DMV/1639 in male and female chickens due to the presence of increased levels of IBV antigen in the kidneys of infected male chickens compared with females at 4 and 11 dpi and in the host immune response due to the presence of comparatively higher levels of CD8+ T cell recruitment in the trachea of infected females compared with males at 11 dpi. However, these findings alone are not sufficient to suggest that chickens of different sexes respond differently to an IBV infection. Moreover, the vast majority of the findings of this study advocate that the sex of a chicken does not play a role in the pathogenesis of IBV or in the host immune response in young chickens up to 18 days of age. Further studies comparing the pathogenesis and immune response in chickens of different ages and breeds challenged with different doses and variants of IBV are essential to conclude if sex plays a role in influencing the pathogenesis of IBV and immune response against IBV in chickens.

The difference in the IBV antigen and CD8+ T cells found in males and females must be investigated in the future to determine if male chickens are more susceptible to IBV DMV1639 infection compared with female chickens, as this could have implications for the transmission of IBV in poultry farms where both male and female chickens are housed together for the purpose of breeding. If males are more susceptible to IBV infection, they could facilitate the transmission of IB in commercial flocks when housed together in both layer and broiler chickens. Hence, an understanding of the gender difference in IBV susceptibility is imperative for the control of IBV in the poultry industry in Canada and globally. The vast majority of IBV genome load, IBV antigen, and histopathology data presented in this study, in addition to the B and T cell recruitment results, suggest that the sex of a chicken does not play an influential role in the pathogenesis of IBV and the host immune response against IBV infection in young chickens. These preliminary data could encourage researchers to use young male chickens for experimental purposes such as infection studies and vaccine efficacy studies instead of or with females and avoid euthanasia of male chickens. Reports from the Food and Agriculture Organization of the United Nations suggest that every year, around 6 billion day-old male chickens are euthanized all over the world as they are considered futile products [37]. This is raising ethical concerns in both the poultry and research industry. Hence, the use of young male chickens instead of or with females for suitable research regarding IBV tropism, IBV pathogenesis, and vaccination trials could be a viable solution to this ethical concern. However, in comparison with the 6 billion day-old male chickens euthanized every year, only a small number of male chickens could be used as experimental animals in studies. Therefore, the use of male chickens in experiments does not completely solve this ethical problem. Moreover, most experiments require adult chickens, and this study assessed a gender difference in IBV susceptibility in older chickens. Hence, future studies must be conducted to compare the pathogenicity of IBV and host immune response against IBV infection in adult male and female chickens.

In conclusion, a marginal difference was observed between the IBV DMV/1639 infected male and female chickens in the viral replication and host responses and these observations agree with previous observations of susceptivity of males for IBV infection [24,44]. Further studies are necessary to elucidate if the increased severity of IBV infection in males is dependent on the infecting IBV strain.

Supplementary Materials: The following supporting information can be downloaded at: https://www.mdpi.com/article/10.3390/v15122285/s1, Figure S1: Immunohistochemical detection of B (Bu-1+) lymphocytes in the trachea (A), lung (B), kidney (C), cecal tonsils (D), spleen (E), bursa of Fabricius (F), and thymus (G) collected at 4 and 11 dpi following infection with the Canadian IBV DMV/1639 strain. Bu-1+ cells were stained with deep brown (indicated with black arrows). Scale bar = 50 μm; Figure S2: Immunohistochemical detection of CD8+ cells in the trachea (H), lung (I), kidney (J), cecal tonsils (K), spleen (L), bursa of Fabricius (M), and thymus (N) collected 4- and 11-days following infection with the Canadian IBV DMV/1639 strain. CD8+ cells were stained with deep brown (indicated with black arrows). Scale bar = 50 μm.

Author Contributions: Conceptualization, M.F.A.-C.; methodology, M.F.A.-C.; formal analysis, I.M.I. and R.M.A.-E.; investigation, I.M.I., R.M.A.-E., M.E.M., S.M.N., H.A.R., A.A., M.S.H.H. and M.F.A.-C.; resources, M.F.A.-C.; writing—original draft preparation, I.M.I.; writing—review and editing, M.F.A.-C., S.C.C. and A.G.; supervision, M.F.A.-C., S.C.C. and A.G.; project administration, M.F.A.-C.; funding acquisition, M.F.A.-C. All authors have read and agreed to the published version of the manuscript.

Funding: This research was funded by Agriculture and Agri Food Canada via Canadian Poultry Research Council Poultry Science Cluster 3 funding (grant number 10025097), Egg Farmers of Canada funding (grant number 10022788) and the Natural Science and Engineering Council of Canada (grant application number RGPIN-2023-03364).

Institutional Review Board Statement: Ethical approval for the proposed work was obtained from the Veterinary Science Animal Care Committee (VSACC) of the University of Calgary (Protocol number: AC19-0011, approved on the 19th of March 2019).

Informed Consent Statement: Not applicable.

Data Availability Statement: The datasets used and/or analyzed within the frame of this study will be provided by the corresponding author upon reasonable request.

Acknowledgments: We would like to thank the University of Guelph for kindly providing us with the IBV-infected samples. We acknowledge the help of staff including Greg Boorman at the Veterinary Science Research Station at Spy Hill campus, University of Calgary for animal management.

Conflicts of Interest: The authors declare no conflict of interest.

References

1. Woo, P.C.Y.; de Groot, R.J.; Haagmans, B.; Lau, S.K.P.; Neuman, B.W.; Perlman, S.; Sola, I.; van der Hoek, L.; Wong, A.C.P.; Yeh, S.H. ICTV Virus Taxonomy Profile: Coronaviridae 2023. *J. Gen. Virol.* **2023**, *104*, 001843. [CrossRef]
2. Schalk, A.F.; Hawn, M.C. An Apparently New Respiratory Disease of Baby Chicks. *J. Am. Vet. Med. Assoc.* **1931**, *78*, 413–423.
3. Cavanagh, D.; Mawditt, K.; Welchman Dde, B.; Britton, P.; Gough, R.E. Coronaviruses from pheasants (*Phasianus colchicus*) are genetically closely related to coronaviruses of domestic fowl (infectious bronchitis virus) and turkeys. *Avian Pathol.* **2002**, *31*, 81–93. [CrossRef]
4. TAFS-Forum. *World Livestock Disease Atlas a Quantitative Analysis of Global Animal Health Data (2006–2009)*; The World Bank: Washington, DC, USA, 2011.
5. Ambali, A.G.; Jones, R.C. Early pathogenesis in chicks of infection with an enterotropic strain of infectious bronchitis virus. *Avian Dis.* **1990**, *34*, 809–817. [CrossRef]
6. Barnard, D.L. Coronaviruses: Molecular and Cellular Biology. *Future Virol.* **2008**, *3*, 119–123. [CrossRef]
7. Wickramasinghe, I.N.; de Vries, R.P.; Gröne, A.; de Haan, C.A.; Verheije, M.H. Binding of avian coronavirus spike proteins to host factors reflects virus tropism and pathogenicity. *J. Virol.* **2011**, *85*, 8903–8912. [CrossRef]
8. Bande, F.; Arshad, S.S.; Omar, A.R.; Bejo, M.H.; Abubakar, M.S.; Abba, Y. Pathogenesis and Diagnostic Approaches of Avian Infectious Bronchitis. *Adv. Virol.* **2016**, *2016*, 4621659. [CrossRef]
9. Ignjatovic, J. Epidemiology of infectious bronchitis in Australia. In Proceedings of the 1st International Symposium on Infectious Bronchitis, Rauischholzhausen, Germany, 23–26 June 1988; p. 84.
10. Isham, I.M.; Hassan, M.S.H.; Abd-Elsalam, R.M.; Ranaweera, H.A.; Mahmoud, M.E.; Najimudeen, S.M.; Ghaffar, A.; Cork, S.C.; Gupta, A.; Abdul-Careem, M.F. Impact of Maternal Antibodies on Infectious Bronchitis Virus (IBV) Infection in Primary and Secondary Lymphoid Organs of Chickens. *Vaccines* **2023**, *11*, 1216. [CrossRef]
11. Najimudeen, S.M.; Abd-Elsalam, R.M.; Ranaweera, H.A.; Isham, I.M.; Hassan, M.S.H.; Farooq, M.; Abdul-Careem, M.F. Replication of infectious bronchitis virus (IBV) Delmarva (DMV)/1639 variant in primary and secondary lymphoid organs leads to immunosuppression in chickens. *Virology* **2023**, *587*, 109852. [CrossRef]
12. Cubillos, A.; Ulloa, J.; Cubillos, V.; Cook, J.K. Characterisation of strains of infectious bronchitis virus isolated in Chile. *Avian Pathol.* **1991**, *20*, 85–99. [CrossRef]
13. Raj, G.D.; Jones, R.C. An in vitro comparison of the virulence of seven strains of infectious bronchitis virus using tracheal and oviduct organ cultures. *Avian Pathol.* **1996**, *25*, 649–662. [CrossRef]
14. Cook, J.K.; Huggins, M.B. Newly isolated serotypes of infectious bronchitis virus: Their role in disease. *Avian Pathol.* **1986**, *15*, 129–138. [CrossRef]
15. Crinion, R.A.; Hofstad, M.S. Pathogenicity of four serotypes of avian infectious bronchitis virus for the oviduct of young chickens of various ages. *Avian Dis.* **1972**, *16*, 351–363. [CrossRef]
16. Albassam, M.A.; Winterfield, R.W.; Thacker, H.L. Comparison of the nephropathogenicity of four strains of infectious bronchitis virus. *Avian Dis.* **1986**, *30*, 468–476. [CrossRef]
17. Chandra, M. Comparative nephropathogenicity of different strains of infectious bronchitis virus in chickens. *Poult Sci.* **1987**, *66*, 954–959. [CrossRef]
18. Cumming, R.B. The control of avian infectious bronchitis/nephrosis in Australia. *Aust. Vet. J.* **1969**, *45*, 200–203. [CrossRef]
19. Hofmann, T.; Schmucker, S.S.; Bessei, W.; Grashorn, M.; Stefanski, V. Impact of Housing Environment on the Immune System in Chickens: A Review. *Animals* **2020**, *10*, 1138. [CrossRef]
20. Animas, S.B.; Otsuki, K.; Tsubokura, M.; Cook, J.K. Comparison of the susceptibility of chicks of different ages to infection with nephrosis/nephritis-causing strain of infectious bronchitis virus. *J. Vet. Med. Sci.* **1994**, *56*, 449–453. [CrossRef]
21. Macdonald, J.W.; Randall, C.J.; McMartin, D.A. An inverse age resistance of chicken kidneys to infectious bronchitis virus. *Avian Pathol.* **1980**, *9*, 245–259. [CrossRef]
22. Bumstead, N.; Huggins, M.B.; Cook, J.K. Genetic differences in susceptibility to a mixture of avian infectious bronchitis virus and Escherichia coli. *Br. Poult. Sci.* **1989**, *30*, 39–48. [CrossRef]
23. Nakamura, K.; Cook, J.K.; Otsuki, K.; Huggins, M.B.; Frazier, J.A. Comparative study of respiratory lesions in two chicken lines of different susceptibility infected with infectious bronchitis virus: Histology, ultrastructure and immunohistochemistry. *Avian Pathol.* **1991**, *20*, 241–257. [CrossRef]
24. Leitner, G.; Heller, E.D.; Friedman, A. Sex-related differences in immune response and survival rate of broiler chickens. *Vet Immunol. Immunopathol.* **1989**, *21*, 249–260. [CrossRef]
25. Younis, M.E.M.; Jaber, F.A.; Majrashi, K.A.; Ghoneim, H.A.; Shukry, M.; Shafi, M.E.; Albaqami, N.M.; Abd El-Hack, M.E.; Abo Ghanima, M.M. Impacts of synthetic androgen and estrogenic antagonist administration on growth performance, sex steroids hormones, and immune markers of male and female broilers. *Poult. Sci.* **2023**, *102*, 102244. [CrossRef]

26. Lockyear, O.; Breedlove, C.; Joiner, K.; Toro, H. Distribution of Infectious Bronchitis Virus Resistance in a Naïve Chicken Population. *Avian Dis.* **2022**, *66*, 101–105. [CrossRef]
27. Taneja, V. Sex Hormones Determine Immune Response. *Front. Immunol.* **2018**, *9*, 1931. [CrossRef]
28. Ansar Ahmed, S.; Penhale, W.J.; Talal, N. Sex hormones, immune responses, and autoimmune diseases. Mechanisms of sex hormone action. *Am. J. Pathol.* **1985**, *121*, 531–551.
29. Schuurs, A.H.; Verheul, H.A. Effects of gender and sex steroids on the immune response. *J. Steroid Biochem.* **1990**, *35*, 157–172. [CrossRef]
30. Foo, Y.Z.; Nakagawa, S.; Rhodes, G.; Simmons, L.W. The effects of sex hormones on immune function: A meta-analysis. *Biol. Rev. Camb. Philos. Soc.* **2017**, *92*, 551–571. [CrossRef]
31. Roved, J.; Westerdahl, H.; Hasselquist, D. Sex differences in immune responses: Hormonal effects, antagonistic selection, and evolutionary consequences. *Horm. Behav.* **2017**, *88*, 95–105. [CrossRef]
32. Gagnon, C.A.; Bournival, V.; Koszegi, M.; Nantel-Fortier, N.; St-Sauveur, V.G.; Provost, C.; Lair, S. Quebec: Avian pathogens identification and genomic characterization: 2021 annual review of the Molecular Diagnostic Laboratory, Université de Montréal. *Can. Vet. J.* **2022**, *63*, 486–490.
33. Hassan, M.S.H.; Ojkic, D.; Coffin, C.S.; Cork, S.C.; van der Meer, F.; Abdul-Careem, M.F. Delmarva (DMV/1639) Infectious Bronchitis Virus (IBV) Variants Isolated in Eastern Canada Show Evidence of Recombination. *Viruses* **2019**, *11*, 1054. [CrossRef]
34. Hassan, M.S.H.; Ali, A.; Buharideen, S.M.; Goldsmith, D.; Coffin, C.S.; Cork, S.C.; van der Meer, F.; Boulianne, M.; Abdul-Careem, M.F. Pathogenicity of the Canadian Delmarva (DMV/1639) Infectious Bronchitis Virus (IBV) on Female Reproductive Tract of Chickens. *Viruses* **2021**, *13*, 2488. [CrossRef]
35. Hassan, M.S.H.; Buharideen, S.M.; Ali, A.; Najimudeen, S.M.; Goldsmith, D.; Coffin, C.S.; Cork, S.C.; van der Meer, F.; Abdul-Careem, M.F. Efficacy of Commercial Infectious Bronchitis Vaccines against Canadian Delmarva (DMV/1639) Infectious Bronchitis Virus Infection in Layers. *Vaccines* **2022**, *10*, 1194. [CrossRef]
36. Reed, L.J.; Muench, H. A simple method of estimating fifty per cent endpoints. *Am. J. Epidemiol.* **1938**, *27*, 493–497. [CrossRef]
37. He, L.; Martins, P.; Huguenin, J.; Van, T.N.; Manso, T.; Galindo, T.; Gregoire, F.; Catherinot, L.; Molina, F.; Espeut, J. Simple, sensitive and robust chicken specific sexing assays, compliant with large scale analysis. *PLoS ONE* **2019**, *14*, e0213033. [CrossRef]
38. Kameka, A.M.; Haddadi, S.; Kim, D.S.; Cork, S.C.; Abdul-Careem, M.F. Induction of innate immune response following infectious bronchitis corona virus infection in the respiratory tract of chickens. *Virology* **2014**, *450–451*, 114–121. [CrossRef]
39. Hussein, E.A.; Hair-Bejo, M.; Adamu, L.; Omar, A.R.; Arshad, S.S.; Awad, E.A.; Aini, I. Scoring System for Lesions Induced by Different Strains of Newcastle Disease Virus in Chicken. *Vet. Med. Int.* **2018**, *2018*, 9296520. [CrossRef]
40. Schindelin, J.; Arganda-Carreras, I.; Frise, E.; Kaynig, V.; Longair, M.; Pietzsch, T.; Preibisch, S.; Rueden, C.; Saalfeld, S.; Schmid, B.; et al. Fiji: An open-source platform for biological-image analysis. *Nat. Methods* **2012**, *9*, 676–682. [CrossRef]
41. Sego, T.J.; Aponte-Serrano, J.O.; Ferrari Gianlupi, J.; Heaps, S.R.; Breithaupt, K.; Brusch, L.; Crawshaw, J.; Osborne, J.M.; Quardokus, E.M.; Plemper, R.K.; et al. A modular framework for multiscale, multicellular, spatiotemporal modeling of acute primary viral infection and immune response in epithelial tissues and its application to drug therapy timing and effectiveness. *PLoS Comput. Biol.* **2020**, *16*, e1008451. [CrossRef]
42. Yang, W.; Liu, X.; Wang, X. The immune system of chicken and its response to H9N2 avian influenza virus. *Vet. Q.* **2023**, *43*, 1–14. [CrossRef]
43. Boonham, N.; Kreuze, J.; Winter, S.; van der Vlugt, R.; Bergervoet, J.; Tomlinson, J.; Mumford, R. Methods in virus diagnostics: From ELISA to next generation sequencing. *Virus Res.* **2014**, *186*, 20–31. [CrossRef]
44. Chousalkar, K.K.; Roberts, J.R.; Reece, R. Comparative histopathology of two serotypes of infectious bronchitis virus (T and n1/88) in laying hens and cockerels. *Poult. Sci.* **2007**, *86*, 50–58. [CrossRef]
45. Klein, D. Quantification using real-time PCR technology: Applications and limitations. *Trends Mol. Med.* **2002**, *8*, 257–260. [CrossRef]
46. Eyzaguirre, E.; Haque, A.K. Application of immunohistochemistry to infections. *Arch. Pathol. Lab. Med.* **2008**, *132*, 424–431. [CrossRef]
47. Awan, M.S.; Irfan, B.; Zahid, I.; Mirza, Y.; Ali, S.A. Comparison of Polymerase Chain Reaction and Immunohistochemistry Assays for Analysing Human Papillomavirus Infection in Oral Squamous Cell Carcinoma. *J. Clin. Diagn. Res.* **2017**, *11*, Xc10–Xc13. [CrossRef]
48. Suárez-Lledó, M.; Marcos, M.; Cuatrecasas, M.; Bombi, J.A.; Fernández-Avilés, F.; Magnano, L.; Martínez-Cibrián, N.; Llobet, N.; Rosiñol, L.; Gutiérrez-García, G.; et al. Quantitative PCR Is Faster, More Objective, and More Reliable Than Immunohistochemistry for the Diagnosis of Cytomegalovirus Gastrointestinal Disease in Allogeneic Stem Cell Transplantation. *Biol. Blood Marrow Transplant.* **2019**, *25*, 2281–2286. [CrossRef]
49. Raj, G.D.; Jones, R.C. Immunopathogenesis of infection in SPF chicks and commercial broiler chickens of a variant infectious bronchitis virus of economic importance. *Avian Pathol.* **1996**, *25*, 481–501. [CrossRef]
50. van Ginkel, F.W.; Padgett, J.; Martinez-Romero, G.; Miller, M.S.; Joiner, K.S.; Gulley, S.L. Age-dependent immune responses and immune protection after avian coronavirus vaccination. *Vaccine* **2015**, *33*, 2655–2661. [CrossRef]
51. Gonzales-Viera, O.; Crossley, B.; Carvallo-Chaigneau, F.R.; Blair, E.R.; Rejmanek, D.; Erdoğan-Bamac, Ő.; Sverlow, K.; Figueroa, A.; Gallardo, R.A.; Mete, A. Infectious Bronchitis Virus Prevalence, Characterization, and Strain Identification in California Backyard Chickens. *Avian Dis.* **2021**, *65*, 188–197. [CrossRef]

52. Farsang, A.; Bódi, I.; Fölker, O.; Minkó, K.; Benyeda, Z.; Bálint, Á.; Kiss, A.L.; Oláh, I. Coronavirus infection retards the development of the cortico-medullary capillary network in the bursa of Fabricius of chicken. *Acta Vet. Hung* **2018**, *66*, 20–27. [CrossRef]
53. Pei, J.; Briles, W.E.; Collisson, E.W. Memory T cells protect chicks from acute infectious bronchitis virus infection. *Virology* **2003**, *306*, 376–384. [CrossRef]
54. Kotani, T.; Wada, S.; Tsukamoto, Y.; Kuwamura, M.; Yamate, J.; Sakuma, S. Kinetics of lymphocytic subsets in chicken tracheal lesions infected with infectious bronchitis virus. *J. Vet. Med. Sci.* **2000**, *62*, 397–401. [CrossRef]
55. Najimudeen, S.; Barboza-Solis, C.; Ali, A.; Buharideen, S.M.; Isham, I.M.; Hassan, M.S.H.; Ojkic, D.; Van Marle, G.; Cork, S.C.; van der Meer, F.; et al. Pathogenesis and host responses in lungs and kidneys following Canadian 4/91 infectious bronchitis virus (IBV) infection in chickens. *Virology* **2022**, *566*, 75–88. [CrossRef]

MDPI AG
Grosspeteranlage 5
4052 Basel
Switzerland
Tel.: +41 61 683 77 34

Viruses Editorial Office
E-mail: viruses@mdpi.com
www.mdpi.com/journal/viruses

www.ingramcontent.com/pod-product-compliance
Lightning Source LLC
LaVergne TN
LVHW072339090526
838202LV00019B/2444